Principles of Pain Management for Anaesthetists

Stephen Coniam MA MB BChir FRCA

Consultant in Anaesthesia and Pain Medicine, Frenchay Hospital, Bristol, UK

Janine Mendham MBChB MRCP FRCA

Consultant in Anaesthesia and Pain Medicine, Frenchay Hospital, Bristol, UK

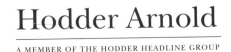

Hodder Arnold

A MEMBER OF THE HODDER HEADLINE GROUP

First published in Great Britain in 2005 by
Hodder Arnold, an imprint of Hodder Education and a member of the
Hodder Headline Group,
338 Euston Road, London NW1 3BH

http://www.hoddereducation.com

Distributed in the United States of America by
Oxford University Press Inc.,
198 Madison Avenue, New York, NY10016
Oxford is a registered trademark of Oxford University Press

British Library Cataloguing in Publication Data
A catalogue record for this book is available from the British Library

Library of Congress Cataloging-in-Publication Data
A catalog record for this book is available from the Library of Congress

ISBN-10   0 340 81648 1
ISBN-13   978 0 340 81648 6

1 2 3 4 5 6 7 8 9 10

Commissioning Editor: Serena Bureau/Clare Christian
Project Editor: Clare Patterson
Production Controller: Jane Lawrence
Cover Design: Nichola Smith

Typeset in 9/12 Minion by Charon Tec Pvt. Ltd, Chennai, India
www.charontec.com
Printed and bound in Great Britain by CPI Bath.

What do you think about this book? Or any other Hodder Arnold title?
Please send your comments to www.hoddereducation.com

Contents

List of Figures

List of Tables

Preface

This book was written in response to a request by trainee anaesthetists about what they could read about pain that would give them the core knowledge required for their training. All anaesthetists need a working knowledge of pain relief in postoperative care, with information about developments in analgesic drugs and the means by which they are administered in particular situations. In addition, many anaesthetists become involved in the management of chronic pain and palliative care; if not always personally involved with the continuing management of these problems, then at least through their anaesthetic management of patients who are receiving treatment for chronic pain. It is important that these anaesthetists, as well as other physicians and paramedical professionals who deal with such patients, have a basic understanding of the medical, physical and psychological approaches to management of these patients.

This book aims to provide an overall view of pain, both acute and chronic, and the ideas upon which treatment is based. Sufficient basic information on drug-based therapy and some of the commonly performed injection techniques with which an anaesthetist may wish to become familiar is provided, but more complex techniques and the details of physical and psychologically based pain management will require further training to gain practical expertise.

We hope that anaesthetists of all grades will find this a useful source of information on the management of pain and that other professional groups will find it a helpful guide to the field of pain and its treatment.

Stephen Coniam
Janine Mendham
Bristol
March 2005

Acknowledgements

Line illustrations contributed by Rose Marriott RGN, Pain Clinic Sister to the Frenchay Hospital Pain Clinic. We would also like to thank Dr Nicholas Ambler for his help with 'Psychological Aspects of Pain Management' and Nicola Mackey RGN, Acute Pain Sister, for her help with the 'Management of Acute Pain'.

Introduction: Pain, Anaesthetists and Pain Teams

Pain is an almost universal human experience. There is surely almost no being in the history of humankind who could claim to have never experienced some pain, and yet its nature and its meaning often defy description and understanding. Pain is a personal experience and we have no absolute means of comparing one person's pain experience with that of another. To be in pain is generally understood to be an unpleasant state, and yet this is not always agreed. Pain may be one aspect of suffering, but may be accompanied by other factors: emotions such as distress, despair and anger, as well as dysfunction and disability, which make up the fuller picture of human suffering.

Acute pain is so often temporally connected with injury or the onset of disease that most people regard pain as part of that injury or disease process. They may not understand the physiological mechanisms behind that sensation of pain, but they feel that they understand the reason for the pain. Cutting, crushing, burning or puncturing of the body's structure produces pain. We like to think that all biological processes have evolved for a specific function and we can rationalize the production of this sensation which we call pain as a highly developed protective mechanism. Injury produces pain so that we try to avoid injury or repeating injurious activity. Pain prevents mobility and so could be seen as an evolved behaviour to allow injured limbs to be rested and heal. It has always been more difficult to explain why sometimes pain persists long after the injury has healed, or even arises when there is no clear injury.

Human beings have always been concerned with trying to relieve pain, or in some situations inflict pain on others. In one form or another it has been one of the forces which have shaped our development. Primitive societies may have associated pain with evil forces and tried to harness magical powers to control pain. Gradually societies have discovered physical interventions or medicines which have some effect on the sensation of pain. The use of stimulation techniques such as acupuncture, or numerous animal, vegetable and mineral derivatives as medicines have at times achieved moderate success in the search for effective pain control. As pain is one of the commonest manifestations of disease and trauma, the relief of pain became a major aim of medical and allied practitioners, with drugs such as opium, cannabis and alcohol being used for many centuries. However, in the late nineteenth century, medicine was developing as a science and theory of disease related to specific pathology became important. Pain as a symptom of disease appeared to be a less important target for medicine and the palliation of pain became subsidiary to medical management of the disease. At the same time, anaesthesia became a developing area of medicine, and the prime aim of anaesthesia was to relieve the pain of surgery.

Anaesthetists increasingly had a role to play in pain relief as this expanded into the postoperative and post-trauma periods. In the mid twentieth century, pain relief was still mainly concerned with acute pain, and the treatment of cancer was mainly disease rather than symptom orientated. In the latter there was a movement for the symptomatic palliation of pain in cancer patients, and the hospice movement and the development of palliative care as a specialty were able to develop the long-term management of pain in disease. Following the second world war a few pioneering surgical practitioners realized that there was an enormous number of injured people who continued to suffer from pain despite the fact that their wounds had healed, and tried to develop techniques of dealing with this chronic pain.

Attempts to deal with cancer pain or post-trauma pain often relied on nerve blocking techniques, following the belief that if a body structure was painful, then it was necessary to destroy its nerve supply to relieve the pain. Many of these attempts to treat pain were therefore delegated to anaesthetists who were seen to be good at performing nerve blocks. Some anaesthetists managed to reserve a little time between their duties in the operating theatre to see patients with chronic pain problems and if possible to offer some form of intervention. The need for this service was gradually accepted by the health service, and eventually separate provision was made for pain relief services through outpatient clinics, inpatient treatment and consultation services. The increasing understanding of the physiology, pathology and psychology of pain resulted in an expansion of chronic pain management from a nerve block service to a more multidisciplinary service exploring the broader use of medication, psychological techniques and physical rehabilitation in the long-term management of pain. This has developed a wider communication between different specialties in an attempt to move from an anaesthetist-orientated service to multidimensional management of the chronic pain sufferer. It is common for the practitioner trained in anaesthesia to act as a coordinator, bringing together the different aspects of management of chronic pain, as well as providing some of the medical interventions that may be appropriate.

The management of acute pain has perhaps surprisingly been slow to evolve over the past decade and a half. Anaesthetists have usually tried to have some input into the postoperative control of pain, but this has often been poorly organized and unable to provide any continuity of care or feedback of response. A report commissioned jointly by the Royal College of Anaesthetists and the Royal College of Surgeons in 1989 considered the poor state of postoperative pain control and recommended improvements. These included the identification of individuals or teams with a special responsibility for monitoring postoperative pain control, applying effective means of pain control, and educating nursing and surgical colleagues directly involved with the postoperative care of patients. At about the same time reports appeared from America and later from the UK and Australia, describing the use of an 'acute pain team' in hospitals who fulfilled these roles. The concept has been developed to include most acute hospitals in the UK with improvements in the pain management of postoperative patients. The pain team may consist of one anaesthetist or nurse – alone, together or in combination with other healthcare staff to provide a daily supervision of pain relief techniques in the hospital, monitor efficacy and provide support and advice for other staff on wards. The closer attention to and monitoring of pain relief has improved the quality of patient care even when using pain relief techniques that have long been available but have not been used for maximum benefit.

Abbreviations Used in this Book

Δ^9 THC	delta-9-tetrahydrocannabinol
5-HT	5-hydroxytryptamine
ACE	angiotensin-converting enzyme
AMP	adenosine monophosphate
AMPA	α-amino-3-hydroxy-5-methyl-4-isoxazolepropionic acid
ASIC	acid-sensing ion channel
ATP	adenosine triphosphate
BDNF	brain-derived neurotrophic factor
BPI	Brief Pain Inventory
CB	cannabinoid
CCK	cholecystokinin
CGRP	calcitonin gene-related peptide
CNS	central nervous system
COX-2	cyclo-oxygenase-2
CPSP	central post-stroke pain
CRPS	complex regional pain syndrome
CSF	cerebrospinal fluid
DBS	deep brain stimulation
DMARD	disease modifying antirheumatic drug
DREZ	dorsal root entry zone
GABA	γ-aminobutyric acid
GDNF	glial cell line-derived neurotrophic factor
HIV	human immunodeficiency virus
IL	interleukin
ICU	intensive care unit
LANR	low-affinity neurotrophin receptor
LMWH	low molecular weight heparin
M-3-G	morphine-3-glucuronide
M-6-G	morphine-6-glucuronide
MAS	multisynaptic ascending system
MCS	motor cortex stimulation
mGluR	glutamate receptor
MPQ	McGill pain questionnaire
MRI	magnetic resonance imaging
MS	multiple sclerosis
MST	slow release morphine
MVD	microvascular decompression
NGF	nerve growth factor
NK	neurokinin
NMDA	N-methyl-D-aspartate
NNH	number needed to harm
NNT	number needed to treat
NOS	nitric oxide synthetase
NRS	numerical rating scale
NSAID	non-steroidal anti-inflammatory drug
$PaCO_2$	partial pressure (arterial) of carbon dioxide
PAG	periaqueductal grey
PaO_2	partial pressure (arterial) of oxygen
PCA	patient controlled analgesia
PCEA	patient controlled epidural analgesia
PET	positron emission tomography
PHN	post-herpetic neuralgia
PID	pain intensity difference
PNS	peripheral nerve stimulation
PO	per oral
PR	per rectum
PRN	as required
SaO_2	arterial oxygen saturation
SCI	spinal cord injury
SCS	spinal cord stimulation
SF-36	Short Form 36
SNS	sympathetic nervous system
SpO_2	oxygen saturation as measured by pulse oximetry
SSRI	serotonin selective reuptake inhibitor
TENS	transcutaneous electrical nerve stimulation
TNF	tumour necrosis factor
trkA	tyrosine kinase receptor A
TRPV	transient receptor potential (vanilloid)
TTX	tetrodotoxin
VAS	visual analogue scale
VPL	ventral posterolateral (nucleus)
VPM	ventral posteromedial (nucleus)
VR	vanilloid receptor
WDR	wide dynamic range (neurones)
WHO	World Health Organization

Section One

1 Pain as a Physiological Process

Pain is an unpleasant sensory and emotional experience associated with actual or potential tissue damage, or described in terms of such damage.
International Association for the Study of Pain (1979)

INTRODUCTION

The word pain is derived from the Latin *poena* meaning 'punishment' from the ancient belief that pain results from some kind of retribution. What is pain? It is difficult to define, ranging from a mild intermittent irritation to severe continuous pain. It is accompanied by emotional and autonomic events and produces a wide range of responses among individuals. The definition of pain applies to acute pain, cancer pain and chronic non-cancer pain.

Acute pain

The International Association for the Study of Pain defines acute pain as 'pain of recent onset and probable limited duration'. It usually has an identifiable temporal and causal relationship to injury or disease.

Chronic pain

Chronic pain is defined as pain lasting for long periods of time and persisting beyond the time of healing of an injury. Often there is no clearly identifiable cause.

Pain can be further classified into **nociceptive pain** (where the normal pain signalling pathways are intact) and **neuropathic pain** (where an abnormality or malfunction at the peripheral or central nervous system level results in pain perception in the absence of tissue damage, i.e. a malfunction of the normal signalling systems). Neuropathic pain and nociceptive pain have different physiological and clinical characteristics, requiring different management strategies.

Why do we need pain?

Nociceptive pain acts as a warning system that protects our bodies from further injury. Flexor motor neurones are also activated by nociceptors. These generate the withdrawal reflex so both the sensation of physiological pain and the flexion withdrawal reflex occur together to protect the body from a potentially hostile environment. The frequent sensation of pain and the withdrawal reflex produce learning behaviour.

Acute pain results from tissue injury or inflammation. Thus, although tissue injury has already occurred, pain aids healing because it tells us to rest. The injured area and surrounding tissue are hypersensitive to all stimuli so contact with external stimuli is avoided.

Some people are born without a sense of pain (congenital insensitivity to pain). Some people are unable to feel pain whereas others may feel pain but lack the affective response that accompanies pain. When the normal response to pain is impaired, many injuries, such as broken bones, are incurred and treatment is often delayed or inadequate. These people may develop pressure sores, damaged joints or missing and damaged fingers, and they usually die young.

THE HISTORY OF PAIN

Direct ascent to the brain

The kneeling figure of Descartes (1596–1650) in Fig. 1.1 depicts a burning sensation irritating the filaments of a nerve in the foot, ascending directly to the brain through that nerve, with the brain being the centre of sensation. It was thought at that time that specific neural pathways mediated pain.

Neural specificity theory

This theory (Von Frey, 1894) became enshrined in the medical texts of the early twentieth century. Von Frey proposed that there were four main senses – warmth, cold, touch and pain – and that each sensation was transmitted by one nerve ending. It is now known that this theory is both anatomically and physiologically incorrect and that nearly any type of stimulus will produce pain if it is intense enough.

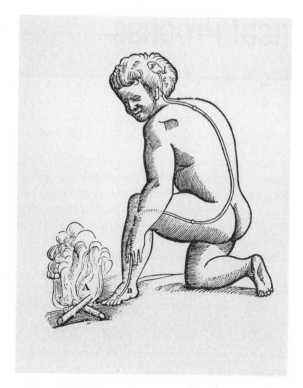

Figure 1.1 *Kneeling figure of Descartes (1664 from Traite de l'homme). © Corbis/Bettmann. A nerve filament in the foot is irritated by the fire and the burning sensation ascends to the brain via that nerve filament*

Pattern theory

According to this theory (Goldschneider, 1896) the intensity and frequency of stimulation (the pattern of stimulation) determines whether the sensation is perceived as pain.

Gate control theory

Modern understanding of pain mechanisms began with the gate control theory of pain proposed by Ronald Melzak and Patrick Wall in 1965 (Fig. 1.2). They published a paper in *Science* entitled 'New theory of pain'. The theory stated that the transmission of pain from the peripheral nerve through the spinal cord is subject to modulation by both intrinsic neurones and descending control from the brain. The sensation of pain is a function of the balance between the information travelling into the spinal cord through large nerve fibres (non-nociceptive) and information travelling to the spinal cord through small nerve fibres (nociceptive). If the relative amount of activity is greater in large nerve fibres, there should be little or no pain. However, if there is more activity in the small nerve fibres, there will be pain.

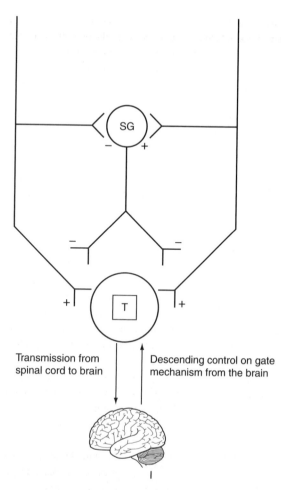

Transmission from spinal cord to brain

Descending control on gate mechanism from the brain

Figure 1.2 *Schematic diagram of the gate control theory of pain. The large diameter fibres excite both substantia gelatinosa (SG) and the transmission (T) cells. The SG cells produce synaptic inhibition by decreasing the membrane potential of the afferent terminals. The small diameter afferent fibres excite transmission cells but inhibit the SG cells turning off the pre-existing presynaptic transmission. The gating mechanism closes in response to normal stimulation of fast conducting 'touch' nerve fibres but opens when slow conducting 'pain' fibres transmit high volume and intensity sensory signals. The gate is closed again by renewed stimulation of the large fibres. This mechanism is also influenced by stimuli descending from the brain. +, excitation; −, inhibition*

The theory does not explain many observations seen in pain, but it was an extremely important development in the investigation of pain mechanisms. Much information is now available about transmitters, receptors and channels involved in the transmission of noxious messages, and there are new potential targets for analgesic therapy and a rationale on which to base their use.

It is now known that the gate control theory is a very simplistic explanation and that many other factors determine how pain messages are interpreted. However, it was an important landmark in helping us to understand the perception of pain. Pain perception involves multiple interacting central and peripheral mechanisms. Pain is multifactorial and involves physical, psychological and environmental aspects in every individual. Perhaps one of the main developments in the understanding of pain has been the acknowledgement that nociception and the experience of pain are not one and the same.

The role of the cerebral cortex – the neuromatrix

More recently (1991) Melzak developed another theory, this time involving the role of the brain in the interpretation of pain. He postulates that 'the brain can generate every quality of experience which is normally triggered by sensory input'. Pain patterns are present in the brain at birth, and genetic specifications are modified by experience. The substrate is a network of neurones or loops between the thalamus and cortex, which he terms the **neuromatrix**. The repeated processing of impulses through the neuromatrix forms a **neurosignature**. A neural centre converts the flow of neurosignatures into a flow of 'awareness', which activates an action neuromatrix – a pattern of movements influenced by the awareness (in this case, pain). In general, our whole body is encoded in the molecular structure of the central nervous system and is constantly modified by external impulses.

Knowledge of anatomical pathways and physiological and biochemical mechanisms of pain transmission remains incomplete and will continue to expand over many years.

PAIN MECHANISMS

Pain threshold

The pain threshold is defined as the minimal stimulus required to produce a sensation of pain on 50 per cent of occasions. It is mediated by Aδ fibres, is relatively constant across subjects and is reproducible. It is a useful scientific tool and temperature (44 °C) is often the stimulus used to measure it.

Pain tolerance

Pain tolerance is the greatest level of pain that a subject is prepared to tolerate. This is the pain patients actually complain about. It is mediated by C fibres. Tolerance is highly variable among subjects and is less reproducible than the pain threshold. It can be measured by the submaximal effort tourniquet test, McGill pain questionnaire or a pain visual analogue scale. Clinically it is more important than the pain threshold.

Nociceptors

Nociceptors are peripheral receptors sensitive to painful mechanical stimuli, extreme heat or cold, and chemical stimuli. They are specific for pain but the pain stimulus is not specific. All nociceptors are free nerve endings. They have small receptive fields and do not adapt to repeat stimulation as do Aβ-mediated low-threshold mechano/thermoreceptors. They can be sensitized by tissue injury.

The quality of the pain perceived on stimulation depends on the site of stimulation and the nature of the fibres transmitting the sensation. Nociceptors are capable of differentiating between innocuous and noxious stimuli. There are two major families of nociceptor.

FIRST PAIN

High threshold mechano-heat receptors respond to thermal and noxious mechanical stimuli and are attached to the thinly myelinated primary afferent Aδ axons. They are associated with the perception of a sharp, pricking pain and localize the pain to a well-defined part of the body surface.

SECOND PAIN

The polymodal nociceptors respond to the three major modalities of tissue damaging stimuli (chemical, thermal and mechanical). These are the receptors of the unmyelinated primary afferent axons (C fibres) and are associated with the perception of burning pain. They exist in many tissues but not in the brain. A dull aching pain lasts long after the termination of the stimulus. Visceral pain is predominantly second pain.

Normally most nociceptors are dormant. Inflammation sensitizes this vast population of nociceptors, making them far more sensitive to stimulation (hyperalgesia) (Fig. 1.3).

SLEEPING NOCICEPTORS

About 15 per cent of C fibre nociceptors are only active under pathological conditions. They are found in visceral as well as cutaneous tissue. They are unmyelinated primal afferent neurones that respond actively only in the presence of chemical sensitization. They cannot be activated by natural stimuli. During inflammation the activation threshold falls so they can be activated by noxious and innocuous stimuli. They are thought to be important in the development of primary hyperalgesia and also thought to play a major role in chronic pain states. These 'silent nociceptors' require further study to determine their exact role in pain transmission.

NOCICEPTION

Nociception results from activation of nociceptors by noxious stimuli (Fig. 1.4) and is the perception of a potentially

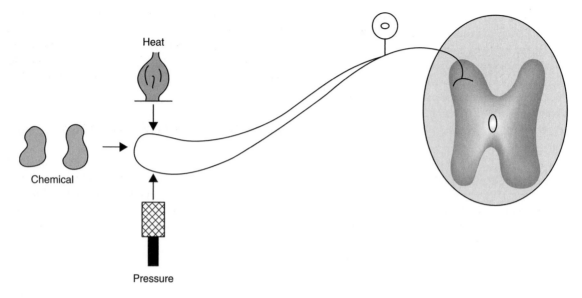

Figure 1.3 *Schematic diagram of a nociceptor*

tissue-damaging stimulus by the receptors attached to the Aδ and C fibres and the subsequent transmission of encoded information to the brain.

Nociceptors → primary afferent fibres → dorsal horn of spinal cord → secondary afferent fibres → tertiary afferent fibres

Tissue injury

Tissue injury stimulates the release of inflammatory mediators from tissues, the immune cells, sympathetic and sensory afferent nerve fibres and blood vessels (Fig. 1.4). The inflammatory mediators activate the arachidonic acid pathway (Fig. 1.5), which then produces prostaglandins and leukotrienes. Prostaglandins are the mediators of fever, pain and inflammation. They can directly activate nociceptors but usually act as sensitizing agents.

KININS – BRADYKININ AND KALLIDIN

Bradykinin is the most potent endogenous algogenic substance known. Bradykinin is formed in the blood and kallidin in the tissues. They are both broken down by kinases. Bradykinin acts at B2 receptors to activate and sensitize the receptors. B2 receptors are located on sensory neurones and are largely responsible for the majority of acute inflammatory events.

Kinins are rapidly generated after tissue injury and they modulate most of the events during the inflammatory process including vasodilation, increased vascular permeability, plasma extravasation, cell migration, pain and hyperalgesia. They activate C fibres and the consequent production of substance P, calcitonin gene-related peptide (CGRP), and release histamine and 5-hydroxytryptamine (5-HT) from degranulation

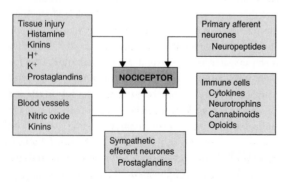

Figure 1.4 *Tissue injury: inflammation and nociceptor sensitization*

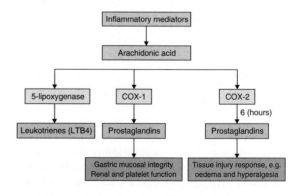

Figure 1.5 *The arachidonate pathway. COX, cyclo-oxygenase*

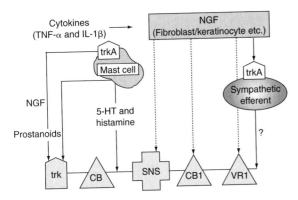

Figure 1.6 *Release of various endogenous inflammatory factors following tissue injury. TNF, tumour necrosis factor; il, interleukin; trk, tyrosine kinase; HT, hydroxytryptamine; NGF, nerve growth factor; CB, cannabinoid receptor; VR, vanilloid receptor; SNS, sympathetic nervous system*

of mast cells. Histamine stimulates sensory neurones by increasing sodium permeability.

Bradykinin antagonists have been developed but they have poor oral bioavailability and most of them display partial receptor agonist effects. B2 receptors also play an important role in other physiological processes especially in the cardiovascular system.

The B1 receptor is normally only present in small numbers but is rapidly induced in inflammatory conditions. It is thought that B1 receptors most certainly have a critical role in the maintenance of the chronic inflammatory disorders and may contribute to hyperalgesia. In the future B1 receptors will be one of the targets for drugs developed to treat inflammation and pain without the side effects of the B2 blockers.

ACTIVATION OF IMMUNE CELLS

Cytokines (Fig. 1.6) are peptides secreted by immune cells that are attracted to the area of damage by leukotrienes. They have potent hyperalgesic effects and stimulate the synthesis and release of other inflammatory mediators. Interleukin (IL)-1β releases prostaglandins from monocytes and fibroblasts and induces B1 receptors. IL-1β and tumour necrosis factor (TNF)-α stimulate the release of nerve growth factor (NGF). There are also anti-inflammatory cytokines (IL-4, IL-10) that may inhibit the release of proinflammatory cytokines and reduce cyclo-oxygenase (COX) expression. Activation of the immune cells also produces bradykinin and kallidin.

BLOOD VESSELS

Nitric oxide is formed from L-arginine by nitric oxide synthetase (NOS) and it sensitizes nociceptors to the effects of bradykinin. There are two isoenzymes: cNOS, which is calcium dependent, and iNOS, which is calcium independent.

The latter is produced by inflammation in macrophages in the microglia. Inducible (i)NOS plays a part in the regulation of COX-2 and prostaglandins activity. Substance P also stimulates the production of nitric oxide from the endothelial layer of blood vessels, causing further vasodilatation.

NEUROTRANSMITTERS OF NOCICEPTION (EXCITATORY)

Neurotransmitters are chemicals that affect nerve transmission; small packets of the chemical form at a synapse. There are receptor sites, or neurone channels, where the neurotransmitters bind to produce an effect on the other side of the gap.

Neuropeptides

Peptides are released by sensory afferent neurones as intercellular messengers. Many neuropeptides are also hormones released by non-neuronal cells. All are synthesized in afferent fibres and released after noxious stimulation. The actions of many are not yet clear.

Tachykinins

Tachykinins are a family of biologically active peptides including substance P (P is for pain), neurokinin A and neurokinin B. Tachykinins increase intercellular calcium (Ca^{2+}) levels by triggering gene transcription. They have diverse pharmacological actions in the central nervous, cardiovascular, genitourinary, respiratory and gastrointestinal systems, and in glandular tissues.

The diversity of activity is due to the existence of three or more subtypes of tachykinin receptor (Box 1.1).

Substance P

Substance P is an 11-amino acid neurotransmitter that appears in both central and peripheral nervous systems. It is involved in transmission of pain and modulates inflammatory and immune responses. Substance P is probably most relevant in signalling persistent pain. Substance P is stored in the periphery and can be released by injury.

Substance P targets are mast cells, blood vessels and immunocompetent cells. It causes degranulation of mast cells and release of histamine, vasodilatation, plasma extravasation and further release of bradykinin, and it activates inflammatory cells – macrophages, monocytes and lymphocytes.

Calcitonin gene-related peptide

Calcitonin gene-related peptide is a neurokinin. It is a primary afferent peptide released by nociceptive afferent fibres in the dorsal horn in response to noxious stimuli. It extends the release zone within the spinal cord for substance P and leads to increased excitability. Sensory neurone neurokinins stimulate sympathetic nerves to release noradrenaline and neuropeptide Y, which in turn produce vasodilation, plasma extravasation, mast cell degranulation and the production of further inflammatory mediators.

Aspartate

Aspartate is an amino acid, which acts as one of the two major neurotransmitters in the dorsal horn.

Glutamate

Glutamate is the other major excitatory neurotransmitter released by primary afferent A and C fibres producing rapid depolarization. It is found mainly in the hippocampus, outer layers of the cerebral cortex, the substantia gelatinosa and the presynaptic nerve terminals. Its most important action in nociception is at the AMPA (α-amino-3-hydroxy-5-methyl-4-isoxazolepropionic acid) receptor. When glutamate is released from the presynaptic terminal it binds glutamate receptors (mGluR) on the postsynaptic membrane. Activation evokes a response via increases in intracellular Ca^{2+} and activation of protein kinases.

Consequences of glutamate receptor activation include production of c-*fos* (see page 20) and spinal production of prostanoids and nitric oxide and it is believed to be a key transmitter in central sensitization.

Somatostatin

Somatostatin is found in small diameter cells of the distal root ganglia and in the afferent terminals in the substantia gelatinosa. It may play an inhibitory role. Analogues of somatostatin, e.g. octreotide, generally show affinity for opioid receptors and may produce analgesia.

Neurotrophins

Neurotrophic factors (or neurotrophins) are endogenous substances that play a role in the development and maintenance of regeneration of the nervous system. They include:

- NGF
- Brain-derived neurotrophic factor (BDNF)
- Neurotrophin-3
- Neurotrophin-4
- Neurotrophin-5

NERVE GROWTH FACTOR

Nerve growth factor is a neurotrophic factor produced by cells in the target organ. It is produced in the periphery by fibroblasts and Schwann cells. It is then transported in a retrograde manner intra-axonally via a high-affinity tyrosine kinase receptor (trkA) to the cell bodies of nociceptors where it plays a central role in the regulation of gene expression. Large numbers of inflammatory mediators increase the production of NGF.

Nerve growth factor is essential for neurone survival and development, and helps with survival of sympathetic fibres. It directly sensitizes nociceptors via the high-affinity trkA receptor, which is expressed almost exclusively on primary afferent nociceptive neurones. Once bound to the receptor, it is taken in and transported in a retrograde manner to the cell body where gene transcription is altered. The excitability of nociceptors is increased by NGF; this also has central consequences in that the hyperalgesic actions of NGF may have an additional central nervous system component, which is dependent upon NMDA (N-methyl-D-aspartate) receptor activation (see below). It also releases histamine from mast cells.

BRAIN-DERIVED NEUROTROPHIC FACTOR

Brain-derived neurotrophic factor is a neuromodulator synthesized in small diameter nociceptive neurones, packed in vesicles and transported in the axons to the terminals of the dorsal horn. It modulates postsynaptic excitability, has potent effects on the spinal cord neurones and is implicated in central

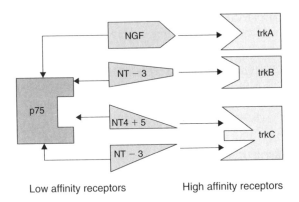

Figure 1.7 *Neurotrophins and their preferred receptors. NGF, nerve growth factor; NT, neurotrophin; trk, tyrosine kinase*

sensitization. It is increased by NGF and inflammation and this increase can be reduced by treatment with antibodies to NGF.

RECEPTORS

Neurotrophin receptors (Fig. 1.7)

There are two classes of neurotrophin cell surface receptor. The p75 receptor (also known as the low-affinity neurotrophin receptor or LANR) is common to all members of the neurotrophin family. The high-affinity receptors include the receptor tyrosine kinase proteins trkA, trkB and trkC. These receptors have different specificities for different members of the neurotrophin family.

THE trKA RECEPTOR

This protein tyrosine kinase receptor is specific for NGF. It plays a crucial role in pain sensation and thermoregulation in humans. Gene mutations that cause loss of receptor function are associated with congenital insensitivity to pain and with anhidrosis.

TRANSIENT RECEPTOR POTENTIAL (VANILLOID) RECEPTORS (PREVIOUSLY VANILLOID RECEPTORS)

TRPV I receptors

Transient receptor potential (vanilloid) (TRPV) 1 receptors are essential for normal thermal nociception and thermal hyperalgesia induced by inflammation. They are normally only found on primary nociceptors (C fibres) but are increased in numbers (up-regulated) on both C and A fibres in persistent inflammatory states. They are stimulated by temperatures above 43°C. Their sensitivity is altered by

capsaicin – the receptor works at lower thresholds, and eventually the receptors will die off if capsaicin use continues. They respond to protons and therefore activity may be enhanced in the acidic environment of inflamed tissues. They also respond to multiple pain-producing stimuli including NGF and bradykinins. They are found mainly in laminae I and II of the dorsal horn, and are mainly postsynaptic to the primary afferents. When a ligated nerve dies the TRPV1 receptors are lost, but are then found on the dorsal root ganglion cells around the ligated nerve and also on non-nociceptive cells.

TRPV3 receptors

These are activated by temperatures between 33°C and 53°C. They are found on Aδ fibres, keratinocytes, dorsal root ganglia and hair follicles. They are considered important because targeting TRPV1 receptors will not relieve pain, but TRPV3 antagonists might.

Tachykinin receptors

These are cell surface proteins that bind tachykinins with high affinity and trigger intracellular changes influencing the behaviour of cells. Three classes of tachykinin receptor have been characterized, NK-1, NK-2 and NK-3, which prefer substance P, neurokinin A and neurokinin B, respectively.

In acute nociception neurokinin A acting on NK-2 receptors plays the major role with NK-1 having a much smaller effect. NK-2 antagonists are effective in acute pain. In pathological pain, NK-1 receptors become increasingly important. They are up-regulated with the increase in substance P released in the spinal cord and produce longlasting depolarization of the dorsal horn neurones and contribute to 'wind-up'.

Purinergic receptors

Purinergic receptors are found on the 30 per cent of nociceptors that depend on glial cell line-derived neurotrophic factor (GDNF) to function. Cell surface proteins bind purines with high affinity and trigger intracellular changes that influence the behaviour of cells. The best known purinergic receptors in mammals are the P1 receptors, which prefer adenosine, and the P2 receptors, which prefer adenosine triphosphate (ATP) or adenosine diphosphate (ADP).

Adenosine triphosphate receptors

Adenosine triphosphate depolarizes sensory neurones. The release of ATP from damaged tissue may augment nociceptor activation. Adenosine, adenosine monophosphate (AMP), ADP and ATP can produce pain. Responses to ATP are enhanced during inflammation. Sympathetic nerves in the vascular endothelium/epithelium may be the source of ATP.

Adenosine exerts a modulatory effect on nociceptive transmission in the periphery and in the central nervous system. There are A1 and A2 adenosine receptors. A2 are mainly excitatory and anti-nociceptive action results from activation of A1 receptors, which exert pre- and postsynaptic inhibitory effects in the dorsal horn. Intravenous adenosine given slowly has been shown to reduce neuropathic pain of many causes but higher doses given quickly may cause pain. Adenosine produces analgesia mediated by adenosine A1 receptors. Higher doses promote pain by actions at lower affinity receptors.

The ATP receptor subfamily (P2X and P2X3) has been shown to be located on small nociceptive neurones. The P2X3 channel may mediate ATP-evoked activation of small nociceptive neurones.

Opioid receptors

Opioid receptors (Table 1.1) are highly prevalent in the spinal cord and are very effective in modulating pain. In lamina I the predominant receptors seem to be mu (μ) and delta (δ), and in laminae II–V, kappa (κ).

Opioid receptor subtypes were originally classified as μ (from the prototypical agonist morphine), κ (from ketocyclazocine) and δ (from the vas deferens). Endogenous peptide ligands that interact with these receptors are classified into four groups: endorphins, dynorphins, encephalins and endomorphins. Dynorphins bind preferentially to κ receptors, encephalins to δ receptors and endomorphins to μ and δ receptors. Endomorphins 1 and 2 were discovered in 1997 and show selectivity for μ receptors that is at least 4000 times greater than for other opioid sites.

Table 1.1 *Types of opioid receptor*

Receptor	Sites found
μ opioid receptor	Widest distribution. Brain: caudate putamen, neocortex, thalamus, periaqueductal grey, superficial layers of the dorsal horn, gut and vas deferens
δ opioid receptor	Olfactory bulb, neocortex, caudate putamen, dorsal horn and vas deferens
κ opioid receptor	Amygdala, hypothalamus, thalamus, caudate putamen

Opioid analgesia occurs by reducing neuronal activity in the following ways:

- closure of voltage-gated calcium channels
- activation of inwardly rectifying potassium currents, thereby stabilizing the membrane potential
- reduction in adenyl cyclase activity.

PERIPHERAL OPIOID RECEPTORS

These are located on the afferent nerve fibres and sympathetic nerve fibres but only in significant numbers in chronic inflammation. The receptors are synthesized in the cell body of the bipolar afferent fibre and transported along the axon centrally to the spinal cord and peripherally to the nociceptor.

Cannabinoid receptors

The major psychoactive constituent of *Cannabis sativa* is Δ^9 tetrahydrocannabinol. Its high lipophilicity and low potency made research on these compounds difficult. The discovery of synthetic cannabinoids such as levonantradol and nabilone aided the discovery of the cannabinoid receptors:

- Neuronal CB1 receptor
- Peripheral CB2 receptor

Cannabinoids exert many of their effects by combining with specific receptors in the brain and periphery. Neuronal CB1 receptors are present in the brain, particularly in areas associated with cognition, memory, reward, anxiety, pain, sensory perception, motor coordination and endocrine function, olfactory areas, cortex, hippocampus, cerebellum, and basal ganglia and spinal cord. There are few in the brain stem, which may account for the lack of respiratory depressant effect. Peripheral CB2 receptors are found in the spleen, macrophages and other peripheral tissues. They are also expressed in peripheral nerve terminals. There is an endogenous system of cannabinoid receptors and anandamines that normally modulates neuronal activity by effects on cyclic AMP, Ca^{2+} and potassium (K^+) ion transport. It is thought to have important interactions with opioid, γ-aminobutyric acid (GABA)ergic, dopaminergic, noradrenergic, serotonergic, cholinergic, glucocorticoid and prostaglandin systems. Exact mechanisms of action of cannabis are not clear.

ION CHANNELS

Voltage-gated ion channels mediate conduction within the nervous system in the first instance. Each type of channel is specific and specialized.

Proton-sensitive channels – acid-sensing receptors

These ion channels are selectively activated by protons and occur widely throughout the nervous system. They are triggered by increased local acidity (ASICs or acid-sensing ion channels), which directly stimulates nociceptors. They are mediators of hyperalgesia in inflamed, poorly perfused tissue that becomes acidotic, and they may be involved in mechanosensitivity.

Sodium channels

The sodium channels of nociceptive sensory neurones are classified as sensitive or resistant to tetrodotoxin (TTX-S or TTX-R). Tetrodotoxin-sensitive, fast acting channels are found on all sensory neurones and are responsible for the initiation of the action potential. Tetrodotoxin-resistant, slow acting channels are found only on small diameter, primary afferent neurones, including polymodal neurones, and they are only expressed after injury. There are two sensory neurone-specific (SNS) TTX-R channels – SNS/PN3 and SNS/NaN. The SNS/PN3 channels are closely associated with the nociceptor population within the dorsal root ganglia and are increased during chronic inflammation. They may play a key role in persistent pain states. Nine different sodium channels have been identified, two on the peripheral nerves (Na 1.9_v and Na 1.8_v). If a peripheral nerve is damaged, the expression is changed: Na_v 1.9 translocates from the dorsal root ganglion to the neuronal tip and Na_v 1.8 disappears and is replaced by Na_v 1.3. Sodium channels are fundamental to the excitability of the neurones so blocking them could provide a good analgesic effect.

Calcium channels

A range of voltage-gated Ca^{2+} channels are involved in transmitter release and prolonged excitatory states of the neuronal membrane. Blocking Ca^{2+} channels with ω-condotoxin (toxin from snails of genus Conus) produces analgesia. Gabapentin has high affinity and specificity for α2δ subunits of these channels and this may be how it eases neuropathic pain.

ANTI-NOCICEPTIVE NEUROTRANSMITTERS (INHIBITORY)

These act by producing local inhibition in the dorsal horn or through descending inhibitory pathways. Forty per cent of inhibitory interneurones use GABA or glycine. The interneurones in laminae I–III are GABA-rich and mediate gate control in the dorsal horn by synapsing on neurones that contain substance P. These substances inhibit the firing of dorsal horn nociceptive neurones by pre- and postsynaptic control. $GABA_A$ is a ligand-gated ion channel that allows chloride ions to leak into the cell. It is modulated by benzodiazepines and is more important at supraspinal than spinal sites. $GABA_B$ activates G-proteins. Baclofen is a $GABA_B$ receptor agonist.

Other inhibitory pathways use endorphins, encephalins and dynorphins, which act by increasing potassium conductance thereby hyperpolarizing neurones. Inhibitory neurotransmitters can also block the release of neurotransmitters from the primary afferent by reducing calcium conductance. The major descending inhibitory pathways use serotonin or noradrenaline.

Opioid systems

The highest concentration of opioid receptors in the spinal cord is around the C-fibre terminal zones in laminae I and II:

- 70 per cent – μ receptors, of which 70 per cent are found in the presynaptic region of the peripheral nociceptive fibres
- 24 per cent – δ receptors
- 6 per cent – κ receptors.

TRANSMISSION OF PAIN SIGNALS

The nociceptor consists of a cell body, dendrites and axons. The dendrites are short, branched processes arising from the cell body that increase the area available for contact with nearby cells. The axon is the filament along which information is conducted. It consists of a central core of axoplasm surrounded by a semipermeable membrane.

The majority of axons lie within a spiral sheath of highly specialized cells known as Schwann cells in the peripheral nervous system and oligodendrocytes in the central nervous system. These cells contain the lipid substance myelin, which acts as an electrical insulator. It influences the rate at which nerve conduction can occur. Nerve conduction is faster in axons with a thick myelin sheath and slowest in axons with a thin myelin sheath. Neuronal conduction velocity is

Table 1.2 *Types of primary afferent axon*

	Aβ	**Aδ**	**C**
Firing threshold	Low	Medium	High
Diameter (μm)	6–14	1–6	0.2–1
Speed (m/s)	36–90	5–36	0.2–2
Myelination	Yes	Yes	No
Receptor type	Mechanoreceptor	Mechanoreceptor – mediates only pain	Polymodal nociceptor – thermal, chemical and mechanical noxious stimuli
Receptive field	Small	Small	Large
Type of signal	Touch	First/fast pain	Slow/second pain

proportional to the square root of the diameter of the neurone and is equal to 6 m/s per micron thickness of myelin. Schwann cells are arranged alongside each other but there are gaps between them leaving bare areas of axon. These areas are called the nodes of Ranvier. When Schwann cells are present, electrical activity occurs only at these nodal areas. Depolarization jumps from node to node (saltatory conduction) making impulse transmission much faster.

AXONS AND THE NERVE IMPULSE

Table 1.2 summarizes the features of the types of primary afferent axon, shown in Fig. 1.8. The firing thresholds of these types of neurone in relation to increasing stimulus strength are illustrated in Fig. 1.9.

In the electrically inactive axon, potassium concentration is greater in the axoplasm than outside. Sodium and chloride concentration is greater outside the cell. Stimulation of the axon alters the permeability of the semipermeable membrane allowing sodium and chloride ions to flow into the cell, while potassium flows out. These depolarization changes occur along the length of the axon and the impulse is conducted along the nerve. When stimulation ceases, the sodium and chloride ions are pumped out of the axon and potassium moves back in so that the nerve is repolarized and nerve conduction ceases.

The synapse

Electrical activity cannot be transferred directly from one nerve to another. Transmission between nerves requires the presence of chemical substances that are released by the process of depolarization at the terminal of the nerve. This transmitter substance (neurotransmitter) crosses the narrow space between the nerves to a receptor site on another nerve and produces depolarization in that neurone. The space across which the neurotransmitter passes is known as the synapse and the membranes before and after the synapse are known as the pre- and the postsynaptic membranes, respectively.

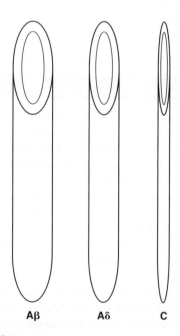

Figure 1.8 *Primary afferent axons*

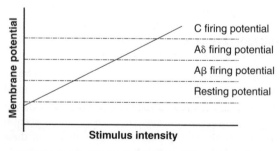

Figure 1.9 *Primary afferent axons: relation between firing thresholds and stimulation intensity*

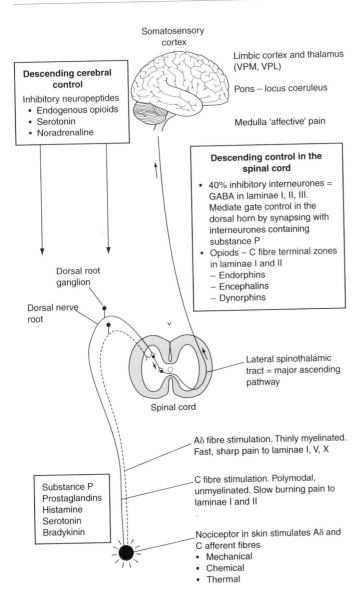

Somatosensory cortex

Limbic cortex and thalamus (VPM, VPL)

Pons – locus coeruleus

Medulla 'affective' pain

Descending cerebral control

Inhibitory neuropeptides
• Endogenous opioids
• Serotonin
• Noradrenaline

Descending control in the spinal cord

• 40% inhibitory interneurones = GABA in laminae I, II, III. Mediate gate control in the dorsal horn by synapsing with interneurones containing substance P
• Opiods – C fibre terminal zones in laminae I and II
  – Endorphins
  – Encephalins
  – Dynorphins

Dorsal root ganglion

Dorsal nerve root

Lateral spinothalamic tract = major ascending pathway

Spinal cord

Aδ fibre stimulation. Thinly myelinated. Fast, sharp pain to laminae I, V, X

C fibre stimulation. Polymodal, unmyelinated. Slow burning pain to laminae I and II

Substance P
Prostaglandins
Histamine
Serotonin
Bradykinin

Nociceptor in skin stimulates Aδ and C afferent fibres
• Mechanical
• Chemical
• Thermal

Figure 1.10 *Pain pathways. GABA, γ-aminobutyric acid; VPM, ventral posteromedial nucleus; VPL, ventral posterolateral nucleus*

Facilitation or inhibition of electrical activity can occur at the presynaptic level or at the postsynaptic membrane. Impulses from a third neurone can form a synapse with the afferent nerve. Impulses from this nerve depolarize the presynaptic membrane, reducing the action potential and hence reducing neurotransmitter release. It is this complex process that is involved in pain modulation.

PAIN PATHWAYS

Very simply, the pain pathway has three components (Fig. 1.10):

1   a first order neurone (cell body in the dorsal root ganglion) which transmits pain from a peripheral receptor

to

2   a second order neurone in the dorsal horn of the spinal cord. This axon crosses the midline to ascend in the spinothalamic tract to the thalamus
    where

3   a third order neurone projects to the postcentral gyrus (via the internal capsule).

Dorsal root

The traditional view is that most of the sensory afferent nerves (first order neurones) enter the spinal cord through the dorsal roots. Their cell bodies lie in the dorsal root ganglia of the dorsal horns. In the root, the thinner fibres are more

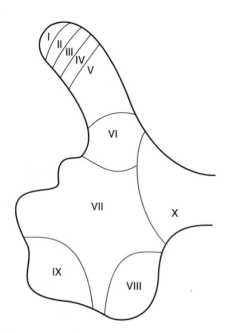

Figure 1.11 *Rexed's laminae*

Table 1.3 *Stimuli associated with Rexed's laminae*

Lamina	Location	Stimulus
I	Marginal zone	Respond to noxious stimuli or both noxious and non-noxious
II	Substantia gelatinosa	
III, IV		Afferent neurones carrying innocuous tactile sensations synapse in the deeper layers
V, IV, VI	Nucleus proprius	Predominantly non-noxious
VII, VIII, X	Intermediate spinal grey matter	

lateral, the myelinated fibres more medial. A rhizotomy (sectioning dorsal root) attempts to section the lateral root preferentially destroying nociceptors and sparing fibres that subserve light touch. However, it is now known that up to 40 per cent of the afferents enter through the anterior (motor) roots and then travel to the dorsal horn.

Bror Rexed classified the grey matter of the dorsal horn into 10 laminae (Rexed's laminae) or layers (Fig. 1.11 and Table 1.3), on the basis of their physiological function and histological appearance. I is the most superficial layer, and X the deepest. The dorsal part is divided into five laminae (I–V), the components of which deal with most of the incoming pain fibres. Lamina VII is in between these laminae and the more

ventral laminae VIII and IX, and X is the grey matter around the central canal of the spinal cord. Lamina VI is related to the innervation of the limbs.

The NGF-dependent peptidergic nociceptors synapse in lamina I and the outer part of lamina II, and the purinergic GDNF-dependent class terminate in the inner part of lamina II. The outermost layer of the cord is lamina I. This is where the marginal cells are found, which are second order neurones. They receive input from C fibres and only fire with high-intensity pain. They are relatively few in number and each cell receives input from a very large area of skin. One cell firing generates only general information about the area of the pain.

C fibres (70 per cent carry nociceptive transmission) predominantly synapse in laminae I (marginal zone) and II (substantia gelatinosa). Aδ fibres synapse in laminae I, V, X (the nucleus proprius). Some Aδ primary afferents move ventrally in lamina V and around the central canal. Some small diameter primary afferents ascend the spinal cord segments 1–2 in Lissauer's tract ipsilaterally, before entering the spinal cord and synapsing on the dorsal horn neurones. The fast Aβ fibres go to lamina V. Usually there is no connection between C fibres and Aβ fibres, but interneurones develop between the two fibres in persistent pain. The second order neurones cross in front of the central canal to the lateral spinothalamic tract and ascend to the thalamus.

Second order neurones

All neurones that receive input from primary afferent fibres are second order neurones. They are the cells of origin of the ascending spinal sensory tracts. Functionally, there are three main groups of dorsal horn cells:

- Nociceptive-specific neurones which respond only to noxious stimuli
- Low-threshold neurones, which respond only to non-noxious stimuli
- Multireceptive or wide dynamic range (WDR) neurones.

Multireceptive neurones are found in layers IV–VI. They respond to a large range of intensity of stimulation, e.g. the neurones in lamina V respond to non-noxious light touch as well as mechanical stimulation and noxious heat. They play an important role in the processing and modulation of nociceptive information. Repetitive stimulation at about one per second via C fibres causes an increase in the response of the WDR cell.

Aβ fibres represent 40 per cent of lumbar dorsal root ganglion cells. The dorsal horn is an area of considerable signal modulation.

Ascending pathways

There are multiple ascending pain pathways including the spinothalamic tract, the different components of the spinoreticular tracts, the spinocervicothalamic tracts, the posterior dorsal column fibres and the visceral nociceptive tracts that run in the posterior columns. Studies underway with new imaging techniques will provide new information and a better understanding of the physiopathological features of these pathways. Current data tend to support the idea that pain is not a unique consequence of impulses in specific, unidirectional hardwired lines that originate in the periphery and terminate in the central nervous system.

SPINOTHALAMIC TRACT (NEOSPINOTHALAMIC)

The major ascending system is the spinothalamic tract (90 per cent). The cells have their origins in the dorsal horn and the intermediate grey matter of the spinal cord. The axons cross to the anterolateral quadrant and ascend to the thalamus. The tract carries fibres mainly from laminae I–V (i.e. first pain). They have small receptive fields and are involved in the localization of pain. This pathway is **monosynaptic** and therefore is responsible for fast pain. Of neurones found in the spinothalamic tract, 54 per cent carry pain messages and 46 per cent carry temperature messages (37 per cent warmth and 9 per cent cold). There are very few opiate receptors in the spinothalamic tract.

SPINORETICULAR TRACT (PALEOSPINOTHALMIC)

This pathway carries the second order neurones from the C fibres. They are found deep in the dorsal horn and ventral horn (laminae VII and VIII). The pathways have larger receptive fields and are responsible for the more diffuse nature of pains. It is a **polysynaptic** ascending pathway and therefore it is a slow pathway. This tract is rich in opiate receptors, which may be why morphine is good for visceral pain.

There is also a pathway arising from the neurones in lamina I of the dorsal horn. These axons ascend in the dorsal part of the lateral funiculus and terminate in the rostral brain stem and the parabrachial nuclei. These pathways may account for the failure of cordotomy because they would not be cut by an anterolateral cordotomy.

Pain afferents also arise in the glossopharyngeal nerve (cranial nerve IX) and the vagus nerve (cranial nerve X) and carry pain from the ear, pharynx and larynx.

Brain pathways

SPINOTHALAMIC TRACT

The spinothalamic tract travels to the ventrobasal lateral thalamus. Connections go to the sensory cortex (postcentral gyrus), which explains the precise location of somatic pain.

SPINORETICULAR SYSTEM

The neurones join the spinal nucleus of the trigeminal nerve and nociceptors from the head. They either cross the midline to nuclei in the thalamus or into the central grey matter and enter the brain stem reticular formation to the thalamus, hypothalamus and the areas of the brain concerned with autonomic activity and emotion.

The emotional and affective responses to pain may be explained by projections that go from the medial nuclei of the thalamus to most of the cortex, especially the frontal cortex and anterior cingulate gyrus. Also, some areas of the brain connect back to the spinal cord – these connections can change or modify information that is coming into the brain. In fact, this is one way in which the brain can reduce pain. Two areas of the brain that are involved in reducing pain are the periaqueductal grey (PAG) and the nucleus raphe magnus.

The fast conducting pain fibres that ascend the spinal cord as the spinothalamic tract are joined by neurones from the sensory nucleus of the trigeminal nerve and pass towards the thalamus as part of the lateral lemniscus and trigeminal lemniscus.

THALAMUS

The pathways eventually converge on the ventrobasal nuclear complex of the thalamus, particularly the ventral posterolateral nucleus (VPL). If this area is stimulated in patients without pain, they do not experience pain but in patients with pain, stimulation of this area produces pain. This phenomenon demonstrates reorganization of the thalamus. Information also passes to the ventral posteromedial (VPM) nucleus and intralaminar nucleus of the thalamus, the hypothalamus and areas connected with autonomic control and emotions. The lateral part of the thalamus is mainly sensory/discriminative and the medial part is responsible for 'affective' pain.

MIDBRAIN

This area carries mainly 'affective' pain connections to the reticular activating system of the brain stem including PAG.

PONS

The locus coeruleus is the major pain area in the pons. It is packed with noradrenaline-containing neurones and projects to a variety of brainstem structures that modulate pain pathways descending to the spinal cord. The parabrachial nuclei receive a vast number of ascending spinoreticular fibres.

CEREBRAL CORTEX

Fibres of the multisynaptic ascending system (MAS) synapse with cells in the reticular activating system and from here fibres radiate to all areas of the cortex. The cerebral cortex is essential in locating the site of pain and for producing the emotional response. Although stimulation of the cortex will not produce pain, positron emission tomography (PET) has identified several cortical regions activated by pain including the anterior cingulate gyrus, insular cortex and somatosensory cortex.

It is likely that the cerebral processing of pain is highly plastic and at present is poorly understood.

Descending control

This control is manifested via pathways from the cortex, thalamus, brainstem (PAG, raphe nuclei) and the locus coeruleus–subcoeruleus complex. There are two descending inhibitory spinal tracts that originate in the brain. The main neurotransmitters are serotonin (5-HT), noradrenaline and endogenous opioids. The serotonergic system has its origins in the rostroventral medulla and the noradrenergic system in the nucleus paragigantocellularis and locus coeruleus of the lateral pons (Fig. 1.12). Both these areas have diverse connections throughout the brain, including the ascending nociceptive systems and the periaqueductal grey, which is the major supraspinal site of opioid analgesia. There are many potential sites at which transmitters might act but as yet the process is poorly understood and all approaches to the study of this area have problems. Stimulation of these pathways leads to inhibition of pain.

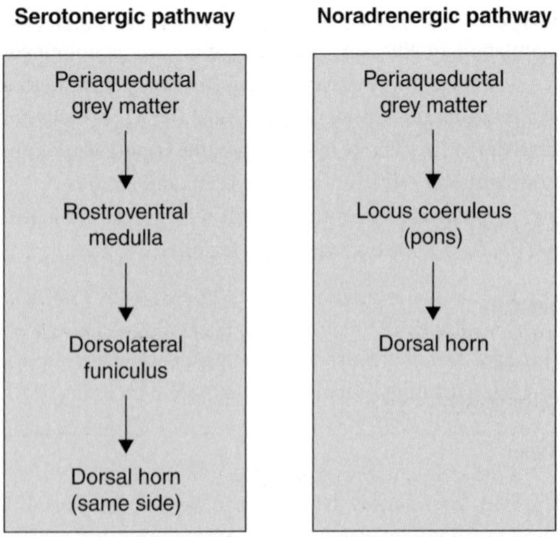

The spinal receptor target for the pathways is the α2 adrenoceptor. Agonists at this receptor, such as clonidine, produce mild anti-nociception and potentiate the actions of morphine. Dexmedetomidine is far more effective but has not been fully evaluated. Opioids are involved in both ascending and descending components of pain modulation. In the ascending pathways μ, δ and κ receptors are involved. In the descending pathway it is mainly the μ and κ receptors. Other transmitters probably include GABA and acetylcholine but their role is disputed.

Currently, there is much interest in developing novel analgesic drugs that exert their effects through these systems.

VISCERAL PAIN

Much less is known about the mechanism of visceral pain, and there are differences in the innervation of the viscera and the skin. The biological role of visceral innervation is to warn of internal threat of disease. The density of visceral nociceptors is less than 1 per cent in comparison with somatic afferents and the cortical mapping is much less detailed. Visceral pain is therefore poorly localized, diffuse and frequently in the midline. Thermal and mechanical stimuli are ineffective in the viscera, but inflammation, ischaemia, distension and contraction of smooth muscle evoke pain.

The pain is often colicky in nature and is associated with nausea and sweating, i.e. autonomic functions. Little pain may be experienced where there is major tissue damage, e.g. neoplasm, but it can be severe when there is little tissue damage, e.g. ureteric colic. The gastrointestinal and urogenital tracts respond rapidly to distension along their entire length. As few as 3 per cent of nociceptors may respond to intraluminal pressure change but this can be increased fourfold in inflammatory conditions, e.g. cystitis. The distending pressures associated with pain are not tissue damaging, and the pressures that produce pain may vary markedly. The area of tissue stimulated may be a crucial determinant of pain threshold. Increasing the area over which a stimulus acts on the skin does not reduce the threshold, but spatial summation may drastically reduce the effective threshold for pain in the viscera. Thus, a localized area of damage may not produce pain, but a small increase in pressure over a large area may do so.

Specific nociceptors have been identified in the viscera but their mechanism of action still remains unclear. Visceral pain generally results in tonic muscular spasm (somatic pain

Serotonergic pathway

Periaqueductal grey matter

↓

Rostroventral medulla

↓

Dorsolateral funiculus

↓

Dorsal horn (same side)

Noradrenergic pathway

Periaqueductal grey matter

↓

Locus coeruleus (pons)

↓

Dorsal horn

Figure 1.12 *Serotonergic and noradrenergic pathways of pain*

usually produces a withdrawal reflex). Acute pain produces stimulation of the high-threshold receptors and the silent nociceptors. Once these are sensitized they begin to respond to innocuous stimuli. Central nervous system mechanisms then amplify and sustain the effect of the peripheral mechanism. Damage and inflammation of the viscus also changes the environment around the nociceptor endings. Visceral pain may persist even after the initial injury is on its way to resolution.

Most visceral afferent fibres seem to belong to the peptide class that express the peptide neurotransmitters and terminate in laminae I and V. The phenomenon of wind-up does not occur in the viscera. The increases in excitability of the spinal cord nociceptive neurones may be due to the properties of the neuronal networks activated by the stimuli and/or the release of certain transmitters. There are two classes of nociceptive sensory receptor in the viscera:

- high threshold to normal stimuli (mainly mechanical)
- intensity-encoding receptors with low threshold (mechanical) to natural stimuli.

There may also be silent nociceptors. See Box 1.2 for a summary of visceral pain.

Referred pain

Visceral pain can be referred to a site far away from the source of stimulation. The origin of the pain is often poorly defined and referred to somatic structures, e.g. cardiac pain felt in the arm.

BOX 1.2 Five characteristics of visceral pain

- Not evoked from all viscera – liver, kidney and lung parenchyma are not sensitive to pain even after gross destruction
- It is not always linked to visceral injury, e.g. stretching of the urinary tract, gastrointestinal tract and gall bladder produces pain
- Diffuse and poorly localized. It is usually perceived as arising from the midline, and either anterior or posterior
- Referred to other locations. The area is usually segmental and superficial, i.e. to muscle, skin or both and innervated by the same spinal nerves as the viscus. The site of referral may also show hyperalgesia
- Accompanied by autonomic reflexes, e.g. nausea, vomiting, lower back muscle tension which may be prolonged

---

Visceral and somatic afferent input converges on the WDR neurones in lamina V. Increased activity of the visceral afferents secondary to injury to the viscera is interpreted by the brain as having arisen from the source of the convergent somatic input so the pain is 'referred' to the somatic site. Local anaesthetic injection of the site of reference can reduce referred pain. Secondary hyperalgesia is also referred to the area where the pain is perceived (e.g. angina produces arm pain; hyperalgesia produces sensitivity in the arm).

Two common principles underlie visceral pain:

- Neurological mechanisms of visceral pain differ from those of somatic pain.
- Perception and psychological processing of visceral pain also differs from that of somatic pain.

Irritable bowel syndrome, functional dyspepsia, etc.

These problems may be the result of visceral hypersensitivity causing patients to become more aware of gastrointestinal activity. There may be increased sensitization of the peripheral nociceptors or altered central processing.

PATHOPHYSIOLOGY OF NEUROPATHIC PAIN

Normal sensory function is the product of an actively maintained equilibrium between neurones and their environment. Any disruption of this equilibrium that results from changes in sensitivity, excitability, transmission, growth status and survival can initiate profound changes in sensory function. A genetic component probably contributes to the diverse phenotype of individuals with apparently similar lesions and would explain, for example, the varied susceptibility to developing post-herpetic neuralgia after shingles. Persistent pain can be subdivided into two different types although both cause profound changes in the spinal cord and brain.

Nociceptive pain

The pain signalling pathway is intact (although it can be up- or down-regulated) and the biological value of the pain is clear.

Neuropathic pain

A disease of the pain signalling system.

There is a central or peripheral malfunction in the pain signalling pathway that permits perception of pain in the absence of tissue damage. It serves no useful biological purpose. It is commoner after insults to the peripheral nervous system. Hyperalgesia and allodynia are the hallmarks of neuropathic pain:

- Hyperalgesia represents an increased response to a normally painful stimulus.
- Allodynia is a painful response to a normally non-painful stimulus.

Neuropathic pain is currently classified on the basis of its aetiology, although it would be better to use an 'aetiology of pain' classification. As yet, there are no means of determining which mechanisms are operating in a particular condition. The following are the commonest causes of neuropathic pain:

- trauma – partial nerve injuries are worse than complete nerve injuries
- phantom limb pain
- spinal cord injury
- ischaemic injury – central pain
- painful diabetic neuropathy
- postherpetic neuralgia
- human immunodeficiency virus (HIV) – glycoprotein 120 on the outer HIV virus interacts with the dorsal root ganglion cells, producing a bilateral sensory neuropathy
- trigeminal neuralgia.

TYPES OF PAIN

Table 1.4 gives an overview of the different types of neuropathic pain.

Other types

- Hyperpathia: Prolonged post-stimulus sensations.
- Dysaesthesia: Evoked or spontaneous altered sensation, discomfort rather than pain.
- Hyperaesthesia: Increased sensitivity of stimulation.
- 'Wind-up': Coined by Mendel in 1966. Prolonged dorsal horn activity after repetitive C fibre stimulation.

Hyperalgesia, allodynia and ongoing pain associated with peripheral nerve injury are due to changes in primary afferent neurones. They reflect the excitability of the neurones. One particularly important change is the development of ongoing ectopic activity. At least two subpopulations of primary afferents develop ectopic activity in the presence of nerve injury: injured afferents and their uninjured neighbours. To elucidate the mechanisms of neuropathic pain it is necessary to examine the plasticity that underlies hyperalgesia and allodynia.

Primary hyperalgesia (peripheral sensitization)

Sensitization is said to have occurred when a receptor or cell responds to a stimulus that would normally be below its threshold. Primary hyperalgesia occurs within the zone of tissue injury and is a local, peripheral phenomenon.

When a stimulus is repeated the nociceptors exhibit sensitization. There can be a reduction in the threshold for activation, an increase in response to a given stimulus or appearance of spontaneous activity. Some molecules excite nociceptors during the physiological events associated with nociception (primary algogens) and some also enhance the sensitivity of nociceptors (e.g. protons, bradykinin and serotonin). It is this sensitizing action that underlies primary hyperalgesia.

Table 1.4 *Types of neuropathic pain*

Type of pain	Mechanism of pain
Paroxysmal, stimulus-independent pain	Activity in sympathetic nervous system
Burning persistent pain	Spontaneous activity in nociceptive C fibres
Stimulus-independent paraesthesia	Spontaneous activity in large myelinated A fibres (and dysaesthesias)
Stimulus-evoked pain (hyperalgesia). An increased response to a normally painful stimulus	Sensitized polymodal nociceptors. There is abnormal processing of nociceptive input
Stimulus-evoked pain (allodynia). A painful response to normally innocuous stimuli	Elements that do not normally signal pain have started to do so. Low threshold myelinated Aβ fibres in altered central nervous system. Decreased threshold of nociceptor terminals in the periphery. Pain threshold lowered. Activation of sensitized mechanoreceptors, test by stroking with cotton wool
Stimulus-independent pain	TTX-S and TTX-R sodium channels in sensory neurones

TTX-S/R, tetrodotoxin-sensitive/resistant.

Some secondary algogens do not excite nociceptors under physiological conditions. However, they do play a role in inflammatory hyperalgesia, often by sensitizing the nociceptor to the actions of primary algogens. These are:

- NGF
- Bradykinin
- Products of arachidonic acid metabolism
  - Prostaglandins
  - Leukotrienes

Protons lower the heat activation threshold of vanilloid receptors (VR1) on nociceptors. The neurotrophin NGF is of major importance in this sensitization process. The electrophysiological characteristics of nociceptors alter during hyperalgesia in that the threshold for excitation falls, predominantly to thermal stimuli. The receptive field and discharge characteristics of cutaneous nociceptors also change, in addition to the development of spontaneous activity. 'Sleeping nociceptors' are also activated during primary hyperalgesia.

Nerve growth factor

Mast cells are important in the NGF-mediated events of primary hyperalgesia as they also express trkA receptors. Mast cells degranulate in response to NGF secreted by a range of connective tissue cells following cytokine stimulation. Degranulating mast cells not only release a 'soup' of molecules that interact with nociceptive neurones, but further NGF is released, thus amplifying the biological signal. NGF may play a different role in the development of chronic pain that results from cell death or atrophy, and failure of adaptation in the spinal cord, e.g. deafferentation pain. This may explain the greater incidence of post-herpetic neuralgia with increasing age after the sixth decade as neurotrophic support to small and large fibres may wane. Changes of NGF expression may, at the early stages of nerve injury or disease, form part of an adaptive response. Failure of this response, or of secondary adaptation in the dorsal spinal cord, may contribute to the development of chronic pain.

TTX channels

Another feature of inflammation currently being revealed by advances in molecular biology is the abnormal pattern of expression of neuronal sodium channels during inflammation. Since sodium channels are the key to the initiation and propagation of action potentials, any change in their characteristics will have profound changes in neuronal excitability.

TTX-S channels are responsible for the initiation of the action potential and exist in all sensory neurones. TTX-R channels are found only on nociceptor sensory neurones. They have much slower activation and inactivation kinetics and are implicated in pathological pain states. After nerve injury, both types of sodium channels begin to accumulate in the axon at the neuroma site and along the length of the axon. This results in foci of hyperexcitability and ectopic action potential discharge in the axon and cell body. After nerve injury, injured and uninjured sensory afferents may display ectopic discharge properties.

Secondary hyperalgesia (central sensitization)

A second and larger zone of secondary hyperalgesia is apparent within and without the zone of injury and is a manifestation of central nervous system plasticity at a spinal cord level. In the skin, secondary hyperalgesia is observed close to the site of injury, whereas in the viscera the secondary hyperalgesia is generally observed in (referred) distant somatic structures.

Inflammation or nerve injury induces profound plastic effects in the spinal processing of nociception. These changes are important in the pathophysiology of chronic pain and can be, to a certain extent, self-sustaining. Once dorsal horn neurones have been sensitized by an injury-induced barrage of afferents their physiological characteristics are altered to an excitable state. They show an enhanced response to subsequent stimuli (wind-up), their receptive fields expand and stimulation thresholds fall. Response in the deep dorsal horn neurones increases dramatically despite a steady input into the spinal cord. It requires a certain frequency of stimulation to occur but it can augment responses in the spinal cord up to 20 times in amplitude and prolong responses even after cessation of the peripheral input.

A number of events have been proposed to account for these changes. These include:

- enhanced excitability of spinal nociceptive systems
- recruitment of 'silent' dorsal horn synapses
- up- and down-regulation of excitatory and inhibitory neurotransmitters and their receptors.

AMPA receptors

AMPA receptors are cell-surface proteins that bind glutamate and directly gate ion channels in cell membranes. AMPA receptors were originally discriminated from other glutamate receptors by their affinity for the agonist AMPA. They are probably the commonest mediators of fast excitatory synaptic transmission in the central nervous system. The resultant receptor channel is primarily a Na^+ channel with rapid activation and deactivation for fast excitatory neurotransmission.

Spinal responses to non-tissue damaging noxious stimuli are mediated by glutamate acting on AMPA receptors. A and C fibre afferent nerve terminals within the substantia gelatinosa of the spinal cord release glutamate and neurokinins in response to noxious stimuli. Glutamate then binds to receptors on the postsynaptic cell. The acute pain response is due to glutamate acting at the AMPA receptors and the neurokinins at the NK1 receptors producing a brief depolarization of the dorsal horn neurones and activation of the central pathways.

More prolonged afferent input leads to NMDA receptor activation.

NMDA receptors

NMDA receptors are a class of ionotropic glutamate receptors characterized by affinity for *N*-methyl-D-aspartate. They also have an allosteric binding site for glycine, which must be occupied for the channel to open efficiently. There is a site within the channel itself to which magnesium ions bind in a voltage-dependent manner and these Mg^{2+} ions block the action of the receptors under normal conditions. Normally, the Mg^{2+} ion block of the NMDA receptor is not removed by glutamate and substance P acts on the NK1 receptor but does not produce pain. However, sustained activity at NK1 and AMPA receptors, for example produced by trauma or inflammation, causes a slow summating depolarization that removes the Mg^{2+} ion block, allowing Ca^{2+} ions to flow into the cell. Once open, there is a massive depolarization because of the Ca^{2+} influx into the cell producing a sudden delayed increase in activity. The neurotrophin BDNF is then released which activates trkB receptors and further enhances NMDA activity. The NMDA receptor channel has much slower kinetics than the AMPA receptor.

Activation of the NMDA receptor ultimately leads to an increased excitability of the dorsal horn. Hyperalgesia, spontaneous pain and some forms of allodynia are mediated by this receptor. The NMDA receptor is responsible for the induction, the setting up of the enhanced response and its subsequent maintenance for prolonged periods of time. There is a clear consensus that the NMDA receptor is only activated when the intensity and duration of the noxious stimulus exceeds a certain level. Thus the NMDA receptor seems implicated in pathological pain states rather than in acute physiological pain.

Calcium ion influx results in the generation of nitric oxide by activation of the enzyme NOS and activation of COX in the spinal cord and these appear to act to further enhance pain signalling (Fig. 1.13). Blockade of the production of nitric oxide abolishes wind-up and reduces hyperalgesia. Central sensitization may be consolidated by protein kinase C-mediated phosphorylation of the NMDA receptor, which reduces the Mg^{2+} gating characteristics of the channel.

Summary

When tissue is damaged:

1 Peripheral chemicals sensitize the sensory endings and excitability changes occur within the nerve itself.

2 Inflammation produces peripheral sensitization in that the system will be driven harder for a given stimulus.

3 The peripheral changes then alter activity in central systems.

4 Marked central changes are likely even when a neuropathy arises from purely peripheral origins.

5 Ongoing ectopic activity in damaged peripheral nerves will continually produce transmitter release into the spinal cord, and this will cause subsequent neuronal activity.

6 After tissue and nerve injury, there are increases in the activity of calcium channels within the spinal cord responsible for both presynaptic transmitter release and postsynaptic neuronal excitability. N-type calcium channels, in particular, become more active and contribute to activity evoked by both low- and high-threshold peripheral stimuli.

7 Following nerve injury, there is an up-regulation of the α2δ subunit of calcium channels, suggesting a greater number of channels are active at any one time.

8 Active calcium channels also produce release of glutamate and peptides into the spinal dorsal horn during inflammation. An increased release of glutamate leads to enhanced activation of the receptors for glutamate, especially the NMDA receptor which is implicated in wind-up and central sensitization.

9 Central sensitization occurs when peripheral sensory neurone activity drives central spinal systems that amplify and prolong the incoming sensory messages. Consequently, this is a mechanism whereby the final sensation of pain becomes dissociated from peripheral activity.

Wind-up

One manifestation of central sensitization is 'wind-up' where repeated constant C fibre stimulation elicits increased spinal neuronal responses in animals and pain reports in patients. As spinal neurones become more excitable, their receptive fields expand and this is thought to be a major factor in secondary hyperalgesia. The AMPA receptor sets the baseline level of activity and, when activated, the NMDA receptor then causes wind-up. This enhances and prolongs transmission and so has been implicated in many states of central hypersensitivity, including hyperalgesia and allodynia seen in postoperative, inflammatory and neuropathic pains.

C-*fos* expression

Genes in the nerve cell produce neurotransmitter proteins. Fluctuations in gene expression that reflect changes in the functional demands on individual neurones are an everyday occurrence.

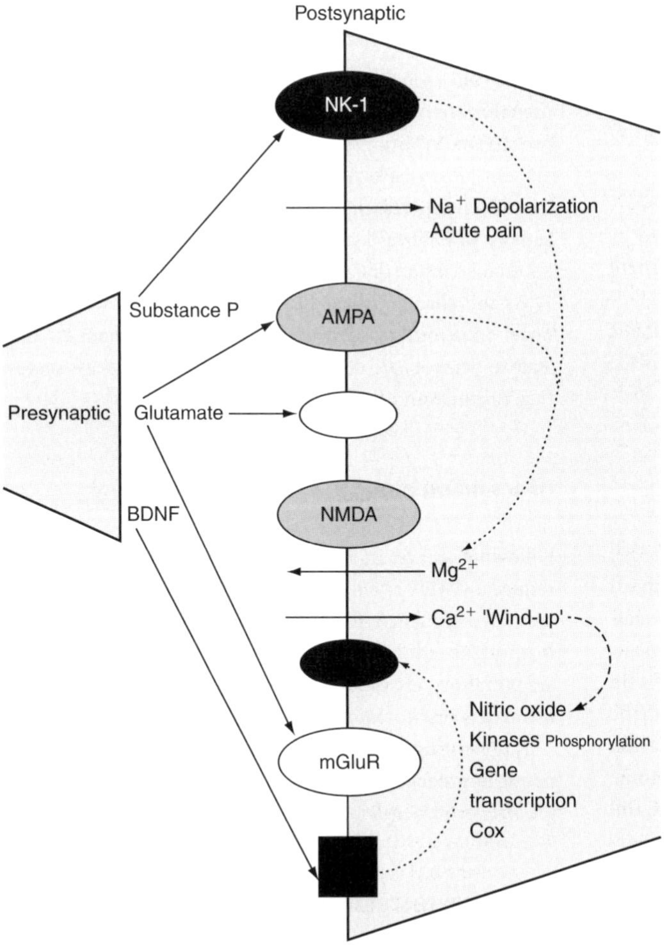

Figure 1.13 *Transmission and NMDA receptors. Sustained activity at NK-1 and AMPA lead to removal of the magnesium block allowing calcium into the cells. This activates nitric oxide and cyclo-oxygenase in the spinal cord. BDNF is then released, activating trkB and enhancing NMDA activity. NMDA receptors are activated by removal of the magnesium channel block and phosphorylation. mGluR, glutamate receptor; NK-1, neurokinin 1 receptor; AMPA, α-3-hydroxy-5-methyl-isoxazolepropionic acid; NMDA, N-methyl-D-aspartate receptor; trkB, tyrosine kinase; BDNF, brain derived neurotrophic factor*

C-*fos* is the gene most studied in the generation of pain. It produces a protein called fos, which is crucial to the central nervous system changes that occur when a person feels pain. Fos is one of the **inducible transcription factors** that controls mammalian gene expression and can promote vast intracellular changes including restructuring and proliferation. Noxious stimulation causes fos to appear in the spinal cord. Even brief stimulation (10 minutes) will produce fos within 30 minutes, peak in one to two hours and disappear within eight hours. This is not seen with non-noxious stimulation. It must therefore be the incoming unmyelinated, polymodal nociceptor C-fibres and Aδ fibres that mediate these effects. Prolonged stimulation causes a many-fold increase in fos expression along with a substantially prolonged expression. C-*fos* is found in: the dorsal horn, sympathetic chain, PAG, locus coeruleus, parabrachial areas, thalamus, hypothalamus and the cerebral cortex.

With prolonged stimulation, c-*fos* disappears from spinal neurones after two to seven days. This disappearance is despite increased neuronal excitability and a marked increase in expression of neurokinin and glutamate receptors and may be because the neuronal changes are so fixed, the transcription factor is no longer needed.

Consequences of fos production include production of neuropeptides and synthesis of a variety of receptors. Too many neurotransmitters are made in the wrong proportions and this causes excess excitation of the pain nerves.

Fentanyl given pre-emptively reduces fos expression up to 50 per cent in a dose-dependent manner but does not abolish it. Morphine given after injury is ineffective in preventing fos expression. Neuraxial block with local anaesthetic agents can almost totally ablate the c-*fos* response but halothane with nitrous oxide does not suppress spinal cord c-*fos*.

The pattern of c-*fos* expression following neuropathic injury is different from that seen in acute pain. Fos is found in laminae III and IV as well as I and II. These are the sites of termination of large diameter non-nociceptive afferents (Aβ) and they do not normally express fos. After sciatic nerve injury, low-intensity Aβ stimulation leads to fos expression. This mechanism may help to explain allodynia but there are still many aspects that are not understood.

Influence of sympathetic nerve activity and catecholamines on primary afferent nerves

Normal primary afferent neurone activity is unaffected by sympathetic outflow but this may change during persistent pain states.

There appears to be two ways in which the sympathetic nervous system influences afferent neurones related to the underlying cause:

- traumatic nerve damage
- peripheral tissue inflammation associated with nociceptor sensitization.

In some patients, injured and uninjured axons begin to express functional α-adrenoceptors and become sensitive to circulating catecholamines and noradrenaline released from postganglionic sympathetic terminals. A peripheral nerve lesion generates plastic changes in both the afferent and sympathetic postganglionic neurones depending on the type of lesion (e.g. complete or partial). Both afferent and postganglionic neurones exhibit degenerative and regenerative changes, and normal neurones may show collateral sprouting in the dorsal root ganglion. The reorganization of peripheral neurones may lead to chemical coupling between sympathetic and afferent neurones. This coupling is responsible for activation of primary afferent neurones by sympathetic neurones. The coupling can occur at different sites on the primary afferent, e.g. at the lesion site, in the dorsal root ganglia or between non-lesioned sympathetic and afferent neurones. Nerve injury induces the sprouting of sympathetic axons into the dorsal root ganglia where they form baskets around the cell bodies of the sensory neurones.

Complete lesion

Sympathetic activity is located in the neuroma and dorsal root ganglia. It is mediated by noradrenaline released from postganglionic neurones and α-adrenoceptors in the membranes of afferent fibres.

Partial lesion

The sympathetic innervation density falls leading to up-regulation of functional α2 adrenoceptors at the membranes of intact nociceptive fibres.

Tissue inflammation

Intact but sensitized primary afferents acquire noradrenaline sensitivity. Noradrenaline induces the release of prostaglandins from sympathetic terminals that sensitize the afferents. Presynaptic up-regulation of neurotransmitter production (i.e. increased production) together with an ongoing activity in C fibres leads to further transmitter release with a sustained influx of Ca^{2+} ions into the dorsal horn neurones.

As the chronic phase becomes established, synthesis of novel transmitters, growth factors and ion channels may lead to phenotypic changes within the nociceptive system (e.g. production of substance P in large fibres).

Descending control

Following nerve injury, inhibitory control may also be reduced. GABA is reduced and GABA and opioid receptors are down-regulated. Expression of cholecystokinin receptors is up-regulated. Interneurones in lamina II, many of which are inhibitory, are thought to die after peripheral nerve injury through an excitotoxic mechanism.

Augmenting central inhibition is therefore a useful therapeutic approach, e.g. tricyclic drugs that act on noradrenergic and serotonergic pathways.

Structural reorganization in neuropathic pain

Following peripheral nerve injury the Aβ fibres sprout and extend from lamina III to lamina II, an area normally occupied by nociceptive C fibres, and then make contact with neurones in this region. This is a plausible explanation of allodynia from normally innocuous Aβ stimulation. Some dorsal root ganglion neurones with Aβ fibres begin to express substance P/CGRP after injury, and spared neurones also show increased expression of substance P/CGRP that may be regulated by NGF.

Sympathetic sprouting occurs around large neurones in the dorsal root ganglia. This confirms that sympathetic efferents and sensory neurones become functionally coupled after nerve injury. Post-injury dorsal column activation has also been described.

The nuclei of the dorsal column neurones are hyperexcitable and display dramatically altered electrophysiological properties in animals with neuropathic pathology. Analysis of activity in the ventro-posterolateral nucleus of the thalamus suggests nociceptive signals from the periphery may shift their afferent pathway from the spinothalamic tract to the dorsal column.

There is a large variation in the type, degree and duration of pain experienced by individuals with the same pathological diagnosis. A better understanding of the multiple mechanisms contributing to neuropathic and inflammatory pain should lead to a more effective use of existing drugs and provide a basis for the development of potential new therapies.

Axonal changes after injury

After axotomy there is an increased coupling of Schwann cells. The Schwann cells wrap themselves around the injured axons when a neurone is injured. The damaged cells down-regulate but the undamaged cells up-regulate and it may be this that is responsible for the development of prolonged pain. Undamaged neurones become less sensitive to TTX and this may explain unresponsiveness to some treatments.

Neurogenic inflammation

Stimulation of C fibres and sympathetic postganglionic terminals causes local vasodilation (redness) and increased capillary permeability (swelling). This is due to retrograde transport along the fibres and the local release of substance P and CGRP. As a consequence, K^+, H^+, acetylcholine, histamine and bradykinin may be released, stimulating further production of prostaglandins and leukotrienes, which then sensitize high-threshold mechanoreceptors. Neurogenic inflammation may spread to surrounding tissue antidromically.

SUMMARY OF THE MAIN PROCESSES IN CHRONIC PAIN

Chronic pain can be a sustained sensory abnormality occurring as a result of ongoing peripheral pathology such as chronic inflammation, or it can be independent of the trigger that initiated it. In the latter case it is the changes in the nervous system that become the pathology and the pain is maladaptive. It may be spontaneous (especially in denervation syndromes) or provoked – a peripheral stimulus produces an exaggerated amplitude or duration of pain.

Mechanical pain sensitivity is largely the consequence of a misrepresentation of normal inputs that are not normally part of the nociceptive or physiological pain system and which never normally generate pain – a consequence of generation of central sensitization.

Table 1.5 shows the important differences between inflammatory and neuropathic pain. Box 1.3 summarizes the main processes in chronic pain.

A change in the function, chemistry and structure of neurones (neural plasticity) clearly underlies the production of

Table 1.5 *Differences between inflammatory and neuropathic pain*

Nerve injury	Inflammation
Ectopic activity	Alterations in structurally intact
Adrenergic sensitivity	neurones
Dorsal root ganglion cell death	Changes in afferent and efferent
Trans-ganglionic atrophy	functions of the peripheral terminals
Trans-synaptic degeneration	

BOX 1.3   Chronic pain – main processes

Primary hyperalgesia
- Sensitization of primary afferents

Secondary hyperalgesia
- Sensitization of spinal cord neurones (dorsal horn)
- Lowered excitation thresholds
- Increased responsiveness to subsequent stimuli (wind-up)
- Receptive field expansion
- Altered gene expression and protein synthesis

Peripheral mechanisms
- Inflammatory mediators + cytokine action on nociceptive nerve terminals → abnormal excitation of the peripheral nociceptive afferent fibres
- Abnormal nociceptor sensitivity
- Spontaneous neuronal activity
- Abnormal ion channel activity: TRPV1; sodium ions
- Catecholamine sensitivity
- Axonal sprouting

Central mechanisms
- Increased C fibre input to the dorsal horn → interaction of two mediators released by C fibres
- Glutamate acting on AMPA and NMDA receptors
- Substance P acting on NK-1 receptors → facilitated transmission in the dorsal horn and higher up in the nociceptive pathway along with involvement of GABA, cholecystokinin, CGRP, somatostatin, neuropeptide Y, adenosine, aminotransmitters, eicosanoids and nitric oxide

---

the altered sensitivity characteristic of neuropathic pain. Similar changes also occur in the brain, especially in the cortex. Only when we have the tools to identify the mechanism responsible for the pain in a particular individual and then the capacity to reverse the mechanism, will the management of neuropathic pain really advance.

2 Assessment of the Patient with Pain

ROLE OF PAIN ASSESSMENT

Patients are usually referred to a pain clinic when other health professionals have been unable to control their symptoms adequately. Pain has many components as well as nociception, including suffering and disability. Any component may cause a patient to seek help and it is important to assess each component separately to know how best to help that patient.

The assessment of the patient may be hindered by patient–physician differences regarding:

- language
- experiences
- expectations of outcome
- frames of reference.

How a physician thinks about pain affects the way he or she assesses the patient who presents with pain. It is therefore important to try to use simple and reliable assessment tools. The purpose of the initial pain clinic assessment is:

- to assess the overall medical condition of the patient
- to diagnose any pathological cause of pain and to identify symptoms and signs that require further investigation
- to identify patients who require a more detailed psychological assessment
- to plan the best method of dealing with the patient's distress
- to assess the response to treatment.

Classification of pain

Pain is not a measurable or definable entity and often the adage 'Pain is what the patient says it is' is the best definition available. Patients with pain are seen by many different specialties. It is necessary for specialists from all disciplines to be able to systematically identify the conditions they are treating, so that aetiology, epidemiology, prognosis and treatment of each disease can be compared.

The understanding of pain physiology and the recognition of pain as part of a disease process has led to the development of a classification of pain syndromes by the International Association for the Study of Pain. The classification allows the standardization of observations by different workers and the exchange of information. The list of pain terms (Table 2.1) was first published in 1979 and was agreed between specialties including anaesthesia, dentistry, neurology, neurosurgery, neurophysiology, psychiatry and psychology. The terms have been developed for use in clinical practice rather than for experimental work, physiology or anatomical purposes.

IMMPACT recommendations for pain assessment

IMMPACT stands for the Initiative on Methods, Measurement and Pain Assessment in Clinical Trials. Many different tools are available for assessment of pain, and when different methods are used in trials it is impossible to compare outcomes of treatment. In order that different treatment methods can be compared, IMMPACT recommends the following six core outcome domains for research purposes.

1 Pain scores – 0–10 numerical rating score and the amount of rescue analgesia used.
2 Physical functioning assessment – e.g. the Brief Pain Inventory (BPI) or measures specific to a disease.
3 Emotional functioning assessment – e.g. the Beck Depression Index.
4 Participant rating of improvement and satisfaction with treatment (global assessment) – patient global impression of change.
5 Symptoms and adverse events as a result of intervention from the trial.
6 Participant disposition – adherence to treatment, reasons for withdrawal.

Patient history

Since pain is the symptom that has led to the consultation, attention to the pain is crucial to establishing a rapport with the patient. Many patients feel their pain is being ignored when they have not been helped by medication, and they are very grateful for being taken seriously and to have someone listen to them.

Table 2.1 *Pain terminology*

Pain	An unpleasant sensory and emotional experience associated with actual or potential tissue damage, or described in terms of such damage
Allodynia	Pain due to a stimulus which does not normally provoke pain
	Allodynia involves a change in the quality of a sensation, whether tactile, thermal, or of any other sort. The original modality is normally non-painful, but the response is painful. There is thus a loss of specificity of a sensory modality
Analgesia	The absence of pain in response to stimulation which would normally be painful
Anaesthesia dolorosa	Pain in an area or region which is anaesthetic
Causalgia	A syndrome of sustained burning pain, allodynia and hyperpathia after a traumatic nerve lesion, often combined with vasomotor and sudomotor dysfunction and later trophic changes
Central pain	Pain initiated or caused by a primary lesion or dysfunction in the central nervous system
Dysaesthesia	An unpleasant abnormal sensation, whether spontaneous or evoked
Hyperalgesia	An increased response to a stimulus which is normally painful. Stimulus and response mode are the same
Hyperaesthesia	Increased sensitivity to stimulation
Hyperpathia	A painful syndrome characterized by an abnormally painful reaction to a stimulus
Hypoalgesia	Diminished pain in response to a normally painful stimulus
Hypoaesthesia	Decreased sensitivity to stimulation
Neuralgia	Pain in the distribution of a nerve or nerves
Neuritis	Inflammation of a nerve or nerve. The term should not be used unless inflammation is thought to be present
Neurogenic pain	Pain initiated or caused by a primary lesion, dysfunction, or transitory perturbation in the peripheral or central nervous system
Neuropathic pain	Pain initiated or caused by a primary lesion or dysfunction in the nervous system
	Peripheral neuropathic pain occurs when the lesion or dysfunction affects the peripheral nervous system
	Central pain may be retained as the term when the lesion or dysfunction affects the central nervous system
Neuropathy	A disturbance of function or pathological change in a nerve: in one nerve, mononeuropathy; in several nerves, mononeuropathy multiplex; if diffuse and bilateral, polyneuropathy
Nociceptor	A receptor preferentially sensitive to a noxious stimulus or to a stimulus which would become noxious if prolonged
Noxious stimulus	A noxious stimulus is one which is damaging to normal tissues
Pain threshold	The least experience of pain which a subject can recognize
Pain tolerance level	The greatest level of pain which a subject is prepared to tolerate
Paraesthesia	An abnormal sensation, whether spontaneous or evoked but not unpleasant
Peripheral neurogenic pain	Pain initiated or caused by a primary lesion or dysfunction or transitory perturbation in the peripheral nervous system
Peripheral neuropathic pain	Pain initiated or caused by a primary lesion or dysfunction in the peripheral nervous system

The initial assessment of a patient in pain begins with a **good history**. It is important to understand not only what the pain feels like but also how it affects the daily activities of the patient.

LOCATION OF PAIN

Patients sometimes have difficulty explaining details about their pain particularly if there are different sensations in different areas. **Pain maps** can be helpful (Fig. 2.1). A picture of a body, both front and back, is given to the patient to mark the areas of pain. Where different types of pain are experienced, different methods of shading can be used. For example, a burning pain could be shown by crosses and a sharp pain by diagonal lines. Pain maps are useful to assess the site or distribution of pain but do not measure intensity. They are not useful for very discrete pain such as a headache.

INTENSITY OF THE PAIN

The only reliable measure of intensity of pain is the patient's report. It is impossible to compare pain intensity among patients. Comparisons can only be made between intensity of pain at a given time for a given patient. Methods of assessing pain intensity are discussed later in the chapter.

Mark these drawings according to where you hurt (if the back of your neck, mark the drawing on the back of the neck, etc.). If you feel any of the following symptoms, please indicate where you feel them by placing the marks shown here on the diagram. Include all affected areas.

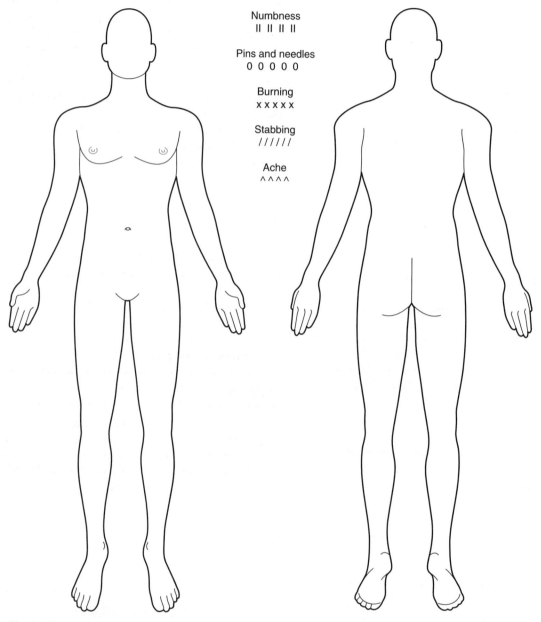

Numbness
‖ ‖ ‖ ‖

Pins and needles
0 0 0 0 0

Burning
x x x x x

Stabbing
/ / / / / /

Ache
^ ^ ^ ^

How bad is your pain now?

Please mark with an X on the body form where the pain is worst now.

Figure 2.1 *Example of a pain map*

CHARACTERISTICS OF THE PAIN

Examples of words used to describe the pain:

- Burning
- Aching
- Shooting.

TEMPORAL ASPECTS OF THE PAIN

Certain pain syndromes have classic temporal patterns, e.g. cluster headaches, rheumatoid arthritis (morning stiffness), osteoarthritis (pain late in day). Ask if the pain is:

- continuous or intermittent
- recurring regularly or irregularly
- paroxysmal
- sustained with superimposed paroxysms.

Ask about the duration of the pain. Are there any specific factors causing the pain? For example, genetic or congenital disorders, trauma, operation, burns, inflammation, neoplasm, or degenerative or mechanical changes.

EXACERBATING AND RELIEVING FACTORS

It is important to establish what increases the pain, e.g. walking will cause claudication pain in spinal stenosis. Often patients will have tried many approaches to relieve the pain and it is important to find out if there is anything they have tried with a successful outcome.

Further assessment

The answers to all of the above questions help to establish both the cause of the pain and the effect it has on the patient's activity levels, and how their life has been affected by the pain. Pain assessment must be multidimensional and should include assessment of the factors given in Table 2.2.

Examination

The examination begins as the patient walks into the room. It is important to see how the patient rises from a chair and how they walk into the room. During discussion of the symptoms it is possible to assess whether they are withdrawn or aggressive and to assess any other relevant emotions. Many patients will have been examined by other healthcare professionals and find the process quite uncomfortable. It is important to examine patients even though this would have been done by others before.

Examination of the patient should take into account the history and relevant systems of the body should be assessed. Where relevant look for:

- pain on palpation, or painful trigger points
- altered temperature
- altered colour
- swelling
- altered sensation such as allodynia or anaesthesia
- range of movement of joints – both active and passive
- curvature of the spine
- how the patient moves, gets out of a chair, etc.

MEASUREMENT OF PAIN

Problems

There are no objective measures of pain. Questionnaires often reflect other experiences as well as pain. Mobility, function and satisfaction are equally as important as pain. There is a large variability in response to pain among patients. The differences in response to pain may be because of:

- sex
- cultural issues

Table 2.2 *Points to consider when taking the history of a patient in pain*

Previous history	Physical difficulties	Role of psychological factors
Previous painful conditions and outcome of treatment	Quality of life	Drug and alcohol use and abuse
Other past and present medical history	Physical difficulties	Effect of pain on family life
Drug history	Effect of pain on sexual function	Effect of pain on social life and work
Allergies		Other behavioural factors
Smoking history		Assessment of mood, anxiety, depression and anger
		Patient's interpretation of symptoms
		Ongoing litigation

- nationality
- environment.

We rarely know how much movement on a particular scale equates to a clinically meaningful change in pain or if the pain relief is adequate for the patient. We need to know how much change constitutes a clinically important difference. Little is known about the meaning to patients of decrease in pain intensity assessed by a 1–10 scale. For example, many studies focus on a 50 per cent improvement in pain scores, whereas many patients are more than happy with a 20 per cent reduction.

Some form of pain measurement is needed to document the severity of the pain and its response to treatment, and to quantify the emotional and psychological aspects influencing the complaints of pain. The usual index is the patient's verbal report, which shows poor correlation between the pathology and the subjective complaint.

There is wide variation in patients' experience of pain, and organic factors cannot explain individual differences in patients' reports. There may be only a slight association between a patient's degree of functional impairment and the severity of tissue damage, thus factors other than tissue injury must contribute to the pain. The patient's appraisal of his or her symptoms is essential in understanding an individual's report of pain and disability.

Different methods of assessment are needed to address the different components of pain. Pain scales can be general and used for all types of pain, or they can be specific to a particular type of pain, for example, the Galer neuropathic pain scale and the Roland Morris back pain and disability scale.

Measuring pain

To be useful, measurement tools need to have the following characteristics, i.e. they must be:

- simple
- easy to understand
- reliable
- consistent for a patient and within a group of patients.

Pain relief scales are perceived as more convenient than pain intensity scales because patients have the same baseline relief (0) whereas they could start with different baseline intensity. A patient with severe initial pain intensity has more scope to show improvement than one who starts with mild pain. Relief scales are thus easier to compare across patients. The theoretical drawback is that a patient has to remember what the pain was like to begin with.

Scales measuring pain alone

VERBAL RATING SCALE

Verbal rating scales can measure either pain intensity or pain relief (Fig. 2.2). They are better for measuring acute pain than a visual analogue scale (VAS).

VERBAL NUMERICAL RATING SCALE

A verbal numerical rating scale (NRS) (Box 2.1) is simple with a high rate of completion. It is more useful than a VAS for postoperative pain. The patient is asked to rate their pain on a scale of 0–10 where 0 = no pain and 10 = worst pain imaginable.

Improvement in pain scores has been related to minimal, moderate and much improvement postoperatively (Table 2.3).

For patients with severe pain, the reduction in the NRS pain score and percentage relief of pain have to be larger to obtain similar degrees of pain relief. So it seems it is the change in the pain intensity that appears to be meaningful to patients, as the severity of the baseline pain increases.

Pain intensity scale		Pain relief scale	
No pain	= 0	Complete pain relief	= 4
Mild pain	= 1	Good pain relief	= 3
Moderate pain	= 2	Moderate pain relief	= 2
Severe pain	= 3	Slight pain relief	= 1
		No pain relief	= 0

Or

1	2	3	4	5	6	7	8	9	10

Figure 2.2 *Types of verbal rating scales*

BOX 2.1 Verbal numerical rating scale

NRS 1–3 = mild pain

NRS 4–6 = moderate pain

NRS >6 = severe pain

Table 2.3 *Assessment of improvement in pain*

Reduction in pain score (units)	Pain improvement
3 (20%)	Minimal improvement
4 (35%)	Moderate improvement
5 (45%)	Much improvement

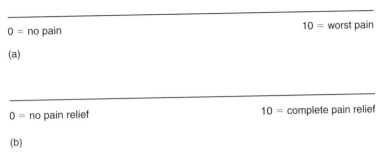

0 = no pain   10 = worst pain

(a)

0 = no pain relief   10 = complete pain relief

(b)

Figure 2.3 *(a) Visual analogue scale; (b) Pain relief scale*

The minimal noticeable change in the NRS ('minimal' improvement) is 20 per cent.

VISUAL ANALOGUE SCALE

The VAS (Fig. 2.3a) is usually a 100 mm line with two words that anchor the two ends of the spectrum (no pain (0) and pain as bad as you can imagine (10)). The patient makes a mark on the 100 mm line and the distance can be measured with a ruler. The VAS is a single dimension scale, valid for patients over 7 years of age. It has a failure rate of about 7 per cent because some patients do not understand how to put a number on their pain.

PAIN RELIEF SCALE

Pain relief scales assess pain before and after an intervention. Any pain scale can be used but before and after measures must be on a different sheet of paper. A scale similar to the 100 mm scale as for the VAS can be used (Fig. 2.3b). A horizontal scale is more reliable than a vertical scale.

ADVANTAGES OF THE ABOVE METHODS OF PAIN MEASUREMENT

- Robust and reproducible
- Simple and easy for the patient
- Understandable
- Rapidly recorded
- Conventional
- 100 mm line fills the central area of the visual field at typical reading distance (45 cm)
- Diagrams avoid anchoring and number/word preferences
- Useful for audit.

DISADVANTAGES OF THE ABOVE METHODS OF PAIN MEASUREMENT

- They are unable to detect subtle differences.
- They are less suitable for research because they are semiqualitative.
- They are not suitable for parametric tests of statistical significance.

- Non-parametric tests must be used, which require larger samples.
- Lines <100 mm are less accurate.
- Response can vary among patients and in the same patient at different times.
- They are subjective measures and can therefore be inaccurate.

If recording two scores at different times, the patient has to remember what the pain was like before an intervention and although this does show some consistency there is a wide variation in response.

PAIN INTENSITY DIFFERENCE

Pain intensity, pain relief and VAS are the measures used most commonly to assess pain relief in trials involving post-operative patients. Pain scores or pain relief scores are recorded over a period of time after the operation. Analgesics are withheld until patients report moderate to severe pain and the study medication is given at a time defined as zero. In most analgesic studies measurements are taken hourly, except for the first hour, during which time more frequent measurements may be taken. Reduction in pain is plotted against time elapsed since administration of medicine. Onset of analgesia will occur before the first reading is taken and peak analgesia will probably occur between readings. The circles correspond to the time of assessment.

SUMMED PAIN INTENSITY DIFFERENCE

To account for differences in baseline pain intensity among patients in the study, pain intensity category and VAS scores are converted into pain intensity difference (PID) scores by subtracting them from the pain score taken at baseline (PID = Pt − P0). Positive scores indicate reduction in pain, making the PID scores analogous to pain relief scores.

Pain intensity difference or relief scores are commonly summed over the observation period, weighted for the time between observations, and the summed scores respectively

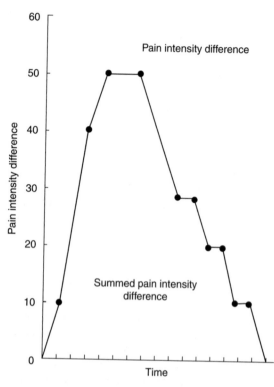

Pain intensity difference (PID)

- PID = pain intensity score at baseline − current pain intensity
- That is, +ve PID = pain relief

Summed pain intensity difference (SPID)

- SPID = area under PID/time curve
- Baseline PID = 0
- That is, higher SPID = greater pain relief

Figure 2.4 *Measuring pain relief*

termed SPID (summed pain intensity difference) or TOTPAR (total pain relief). These summary variables are estimates of the area under the time–effect curve (AUC). The maximum possible SPID is the value of SPID that would be obtained if a patient was pain-free for the total period of observation. This adjustment may partly correct for the bias that patients who start off with higher pain scores tend to have larger pain reductions – higher PID scores – if pain is reduced to zero or any other fixed endpoint (Fig. 2.4).

PAIN DIARIES

Detailed information can be obtained about pain when the patient is asked to keep a diary of when they have pain, what it was like, what they did about it and did any medication relieve it? It can be a useful research tool.

Syndrome-specific pain scales

Many pain scales have been developed to measure pain in specific diseases and are only validated in these syndromes, for example neuropathic pain, pain in rheumatoid arthritis and back pain. Some scales are specifically meant for recording pain and others include symptom or disability scores, such as the Oswestry disability questionnaire. For many patients, problems arise not simply because of the pain they experience but also because of the accompanying disability that their pain causes. It is important to assess the difficulties caused by the pain as well as the pain itself.

GALER NEUROPATHIC PAIN SCORE

After studying 288 patients with neuropathic pain, researchers identified eight common qualities of neuropathic pain: sharp, hot, dull, cold, sensitive (like raw skin or sunburn), itchy, and deep and surface pain. Each item is rated on a 0–10 scale (0 = none, 10 = worst imaginable). It takes about five minutes to complete and is sensitive to the effects of treatment. This pain scale may be a useful tool in the initial assessment of patients with chronic pain and to evaluate effectiveness of treatment.

OSWESTRY DISABILITY QUESTIONNAIRE

The Oswestry disability questionnaire is a brief self-report instrument specifically designed to assess the perceived degree of disability in a patient with back pain. It is clear, brief and easy to administer and interpret. It is one of the scales that is recommended as an assessment tool in all back pain research.

PAIN MEASUREMENT IN RHEUMATOID ARTHRITIS

The standard method of assessing response to treatment by patients with rheumatoid arthritis is the American College of Rheumatology response criteria. A core set of variables is measured at baseline and at set intervals after commencement of therapy.

OSTEOARTHRITIS

Arthritis Impact Measurement Scales

The Arthritis Impact Measurement Scales (AIMS) are a combination of previously studied and newly created health status scales which assess physical, emotional and social wellbeing. They consist of a self-administered questionnaire for patients with osteoarthritis, and are practical and generate reliable and valid measures. The AIMS approach to health status measurement should prove useful for evaluating the outcomes of arthritis treatments and programmes.

WOMAC

The Western Ontario and McMaster Universities (WOMAC) Osteoarthritis Index is a disease-specific, self-administered health status measure. It probes clinically important symptoms in the areas of pain, stiffness and physical function in patients with osteoarthritis of the hip and/or knee.

Multidimensional pain scales

Mobility, function and satisfaction are important in chronic pain. Any intervention that improves pain by as little as 10 per cent may be very important to the patient because the small shift in pain allows an important shift in function. Measured solely as pain reduction, this might be missed.

The validity of some of the measures is questionable, but they are economical and efficient. Global quality of life scores have been designed to pick up changes in other significant factors related to the pain experience, e.g. the short form (SF)-36, but when assessing function, a scale designed for a particular disease produces better outcomes.

GLOBAL IMPRESSION OF CHANGE SCALE

This scoring system is completed by both the patient and the clinician. The patient is asked to tick the box they feel most closely describes any changes which they have experienced since beginning the study medication. The scale takes into account all changes, whether or not one believes these are entirely due to drug treatment. Only ONE response is chosen from the list shown in Box 2.2 below.

BRIEF PAIN INVENTORY

The purpose of the BPI is to assess the severity of pain and the impact of pain on daily functions in patients with cancer pain and pain due to other chronic diseases. It is usually a

---

BOX 2.2 Global impression of change scale

Since the start of the study, my overall status is:

- Very much improved – 1
- Much improved – 2
- Minimally improved – 3
- No change – 4
- Minimally worse – 5
- Much worse – 6
- Very much worse – 7

---

self-report questionnaire but some patients require help completing it. The BPI includes:

- severity of pain
- impact of pain on daily function
- location of pain
- pain medications
- amount of pain relief in the past 24 hours or the past week.

This method of assessment has been used extensively in research. It is reasonable in its validity and reliability and useful in a variety of clinical settings. It takes about 15 minutes to complete and has been translated into many other languages.

SHORT FORM – 36 PHYSICAL FUNCTION SCALE

The SF-36 was originally developed in the USA to help understand how the healthcare system affects health. It now has a much wider application, being used to measure the general health of populations as well as to compare the health of patients with different medical conditions. It is a general measure that is intended to capture quality of life as well as whether an individual is healthy or not. The SF-36 consists of eight scales. These cover ability to function and complete everyday activities, including physical activities and social activities. The scales also capture wellbeing such as energy or fatigue and mental health over a 4-week period. It was developed from the sickness impact profile.

ROLAND MORRIS QUESTIONNAIRE

This questionnaire consists of 24 questions asking about the effect of back and/or leg pain on certain activities.

HEALTH ASSESSMENT QUESTIONNAIRE

Patients are asked to rate activities according to how difficult they find them.

PSYCHOLOGICAL ASSESSMENT

Some patients require a full psychological assessment by a trained clinical psychologist, and in many clinics specific psychological assessment is not done by the pain clinician but by the psychologist. Questionnaires are usually completed either to assess the outcome of an intervention or for research purposes and generally do not change the management of the patient.

McGill pain questionnaire

This is a multidimensional questionnaire that was developed by Ronald Melzak and colleagues at McGill University, Canada, in 1975 for use in acute, chronic or cancer pain. The McGill pain questionnaire (MPQ) was developed to indicate the extent of change in pain quality and intensity as a result of an intervention. The questionnaire was an attempt to produce a standard measurement that would assess many of the different phenomena associated with pain. The first form was cumbersome and time consuming, and it was difficult to understand the words. Explanation of the words invalidates the measures.

A short form of the McGill Pain Questionnaire (SF-MPQ) has been developed that is easier to use. The short form contains 15 questions (Box 2.3) and categorizes pain under the three psychological dimensions using verbal rating scales. Each descriptor is ranked on a 4-point intensity scale (0 = none, 1 = mild, 2 = moderate, 3 = severe).

The SF-MPQ also includes:

- a numerical rating scale for intensity and distribution of pain
- present pain intensity scale
- a picture to mark location of pain.

BOX 2.3 The SF-MPQ

Sensory – physical dimensions of pain
- Throbbing
- Shooting
- Stabbing
- Sharp
- Cramping
- Gnawing
- Hot/burning
- Aching
- Heavy
- Tender

Affective – feelings associated with pain
- Splitting/tiring
- Exhausting
- Sickening
- Fearful

Evaluative – the meaning of the pain experienced
- Punishing/cruel

Beck's Depression Inventory

Depression may play a large role in the pain experience either as a cause or as a result of the pain. Many different scales are used in depression. Patients suffering from depression experience pain. Treatment of depression can sometimes alleviate pain without any further intervention.

Beck's Depression Inventory is a 21-item self-rating scale that measures the severity of key symptoms associated with clinical depression but not with other psychological factors aggravating pain. It takes about five minutes to complete and includes 20 questions. Low scores indicate mild depression and high scores more severe depression.

Sickness impact profile

This assessment system has been best studied in the population with chronic back pain. It is a general indicator of health status and health-related dysfunction rather than pain and can be administered by an interviewer or the patient. It has not been validated in other populations. It is a 36-item self-report questionnaire that includes 12 categories grouped into physical, psychosocial and independent dimensions. The physical dimensions are ambulation, mobility and body care/movement. The psychosocial dimensions are social interaction, alertness, emotional behaviour and communication and the independent dimensions are sleep and rest, eating, work, home and recreation.

Minnesota multiphasic personality inventory

This is a self-administered true–false test. The questionnaire consists of 567 items including a post-traumatic stress scale and a gender role scale. It does not discriminate between scores that were elevated prior to or as a result of the pain and is time consuming to complete. The scale is designed to place patients in one of four groups: hypochondriacal, reactively depressed, 'somaticisers' and manipulators.

OBJECTIVE METHODS OF ASSESSING PHYSICAL CHANGES IN NEUROPATHIC PAIN

Most of the objective methods of assessing physical changes in neuropathic pain are currently used more for research purposes than in clinical situations. They do not usually affect the management of the symptoms.

Temperature discrimination

A change in temperature sensation can be used to check small nerve fibre dysfunction. One method of testing temperature sensation uses two rollers, one set at 40°C (8°C above normal skin temperature), and the other at 25°C (7°C below normal skin temperature). Moving the rollers in contact with the skin identifies areas with abnormal temperature sensibility.

Vibration

Vibration is detected by pacinian corpuscles and is mediated through the Aβ fibres. A tuning fork used to be the standard method for testing vibration sensation but machines are now available that provide a well-defined 100 Hz vibratory stimulation whose amplitude is manually controlled. This machine can be used to find the vibration perception threshold. This correlates well with the function of the thick myelinated sensory nerves and can be used to trace Aβ nerve fibre pathology.

Light touch

A set of Von Frey hairs consist of a series of filaments of increasing diameter that produce increasing sensations of touch when applied to the skin. Today, hairs are mostly manufactured from nylon monofilaments. A set of 20 monofilaments with varying diameters and constant length produce a characteristic force perpendicular to the contacting surface. The downward force does not depend on the degree of bend of the monofilament.

Von Frey hairs are used in the diagnosis of allodynia. Allodynia is often tested with a cotton wool ball or a pin but cotton wool is often too gross to test for subclinical loss of touch. Because allodynia is pain from a non-painful stimulus, a pin prick, which is painful, cannot be used in the diagnosis of allodynia.

Pressure

The algometer is a valuable tool in the diagnosis of diseases like fibromyalgia, tension headache and arthritis. It is used to measure the pressure level for pain at points relevant for the disease. During the pressure application, the operator is guided by the algometer to keep the application rate constant, which reduces operator-induced variability. Pressure-induced pain levels can be quantified and treatment effects evaluated.

SPECIFIC TESTS

The tests listed in this section should be considered if indicated by the history and examination. Many patients attending a chronic pain clinic will have had relevant investigations completed but it may be necessary to consider the following depending on the history and examination:

- Blood tests
- Radiographs
- Magnetic resonance imaging (MRI) or computed tomography scanning
- Nerve conduction studies.

MEASUREMENT OF PAIN IN PATIENTS WITH COGNITIVE IMPAIRMENT

Cognitive impairment can be congenital or acquired and includes:

- Dementia
- Head injury
- Learning disability.

When children or adults are unable to communicate their pain a normal way, assessment of pain and the effects of treatment can be very difficult. It is also unclear whether the experience of pain of the patient with severe cognitive impairment from whatever cause is the same as that of a patient without cognitive impairment, or with mild cognitive impairment. Many pain scales have been developed for use in these patients but several are time consuming and have been tested mainly in a nursing home setting in chronic pain. There are fewer methods of assessing acute pain in the cognitively impaired and there are none for acute trauma and head injury.

Parents or carers can be helpful because they are better at identifying signs of distress but it may be difficult to distinguish pain from other causes of distress. Often administering analgesia and observing the outcome is the only way of assessing whether the patient is in some degree of pain.

Biological measures

Patients with cognitive impairment may exhibit some or all of the signs of distress shown in Box 2.4 when they are in pain.

Biological measures are not effective for long-term pain but in the acute setting they may be helpful.

BOX 2.4 Signs of distress

Vocal
- Crying
- Moaning
- Screaming
- Specific sound

Eating/sleeping
- Eats less
- Increased sleep
- Decreased sleep

Social personality
- Not cooperative
- Less interaction
- Seeks comfort
- Difficult to distract

Facial expression
- Cringe
- Grimace
- Furrowed brow

Pain assessment in the patient with dementia

Several scales have been developed to try to assess pain in cognitive impairment but most of them are used in the nursing home setting rather than hospital. Many rely on assessing changes from normal behaviour and so are not appropriate when a patient presents to hospital. Many also take a considerable amount of time to complete. A record of normal behaviour prior to admission or review is useful and this should be discussed with relatives or carers.

Some of the following assessments can be used and those most appropriate to monitor a patient should be chosen. They are not all necessary.

- Folstein's Mini-Mental State Examination
- Geriatric depression scale
- Pain maps
- Faces scale
- VAS (vertical not horizontal)
- Pain on rest and movement
- Body language (Hurley)
- Functional pain scale (Gloth)
- Assessment of discomfort in dementia protocol
- Non-verbal VAS
- Philadelphia pain intensity scale
- Coloured analogue scales
- Facial affective scale

PAIN IMAGING

Different types of pain activate different areas of the brain and increased activity is associated with increased blood flow. The imaging methods discussed in this section should therefore show areas that are active when a patient is experiencing pain and help identify the areas of the brain involved in pain processing. Pain imaging may also be useful for the assessment of outcome of treatment in painful conditions.

Positron emission tomography

Positron emission tomography, also called PET imaging or a PET scan, is a diagnostic examination that involves the acquisition of physiological images based on the detection of positrons.

A radioactive substance is attached to a natural body compound, most commonly glucose, but sometimes water or ammonia. One example of such an agent is 2-fluoro-2-deoxy-D-glucose, which is similar to a naturally occurring sugar, glucose, with the addition of a radioactive fluorine atom. The radioactive substance is given as an intravenous injection. It takes approximately 30–60 minutes for the substance to travel through the body and be absorbed by the tissue under study. Scanning takes an additional 30–45 minutes.

Gamma radiation produced from collisions between positrons and electrons is detected by the PET scanner and shows in fine detail the metabolism of glucose in the brain. A computer converts the detected radiation into a complex picture of the patient's working brain. Different colours or degrees of brightness on a PET image represent different levels of tissue or organ function. The images generated by PET are produced as a result of the metabolic activity of the cell – therefore these images represent the function of cells rather than their anatomical structure.

Positron emission tomography scans have revealed that it is the prefrontal and anterior cingulate cortex that responds to the suffering components of acute and chronic pain and that the changes are bilateral.

ADVANTAGE

Positron emission tomography is a non-invasive alternative to biopsy.

DISADVANTAGES

- Limited resolution (detection limited in lesions under 1 cm).
- Limited but growing availability.

Functional magnetic resonance imaging

Functional MRI (fMRI) is a new use of existing MRI technology. It is used to visualize brain function, by visualizing changes in chemical composition of brain areas or changes in the flow of fluids that occur over seconds to minutes. In the brain, blood perfusion is related to neural activity, so fMRI can be used to find out what the brain is doing when a patient carries out specific tasks or is exposed to specific stimuli.

The term 'fMRI' is usually used to denote techniques involving fast MRI scans, which can allow imaging of a complete brain slice in 20 ms. The main advantages of fMRI as a technique to image brain activity related to a specific task or sensory process include:

- signal does not require injections of radioactive isotopes
- total scan time required can be very short, i.e. in the order of 1.5–2.0 min/run
- in-plane resolution of the functional image is generally about 1.5×1.5 mm although resolutions less than 1 mm are possible.

ROLE OF fMRI IN PAIN MANAGEMENT

Studies in patients with post-herpetic neuralgia indicated that the cortical representation of sympathetically maintained pain involves specific and identifiable cortical activity, as does the relief of that pain achieved by a peripheral nerve block procedure. Continuing investigations will extend these findings to other pain treatments to determine the extent to which this finding is seen with other pain relief mechanisms. The preliminary studies suggest a wide range of other approaches using fMRI to investigate cortical representations of specific pain types, and therefore, new specific therapeutic options.

Other neurological conditions currently under investigation using fMRI include phantom limb pain.

Single proton emission computed tomography

Single proton emission computed tomography (SPECT) also shows blood flow through different areas of the brain. It indicates areas that are not functioning normally. Radioactive isotopes are bound to neuro-specific drugs and are injected into a vein. The radioisotopes are taken up by areas of the brain where blood is flowing. Areas of increased blood flow have more isotopic labelling. The isotope commonly used is technetium-99 which emits γ rays that are then detected by a 4-headed SPECT gamma camera. This technique can also be used to highlight areas involved with pain sensation and response to treatment.

SUMMARY

It is important to establish as much information as possible about the pain itself and its effects on the life of the patient. The most effective treatment plan can then be made, depending on the outcome of an accurate assessment. An accurate history is the most important aspect of the assessment and the examination should help in understanding the effect the pain has upon the patient.

The treatment plan will usually depend on the findings from the history and examination. Many other questionnaires have been developed to assess quality of life, disability and psychological status of the patient. They rarely alter any planned treatment in a pain clinic. Some questionnaires are general and some are disease-specific but they are mainly used as a means of assessing outcome of treatment. The IMMPACT guidelines on use of these methods for research purposes will hopefully simplify the tests used to measure outcome in clinical trials and make it easier to compare treatment effects.

CASE SCENARIO

Neck pain assessment

A 46-year-old man presented with pain and stiffness in his neck of two years' duration following a road traffic accident when his car was hit from behind. There had been a previous similar incident five years previously but this had not resulted in any long-term problems.

HISTORY

The descriptive terms used by the patient will be a guide to how much the pain is affecting the patient in many ways. It is necessary to ask about exacerbating factors and the situations where the patient is most comfortable. The following are all relevant questions:

- Sleep
- Drug history
- Effect of pain on lifestyle
- Work history
- Social history
- Litigation
- Meaning of pain to the patient

LOCATION OF PAIN – PAIN MAP

The pain was constant in his neck and right shoulder. It kept him awake every night. He was unable to continue his manual job and had been asked to leave. He had very few hobbies and his life mainly revolved around the television. He was unable to play with his two boys aged 10 and 11 and he could see no future for himself. He had consulted neurosurgeons, physiotherapists and chiropractors. He could no longer afford to pay for acupuncture, which only gave him pain relief for about five days. His general practitioner had prescribed many painkillers and he had tried anticonvulsants and antidepressants.

EXAMINATION

He was tender to palpation over the neck mainly on the right side and had painful muscles around the right shoulder. There were no specific trigger areas. Movement of the neck was reduced in all directions – it was limited by pain but his neck had also become very stiff. There was no change in sensation and there were no abnormal neurological findings.

Other assessment tools that may help in evaluating the patient or assessing outcome of treatment include:

- Brief Pain Inventory
- Pain intensity, e.g. VAS score
- Beck Depression Inventory
- Sickness impact profile

A neck X-ray showed changes expected in a patient of his age. An MRI scan was not indicated as there were no radicular signs.

3 Pharmacology of Pain Relief

INTRODUCTION

Many drugs are used in the management of acute and chronic pain with variable degrees of success. Complete pain relief from a single drug is unlikely given the complexity of the causes of pain, however, research continues into new analgesic agents because pain is common and pain relief difficult to achieve.

Analgesic drugs are often used incorrectly and inappropriately. Better pain control can be obtained by rationalizing the use of available drugs and using combinations of drugs to achieve the desired effect. Different drugs act on different parts of the pain pathway and combining different agents often has a synergistic effect.

Although antidepressants, anticonvulsants and NMDA (*N*-methyl-D-aspartate) receptor antagonists are usually considered to play a role in the management of chronic neuropathic pain, it is becoming more obvious that neuropathic pain also plays a part in severe acute pain and these drugs are being used increasingly in the postoperative period.

THE OXFORD LEAGUE TABLE OF ANALGESICS IN ACUTE PAIN

Although there is a large number of drugs on the market for the management of acute pain, and despite many years' experience of their use, it remains uncertain which group of drugs or which drug within a group is the most appropriate for use in a particular situation.

The Oxford league table (Table 3.1) has been constructed from information taken from systematic reviews of randomized, double blind, single dose studies in patients with moderate to severe pain. The outcome is at least 50 per cent pain relief over four to six hours. The pain measurements are standardized and have been validated. The aim is to pool the information from several studies to produce a guide to the effectiveness of various analgesic agents in the management of acute pain.

NUMBER NEEDED TO TREAT

There are a number of statistical ways to examine results of clinical trials, but they are difficult for the non-specialist to interpret. The number needed to treat (NNT) is an attempt

Table 3.1 *The Oxford league table of analgesic efficacy*

Analgesic	NNT
Valdecoxib 40 mg	1.6
Diclofenac 100	1.9
Paracetamol 1000 + Codeine 60	2.2
Parecoxib 40 mg (IV)	2.2
Diclofenac 50	2.3
Ibuprofen 400	2.4
Ketorolac 10	2.6
Ibuprofen 200	2.7
Pethidine 100 (IM)	2.9
Morphine 10 (IM)	2.9
Ketorolac 30 (IM)	3.4
Paracetamol 500	3.5
Paracetamol 1000	3.8
Paracetamol 650 + Dextropropoxyphene	4.4
Tramadol 100	4.8
Tramadol 75	5.3
Tramadol 50	8.3
Codeine 60	16.7

NNT, number needed to treat; IV, intravenous; IM, intramuscular. By kind permission of Oxford University Press. Adapted from Moore A, Edwards J, Barden J and McQuay H (2003) *Bandolier's Little Book of Pain*, p. 91. Oxford: OUP.

to overcome these problems. It is an estimate of the number of patients that would need to be given a treatment for one of them to achieve a desired outcome. The NNT should specify:

- the patient group
- the intervention
- the outcome.

Using postoperative pain as the example, the NNT describes the number of patients who have to be treated with an analgesic intervention for one of them to have at least 50 per cent pain relief over four to six hours, and who would not have had pain relief of that magnitude with a placebo. However, that does not mean that pain relief of a lower intensity will not occur. For an analgesic trial, the NNT is calculated very simply as:

NNT = 1/(proportion of patients with at least 50 per cent pain relief with analgesic − proportion of patients with at least 50 per cent pain relief with placebo).

For example, 50 patients are given placebo, and 10 of them have more than 50 per cent pain relief. Another 50 patients are given an analgesic agent, and 27 of them have more than 50 per cent pain relief. Therefore, NNT = 1/(27/50) − (10/50) = 1/0.54 − 0.20 = 1/0.34 = 2.9.

The best NNT would be 1, that is, every patient given treatment benefited, but none of the controls. Generally NNTs between 2 and 5 are indicative of effective analgesic treatments.

For adverse effects, the number needed to harm (NNH) is calculated the same way as an NNT. For an NNH, large numbers are better than small numbers.

The tables will change if different trials indicate different outcomes and can only be used as a guide to treatment.

PARACETAMOL

The mode of action of paracetamol is not completely understood but it is thought to act in the brain, with only weak action in the peripheral anti-inflammatory systems.

Current theories of action

- Weak effects on the cyclo-oxygenase (COX)-1 and COX-2 enzymes
- Central nervous system (CNS) prostaglandin inhibition
- Serotonergic pathway activation or inhibition of injury-induced hyperalgesia
- Via mechanisms involving substance P or nitric oxide
- NMDA antagonism
- COX-3 mechanism

Metabolism

Paracetamol is metabolized by the liver where it is conjugated to:

- 60–80 per cent glucuronide
- 20–30 per cent sulphate
- Cysteine
- 3–10 per cent is metabolized by cytochrome P-450 into N-acetyl-p-amino-benzoquinone imine (NAPQI). Under normal conditions this is rapidly detoxified by reduced glutathione and eliminated in the urine after conjugation with cysteine and mercapturic acid. It is potentially hepatotoxic and the level increases significantly with overdose.

An overdose of paracetamol exhausts stores of hepatic glutathione or N-acetylcysteine and toxicity occurs. Metabolites are mainly excreted in the urine within 24 hours.

Dose

Blood levels of paracetamol required to produce analgesia are thought to be 10–20 mg/L. The dose prescribed for adults is usually 1 gm four hourly but therapeutic blood levels may not be reached with this dose in many adults or children over 50 kg. Recent trials with 1500 mg paracetamol have shown improved pain relief, but the likelihood of increasing the risk of liver toxicity is not yet known. Further studies are underway to find the optimum dose of paracetamol. An overdose of 7.5 g or more in adults or 140 mg/kg in children in a single dose usually causes hepatic cytolysis likely to induce complete and irreversible necrosis unless treatment is started as soon as possible. Rectal bioavailability is 25–98 per cent so the loading dose in children should be 20–40 mg/kg. Thereafter doses of 20 mg/kg eight hourly are recommended.

In neonates, the plasma half-life is longer (3.5 hours versus 2.7 hours in adults). In infants the plasma half-life is shorter (1.5–2 hours). Neonates, infants and children up to 10 years excrete significantly less glucuronide and more sulphate conjugates than adults.

Rectal paracetamol

The bioavailability of paracetamol suppositories is variable. It is approximately 80 per cent of that of the tablets and the rate of absorption is slower, with maximum plasma concentrations achieved about two to three hours after administration. It is not optimal to administer rectal paracetamol at the induction of anaesthesia in procedures lasting only 0.5–1 hour or to administer rectal paracetamol after surgery. It has to be taken into consideration that the vehicle base of the suppository has been shown to have an effect on the absorption of poorly soluble drugs such as paracetamol. A lipophilic base produces higher plasma paracetamol concentrations than a hydrophilic base. Higher doses than used orally are required to produce equivalent analgesia. Studies using 40–60 mg/kg paracetamol showed better analgesia than studies using lower doses.

Intravenous paracetamol

Propacetamol, an injectable prodrug of paracetamol, is completely hydrolysed within six minutes of administration and 1 g of propacetamol yields 0.5 g of paracetamol. There are still surprisingly few eligible randomized studies of oral versus rectal versus intravenous paracetamol. Intravenous paracetamol may, however, have greater analgesic effect than equivalent doses of oral paracetamol.

> **BOX 3.1   Intravenous paracetamol**
>
> - 10 mg/mL paracetamol is contained in a vial of 100 mL (1000 mg)
> - Clear and slightly yellowish solution
> - For use when other routes of administration are not possible

In a comparison of parenteral and oral administration, paracetamol 1 g was given after surgery in both study groups. Pain scores were significantly lower up to four hours after surgery and time to first analgesic request was significantly increased, by 34 minutes in the parenteral group. In conclusion, 1 gm of intravenous paracetamol appears to provide a significantly greater and longer analgesic effect than the same dosage in oral form (see Box 3.1).

More studies are needed to test the evidence for any difference in analgesic efficacy of paracetamol given by different routes. Until such data are available, the route of administration in the postsurgical setting should probably depend on factors such as the presence or absence of gastrointestinal paralysis, nausea and vomiting and sedation.

DOSE

The dose of intravenous paracetamol is 15 mg/kg four hourly, not exceeding 60 mg/kg per day to be given over 15 minutes. It is recommended that with creatinine clearance <30 mL/min the dose interval be increased to six hourly.

CONTRAINDICATIONS

- Hypersensitivity to paracetamol
- Severe hepatocellular insufficiency

There are no known undesirable effects in pregnancy on the health of the fetus or neonate. It can be used during breastfeeding but is excreted into breast milk and where possible all drugs should be avoided in both pregnancy and breastfeeding.

SIDE EFFECTS (ALL RARE)

- Hypersensitivity ranging from rash or urticaria to anaphylactic shock
- Malaise
- Hypotension
- Dehydration
- Thrombocytopenia
- Injection site pain
- Headache
- Vomiting

OVERDOSE

Overdose is more commonly seen in:

- Renal insufficiency
- Dehydration
- Chronic therapy
- Elderly
- Young children
- Liver disease
- Chronic alcoholism
- Chronic malnutrition (reduced glutathione levels)
- Patients receiving concomitant enzyme-inducing drugs (P-450 enzyme induction)

NON-STEROIDAL ANTI-INFLAMMATORY DRUGS

The strongest oral analgesia for acute pain is provided by a non-steroidal anti-inflammatory drug (NSAID) given with a paracetamol and opioid combination. For patients unable to tolerate NSAIDs, a combination of paracetamol and opioid is the next best choice. There is no evidence that NSAIDs given rectally or by injection perform better than the same drug at the same dose given by mouth. Ibuprofen is the safest when gastric bleeding is the main worry but all NSAIDs produce pain relief. They decrease or eliminate the need for opioids thereby reducing opioid side effects. Not all patients will have the same degree of pain relief from all NSAIDs so if pain relief from one drug is poor it is worth trying a different NSAID. If pain relief continues to be poor then further NSAIDs are unlikely to be effective.

Mechanism of action

NSAIDs inhibit the enzyme cyclo-oxygenase (COX). COX is the main enzyme that converts arachidonic acid to prostaglandins, thromboxane and prostacyclins. There are two forms of COX enzyme: COX-1 and COX-2. Most of the older NSAIDs block both forms of the enzyme (Table 3.2), but the newer COX-2 inhibitors are more specifically designed to block only COX-2. COX-1 is thought to be mainly concerned with constitutive processes such as gastric and renal reactions, whereas COX-2 is mainly produced during the inflammatory process. Blocking COX-2 alone should reduce the unwanted effects of NSAIDs. Unfortunately the COX-2 drugs still have some of these effects even though the incidence is reduced. They may also display some unwanted effects unique to the COX-2 group such as increased platelet stickiness and an increased risk of myocardial infarction.

Table 3.2 *Ratio of COX-2 to COX-1 selectivity*

NSAID	COX-2:COX-1 ratio
Rofecoxib (withdrawn)	35:1
Celecoxib	7.6:1
Meloxicam	2:1
Diclofenac	3:1
Ibuprofen	0.4:1

NSAID, non-steroidal anti-inflammatory drug; COX, cyclo-oxygenase.

Royal College of Anaesthetists clinical guidelines on the use of NSAIDs

- NSAIDs may decrease opioid requirement.
- They may be effective alone for some procedures.
- Preoperative administration is more effective perhaps because they require time to act on the arachidonic cascade to inhibit the pain pathways.
- They should be given postoperatively because of the risk of bleeding in high-risk procedures. They should be avoided in tonsillectomy and in patients where blood loss or platelet function poses particular risks. Increased bleeding has been demonstrated but only ketorolac has been associated with a significantly increased risk of bleeding.
- Avoid intramuscular diclofenac.

Postoperatively the main concerns regarding the use of NSAIDs are their renal and coagulation properties. Acute renal failure can be precipitated with pre-existing heart failure, pre-existing kidney disease, in those taking loop diuretics and where blood loss has exceeded 10 per cent of the blood volume. Stop NSAIDs if urea, creatinine or K^+ rise or urine output falls.

Caution should be exercised when using NSAIDs in the following situations:

- considerable dissection of tissues
- where a reduction of haemostatic function could be a risk
- where outcome could be adversely affected by bleeding, e.g. intracranial or neck surgery
- with a coagulopathy
- patients over 65 years (because of possible renal impairment)
- diabetes
- widespread vascular disease
- hepatobiliary, cardiac or major vascular surgery (because of the possibility of acute renal failure)
- angiotensin-converting enzyme (ACE) inhibitors
- potassium-sparing diuretics (triamterene)
- β blockers.

Avoid NSAIDs in:

- Renal impairment
- Hyperkalaemia
- Hypovolaemia
- Systemic inflammatory response syndrome
- Circulatory failure – hypotension, heart failure
- Severe liver dysfunction
- Renal transplantation
- Pre-eclampsia

Meloxicam and COX-2 inhibitors show no real improvement over COX-1 drugs.

Interactions

- Warfarin – increased bleeding tendency.
- Lithium – impaired clearance of lithium.
- The effect of oral hypoglycaemic agents may be enhanced by NSAIDs including azapropazone and salicylates.
- Phenytoin – displaced from the albumin-binding site – increased levels.
- Methotrexate – increased concentrations of methotrexate.
- Ciclosporin – avoid.
- Care with anti-hypertensives – may antagonize or potentiate sodium and water retention.
- Care with digoxin and aminoglycosides because they interfere with renal function.

Bleeding and NSAIDs

NSAIDs lengthen bleeding time (about 30 per cent) but usually still within the normal range. This action lasts days with aspirin but hours with the other drugs. It remains unknown whether they increase blood loss. Haemorrhagic events do occur in the postoperative period but the relationship with NSAIDs remains unclear.

Reports of significant bleeding with ketorolac have led to its being withdrawn from some European countries, and its use limited by others.

Gastrointestinal side effects and NSAIDs

NSAID-induced gastroduodenal lesions are asymptomatic in 50 per cent of patients. Long-term therapy with azapropazone and piroxicam has the highest risk of ulcer complications, ibuprofen has the lowest. The risk increases with age and with the use of anticoagulants. Among those over the age of 65 years 1:1200 patients on long-term NSAIDs

Table 3.3 *Non-steroidal anti-inflammatory drugs: associated risk factors*

Gastrointestinal risk factors	Renal risk factors
Age >65 years	Existing renal disease
Previous gastrointestinal bleed	Hypertension
Peptic ulcer disease	Heart failure
Concurrent use of glucocorticoids	Concurrent use of diuretic
Concurrent use of anticoagulants	Concurrent use of ACE inhibitor
Smoking	
Significant alcohol use	

ACE, angiotensin-converting enzyme.

will die from the gastrointestinal effects of the drugs. The risk is dose related.

The gastrointestinal and renal risk factors associated with NSAIDs are summarized in Table 3.3.

d wound healing

Bone metabolism and repair involves prostaglandins produced by osteoblasts. Interfering with osteoblast activity therefore may influence bone healing. NSAIDs have been used to reduce heterotopic bone formation. Cyclo-oxygenase-1 drugs have been shown in animal studies to reduce osteoblast activity and delay the formation of new bone and this has given rise to concern that they may be responsible for non-union of fractures in humans. Most studies do not confirm this finding but there is some evidence that ketorolac delays healing in spinal surgery and indomethacin increases the risk of non-union in long-bone fractures. Similar studies using COX-2 drugs in animals show no new bone growth at all and they may therefore delay wound healing more than COX-1 drugs. Work in humans relating to the use of COX-2 drugs and bone healing is not available. Many orthopaedic surgeons avoid the use of NSAIDs perioperatively.

COX-2 inhibitors

Celecoxib, valdecoxib, parecoxib, etoricoxib and meloxicam are examples of COX-2 inhibitors. These new drugs are thought to act only on the COX isoenzyme responsible for the inflammatory pathway with no effect on COX-1 isoenzymes. These are physiological enzymes found in the stomach, the lung and on platelets which, when blocked, cause the problems with bleeding, ulceration, bronchoconstriction and renal function. Cyclo-oxygenase-2 is expressed constitutively in the CNS and the kidney. Its byproducts exert a protective effect on the tubular cells. Part of the adaptive regulation of the kidney function is mediated by COX-2

products released from the juxtaglomerular cells and epithelial cells in the renal cortex and medulla. Celecoxib reduces the excretion of prostaglandin metabolites.

All coxibs show dose- and pharmacokinetic-dependent increases in systolic blood pressure and fluid retention, thus care must be taken when using these drugs in patients with hypertension, those on ACE inhibitors and patients with reduced renal function. More recently they have been associated with an increased incidence of myocardial infarction and rofecoxib has been withdrawn for this reason. There may be a similar effect with the other COX-2 inhibitors and care should be taken when prescribing these drugs to patients at risk. It is currently felt that these drugs have very little advantage over the non-selective NSAIDs. Diuretics and β blockers interact with the coxibs.

NSAIDs in pregnancy

It has been shown that taking NSAIDs in the first half of pregnancy is associated with an 80 per cent increased risk of miscarriage especially with ibuprofen. There is no risk of congenital malformation, low birthweight or preterm birth but there is a risk of failure of ductus arteriosus closure when NSAIDs are taken regularly in the third trimester.

NSAID use in children

When rectal medications are to be used, consent must be obtained from the parents and the child. Care must be taken when NSAIDs are used in children under 1 year of age because of the immaturity of renal function. Avoid NSAIDs in the following conditions:

- previous hospitalization for asthma especially if the child required intensive care
- nasal polyps with asthma
- severe eczema or atopy.

Combination of paracetamol and ibuprofen

Immediate postoperative pain relief may be no better when both drugs are given together than when either paracetamol or ibuprofen are given alone but it has been shown that children undergoing adenoidectomy who received both drugs required much less analgesia at home after discharge (49 versus 74 per cent) than when either drug was given alone. This may be because of the slow absorption of drugs administered rectally. Ibuprofen results in less sedation and faster discharge than paracetamol.

Topical NSAIDs

Topical NSAIDs do have an effect in some patients with an NNT for osteoarthritis of 3.2 (2.6–4.1). There is no evidence that topical NSAIDs cause gastrointestinal problems.

OPIOIDS

Morphine

Morphine is the 'gold standard' against which all other analgesic agents are assessed.

RESPIRATORY EFFECTS OF OPIOIDS

In healthy subjects $PaCO_2$ is a more important determinant of respiratory drive than PaO_2. Acute pain stimulates respiratory drive and antagonizes the effects of opioids. Systemically administered opioids diminish the respiratory rate and tidal volume. Appropriate doses of opioids result in significant depression of the carbon dioxide response curve but there is only a mild increase in $PaCO_2$. If the opioid analgesic action is longer than the pain stimulus the patient may get respiratory depression. The patient should be woken and encouraged to breathe until the effect wears off.

During normal respiration, subatmospheric pressure in the pharynx draws the tongue against the palate narrowing the airway. Finely coordinated contraction of the tongue (especially genioglossus) and the pharyngeal musculature helps maintain the airway patency and prevents snoring or inspiratory collapse of the airway. Sleep and opioids depress genioglossus and the pharyngeal muscle tone and reduce airway protective reflexes.

Critical incidents from opioid-induced respiratory depression occur more frequently between midnight and 6 am. Respiratory depression is almost always preceded by sedation. Sleep disturbance and episodic hypoxaemia are extremely common in patients receiving opioids after surgery. Rapid eye movement (REM) sleep is initially suppressed with a rebound in REM sleep on the second and third postoperative nights; opioids may contribute to this. Methods to reduce postoperative sleep disturbance, fatigue and disability include:

- minimally invasive surgery where possible
- reduce postoperative opioids by using NSAIDs and local/regional techniques
- early enteral feeding
- early postoperative mobilization.

The key principle in avoiding respiratory depression with opioids is to titrate the dose to achieve the effect required.

METABOLISM

Morphine is metabolized by uridine 5′-diphosphonate glucuronosyltransferase (UGT2B7) to morphine-6-glucuronide (M-6-G) (active) and morphine-3-glucuronide (M-3-G). Analgesia is the result of a balance between how much M-6-G and M-3-G are produced by the separate enzymes that control the amount of each metabolite. Some individuals produce a lot of M-6-G and are very sensitive to morphine whereas others produce more M-3-G causing relative morphine resistance.

Altered metabolism of morphine may increase the ratio of M-3-G to M-6-G and this has been associated with uncontrolled nociceptive pain. It has been considered that M-3-G may act as an antagonist in high concentrations, so increasing doses of morphine may actually produce less pain relief, but there is little evidence for this theory.

DOSE

Oral

The oral bioavailability of morphine is 20–50 per cent. Because of this variability, it is difficult to predict the dose of morphine required in a particular patient. It is best to start with a 10 mg dose, which can be given hourly. This dose can then be adjusted depending on the response.

Intramuscular

The time taken for an intramuscular dose to have a full effect is 40 minutes. If the patient still has pain after this time a further dose should be given. Again the starting dose should be 10 mg.

Intravenous

If morphine is given intravenously the dose should be titrated to the pain relief; 2 mg boluses can be given at 5-minute intervals until the patient is comfortable or morphine can be given by patient controlled analgesia (PCA).

SIDE EFFECTS

Minor adverse effects are seen in 34 per cent of patients:

- Daytime drowsiness, dizziness or mental clouding occur commonly at the beginning of treatment but resolve when the dose is stabilized, usually within a few days.
- Nausea and vomiting may occur in up to 60 per cent of patients when morphine is started but usually resolve.
- The main adverse effect of morphine is constipation. It usually persists and requires treatment. A stool-softening agent and stimulant are often required, e.g. sodium docusate.
- Itching, which can often be managed with ondansetron.

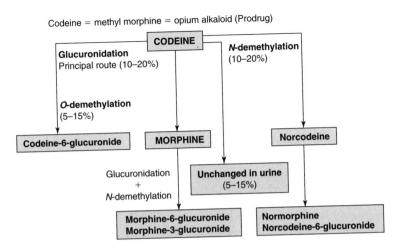

Codeine = methyl morphine = opium alkaloid (Prodrug)

Figure 3.1 *Metabolism of codeine*

- Cognitive and psychomotor effects may occur in the first few days of treatment but in the long term there are not usually any adverse effects.
- Long-term endocrine and immunological effects: the clinical significance of these is unknown.
- Tolerance is uncommon.
- Physical dependence is common but tapered withdrawal will usually work without too many problems.
- Psychological dependence (compulsion to use) is rare in patients on a stable therapeutic dose.
- Addiction is compulsive use to the detriment of the user's physical and/or psychological health and/or social function. This is rare.

Recent research promises new approaches, including opioid analgesics acting outside the CNS, targeting of opioid peptide-containing immune cells to peripheral damaged tissue, and gene transfer to enhance opioid production at sites of injury.

MORPHINE AND RENAL DYSFUNCTION

Morphine-6-glucuronide accumulates with poor renal function but if the dose is titrated against effect this will not matter because the patient will simply require less morphine. Accumulation becomes a problem when the patient is sedated or unconscious in the intensive care unit. If the patient is being dialysed M-6-G will not be removed by dialysis and may accumulate.

With renal impairment the ratios of morphine glucuronides to morphine increases significantly whether given intravenously or orally. Thus active metabolites will be higher in patients with impaired renal function producing greater analgesia for a given dose of morphine and increased side effects.

Codeine phosphate

METABOLISM (FIG. 3.1)

- 50 per cent pre-metabolized in liver and gut.
- Glucuronidation at 6-OH position to codeine-6-glucuronide.
- *N*-demethylation to nor-codeine (10–20 per cent).
- 5–15 per cent undergoes *O*-demethylation by CYP2D6 (cytochrome P-450 enzyme) into morphine (minor metabolite).
- 5–15 per cent excreted unchanged.

The analgesic effect of codeine is either wholly or mostly dependent on its metabolism to morphine. Codeine has a variable analgesic effect due to genetic polymorphism producing variable expression of the enzyme CYP2D6. There are approximately 60 unique p450 genes but only about 12 are concerned with drug metabolism. The enzyme is found in the liver and in other organs and tissues including the brain. Enzyme activity is absent *in utero* but increase rapidly after birth. However, it may remain at 25 per cent of adult levels up to the age of 5 or more and is particularly low in neonates. There are over 50 different genetic variants for CYP2D6.

People are usually classified as poor metabolizers or extensive metabolizers. Incidence of poor metabolizers is as follows:

- About 9 per cent in UK Caucasians
- 1 per cent in Arabs
- 30 per cent in Hong Kong Chinese

This is a gross oversimplification and effects vary significantly among people. Extensive metabolizers convert up to 15 per cent of codeine to morphine, poor metabolizers convert nothing.

There is no clear relation between plasma morphine and phenotype. In a study of 96 children, 47 per cent had genotypes associated with reduced enzyme activity. Morphine and its metabolites were not seen in 36 per cent of children. In 100 per cent of poor metabolizers no morphine was detected. At two hours 17 per cent of patients receiving codeine needed more analgesia. Both poor and extensive metabolizers still have the same side effects!

DOSE

- 170 mg codeine ≡ 20 mg morphine but the usual dose given is 30–60 mg codeine
- Children: 1–3 mg/kg per day

Codeine can be given orally, intramuscularly or rectally but not intravenously because of severe hypotension due to histamine release. Peak plasma concentrations are usually seen at one hour when given orally and 30 minutes after an intramuscular dose. However, at one hour 50 per cent of patients will not have full effect and many will have subtherapeutic levels. When used rectally, there is a lower plasma level because of reduced bioavailability.

SIDE EFFECTS

There is little evidence to confirm that the side effects of codeine are significantly fewer than other opioids at equipotent doses. The side effects include:

- drowsiness
- constipation
- codeine-induced headaches requiring slow withdrawal of the drug.

Side effects = codeine > morphine > placebo

Codeine rapidly penetrates the blood–brain barrier. Expression of CYP2D6 in the brain may lead to higher levels in the CNS and this may produce different levels of analgesia in different people. Efficacy of codeine is low and it has a ceiling effect above which the side effects increase but the analgesia does not.

Adding codeine to paracetamol significantly increases the effect, particularly over a period of time. This has been ascribed to accumulation of morphine.

CONCLUSION

Codeine does not seem a suitable prodrug in analgesic therapy as it possesses most of the disadvantages of morphine without the analgesic effects. The problems could be avoided by using small doses of morphine.

Tramadol

Tramadol is (+)cis-2[(dimethylamino)methyl]-1-(3-methoxyphenyl)-cyclohexanol hydrochloride.

MECHANISM OF ACTION

Tramadol has weak affinity for μ opioid receptors: 10 000 × lower than morphine and 10 × less than codeine. There is monoaminergic spinal modulation of pain through indirect activation of postsynaptic α2 adrenoceptor blocking impulses from reaching the brain. Tramadol enhances the function of the spinal descending inhibitory pathway by inhibition of reuptake of 5-hydroxytryptamine (5-HT) and noradrenaline and presynaptic stimulation of 5-HT release. It may work better when given with paracetamol; 100 mg tramadol ≡ 1000 mg paracetamol.

METABOLISM

Tramadol is rapidly absorbed when given orally. There is 69 per cent bioavailability after 1 dose and 90–100 per cent with multiple doses. It is metabolized by cytochrome P-450 enzyme in the liver to form 11 metabolites of which O-desmethyltramadol predominates. This metabolite has a higher affinity than tramadol for opioid receptors. The O-demethylation depends on CYP2D6 and poor metabolizers show evidence of reduced analgesic activity. Metabolism also requires the enzyme sparteine oxygenase which is absent in 7 per cent of Caucasians. If absent there is a decreased effect but there is still some analgesia, unlike codeine. Ninety per cent is excreted by the kidneys.

DOSE

- Maximum dose is 1000 mg by any route.
- There is no correlation between plasma level and tramadol's analgesic effect but generally there is better analgesia with larger doses.

Oral

- Usual dose 400 mg per day in four divided doses (100 mg four times daily).
- Maximum dose is 600 mg in 24 hours.
- If creatinine clearance is below 30 mL/min the dose should be reduced to a maximum of 200 mg/day 12 hourly.

Intravenous

- 0.5–2 mg/kg to a maximum of 100 mg given regularly.
- 3 mg/kg bolus dose given at induction.

- 3 mg/kg bolus at wound closure ≡ 10 mg morphine but up to 6 mg/kg may be needed for good analgesia.
- Infusion = 600 mg over 24 hours.
- PCA = 20 mg bolus with 5-minute lock-out.

ADVANTAGES

- Reduces postoperative shivering – 1 mg/kg can treat the shivering due to anaesthesia or in obstetrics.
- It has been shown to be better for day-case hernias than fentanyl and cocodamol.
- It may prove particularly useful in patients with poor cardiopulmonary function, including elderly patients, obese patients, smokers, those with impaired hepatic or renal function and in patients in whom NSAIDs are not recommended.
- It causes less constipation than opioids.
- It may have a specific effect in neuropathic pain.
- It is not a controlled drug.

SIDE EFFECTS

Around 19–30 per cent of patients discontinue use because of side effects. It causes at least as much nausea and vomiting as other opioids, plus mood changes and sweating. Other side effects include:

- Headache – 18–32 per cent
- Nausea – 24–40 per cent
- Vomiting – 9–17 per cent
- Dizziness – 26–33 per cent
- Somnolence – 16–25 per cent
- Constipation – 24–46 per cent
- Dry mouth
- Sweating
- Cirrhosis: t1/2 doubled. Maximum dose 50 mg twice daily.

Avoid tramadol in epilepsy and take care with other drugs that may lower seizure threshold. The slow release form has fewer side effects and there is now a once daily formula available. It has a very low abuse potential but there does remain a small potential for physical dependence. Withdrawal is less severe than with opioids.

INTERACTIONS

- Coumarin anticoagulants – increased international normalized ratio (INR)?
- Monoamine oxidase inhibitors (MAOIs) – hypertensive crisis.
- If given with carbamazepine the dose of tramadol can be doubled because of increased hepatic clearance.
- Ondansetron is metabolized by the same system and concurrent use may reduce the action of each.

Dihydrocodeine

Dihydrocodeine is a weak opioid drug. There are few studies on its efficacy and no studies comparing 30 mg with 60 mg.

Oxycodone

When given orally oxycodone is twice as potent as morphine because of better bioavailability which is between 60 and 80 per cent. It has a basic morphine structure apart from an additional side chain.

Oxycodone appears to cause less nausea and vomiting, fewer hallucinations and is less sedating than morphine. It is often tolerated when morphine is not. Normal and slow release forms are available.

Metabolism of oxycodone is CYP2D6-dependent and drugs which inhibit CYP2D6 such as celecoxib, chlorphenamine, metoclopramide and ranitidine may reduce effectiveness of codeine and oxycodone.

Pethidine

Pethidine is metabolized by the liver. It undergoes demethylation to norpethidine which has a half-life of up to 20 hours. Oral bioavailability of pethidine is 30–60 per cent. Pethidine should be avoided in:

- impaired renal function – it is not removed by haemodialysis
- high opioid requirement
- concurrent use of phenytoin.

DOSE

- 50 mg is not sufficient to produce adequate analgesia in most patients.
- Intramuscular pethidine 100 mg – NNT = 2.9 (2.3–3.9) ≡ 10 mg morphine.
- Maximum dose 10 mg/kg per day.
- It has a quicker onset but shorter action than morphine.

Pethidine does not have less effect than morphine on the sphincter of Oddi and pethidine and morphine cause a similar rise in pressure in the common bile duct. Nor is it better in colicky pain. Other opioids are just as effective as pethidine for renal colic and NSAIDs are better than opioids.

PROBLEMS WITH PETHIDINE

- Norpethidine toxicity:
  - tremor
  - disorientation

- myoclonus
- fits
- hallucinations.

■ Pethidine seems to pose a higher risk than other opioids of iatrogenic drug dependence and addiction.

■ It is sought after by addicts and it is often involved in drug addiction in health professionals.

The use of pethidine has been declining over recent years and it should not be used as a first line analgesic agent. With the development of newer and safer opioids the need for pethidine should rarely if ever arise.

Fentanyl

Fentanyl is a synthetic lipid-soluble opioid with high potency (100 × morphine). It is most commonly used peroperatively but it is also used in epidural infusions and occasionally in PCAs. When used for PCA the loading dose is 0.5 µg/kg. The concentration should be 10 µg/mL with a 1 mL bolus and a 5-minute lock-out.

CONTRAINDICATIONS

■ Allergy to fentanyl (rare).

ADVANTAGES

■ Rapid onset (three to five minutes).
■ No active metabolites so it can be used in renal and hepatic failure.

DISADVANTAGES

■ Cost.
■ Side effects similar to opioids.

FENTANYL PATCHES

To penetrate the stratum corneum of the skin, drugs need to be of small molecular weight, and they need to be lipophilic, uncharged and potent like fentanyl and glyceryl trinitrate (GTN). Transdermal delivery avoids first pass metabolism, and is simple and continuous.

A deposit of fentanyl is formed in the skin and surrounding tissue and the drug is delivered slowly into the circulation. Each patch lasts up to 72 hours but occasionally patients need to change it every 48 hours. The patches are designed for chronic, stable pain, and because of their long action they are not good for acute pain. The patch should not be cut in half or damaged in any way. Skin reactions to the patch are not uncommon (41 per cent).

Fentanyl patches may provide better analgesia and less constipation than morphine. Fentanyl may be better for neuropathic pain.

FENTANYL LOLLY

Fentanyl is available as 200/300/400 µg lollies. Only 50 per cent of each lolly is absorbed into the circulation and the effects of the drug last for up to two hours. Uptake is partly from the mucosa of the mouth and partly from the stomach. It is rapid but the effect depends on how much of the drug is swallowed because then it is inactivated. They are useful in the management of breakthrough pain in patients with malignant disease.

SIDE EFFECTS

■ Pruritus in 44 per cent.
■ Nausea and vomiting in 15–20 per cent; not prevented by antiemetics.
■ Respiratory depression with $SpO_2 < 90$ per cent in 5 per cent; must use pulse oximeter even if awake.
■ Sedation within 15–30 minutes.

Buprenorphine

Buprenorphine has been available for many years and was at first thought to be a partial agonist drug. Given sublingually it is associated with many side effects especially nausea and vomiting. It is now being produced as a transdermal formulation and recent studies have suggested that in the normal clinical range buprenorphine is a full agonist; 10 mg morphine = 0.3 mg buprenorphine.

DOSE

■ 200 µg sublingual tablet.
■ The transdermal 3-day release patch comes in three sizes – 35 µg/h, 52.5 µg/h, 70 µg/h. The patch can be cut in half.

Methadone hydrochloride

Methadone is a synthetic opioid that has been in use since the second world war. It has less κ action but more µ action than morphine and is less sedating. It inhibits uptake of 5-HT and noradrenaline.

Methadone has a very long elimination half-life (3–128 hours) although its analgesic effect may not last that long. For the treatment of withdrawal from opioid addiction it is usually given as a once-a-day dose but it may need to be given more frequently (up to six hourly) for the control of pain.

It can be a useful analgesic agent for neuropathic and cancer pains and is a safe drug when used properly. Its use should be considered when a patient does not achieve adequate pain relief with conventional opioids or when there are unacceptable side effects with other opioids. NSAIDs and other adjuvant drugs should be used as well.

Methadone is thought to be equipotent with morphine but it has a very high bioavailability and many conversion tables underestimate the potency of methadone. It can be difficult to convert a patient from a stable dose of morphine to methadone because of the differences in bioavailability, tissue accumulation and large inter-patient variations. Conversion of opioids should only be done within a hospital setting because of the risk of increased pain or increased effect.

DOSE

The starting oral dose in an opioid-naive patient should be 2.5 mg eight hourly increasing every five to seven days as necessary. When patients reach a stable dose they should be reviewed monthly. Effects of methadone will increase over at least one week after increasing the dose. It should not be used for breakthrough pain because of its long action.

Methadone infusion

- 0.1–0.2 mg/kg per hour for two hours followed by 0.01–0.02 mg/kg per hour.

AGENTS THAT REDUCE METHADONE CONCENTRATION

- Anticonvulsants (except sodium valproate and gabapentin)
- Antipsychotics (risperidone)
- Antiretrovirals
- Antitubercular drugs (rifampicin).

AGENTS THAT INCREASE METHADONE CONCENTRATIONS

- Antidepressants (amitriptyline, serotonin selective reuptake inhibitors (SSRIs))
- Antifungals.

AGENTS THAT INCREASE THE ADVERSE EFFECT OF METHADONE

- Benzodiazepines
- St John's wort.

Opioids in acute pain: summary

- Do not use delayed release formulations in acute pain because the delayed onset and offset can be dangerous.
- There is no evidence that one opioid is better than another.

- Pethidine has a major disadvantage in that a metabolite, norpethidine, has a long half-life and is toxic and should not be used when multiple injections are needed.
- Pethidine is not better than morphine at dealing with colicky pain.
- If the patient requests more opioid they have inadequate pain control because of:
  - too little drug
  - too long between doses
  - too little attention being paid to the patient
  - too much reliance on rigid (inadequate) prescriptions.

Table 3.4 provides a summary of opioid equivalent doses.

Peripherally acting opioids

A new generation of opioid drugs selectively activate opioid receptors outside the CNS, avoiding all centrally mediated, unwanted effects. Opioid receptors have been identified on peripheral processes of sensory neurones and there are opioid receptors on C and A fibres.

The relative contribution of peripheral, spinal and supraspinal opioid receptors after the systemic administration of an opioid agonist has not been examined thoroughly. Systemically and centrally injected opioid agonists may act predominantly through peripheral opioid receptors.

POSSIBLE MECHANISMS OF ACTION

The modulation of calcium channels seems to be the primary mechanism that leads to the following:

- inhibition of adenylyl cyclase suppresses tetrodotoxin-resistant sodium selective and non-selective cation currents stimulated by the inflammatory agent prostaglandin E_2
- attenuation of the excitability of peripheral nociceptor terminals
- attenuation of the propagation of action potentials
- attenuation of the release of excitatory proinflammatory neuropeptides (substance P, calcitonin gene-related peptide) from peripheral sensory nerve endings
- attenuation of the vasodilation evoked by stimulation of C fibres.

All these mechanisms result in analgesia or anti-inflammatory actions. Pain relief has been reported in the following situations:

- intra-articular administration of morphine postoperatively.
- local morphine injection at the iliac bone harvest site in spinal fusion surgery significantly reduces pain up to one year.
- submucous injection of morphine for chronic inflammatory tooth pain.

Table 3.4 *Opioid equivalent doses*

Drug	Dose (mg)*	Half-life (h)	Duration (h)	Comment
Morphine	20–30	2–3	2–4	
Controlled-release morphine	20–30	2–3	8–12	Various formulations are not bioequivalent
Sustained-release morphine	20–30	2–3	24	
Oxycodone	20	2–3	3–4	
Controlled-release oxycodone	20	2–3	8–12	
Hydromorphone	7.5	2–3	2–4	Potency may be greater during long-term use. Hydromorphone:morphine is 3:1 rather than 6·7:1
Methadone	20	12–190	4–12	Although 1:1 ratio with morphine in single dose, there is a change with chronic dosing and large dose reduction (75–90%) is needed when switching to methadone
Oxymorphone	10	2–3	2–4	Available in rectal and injectable formulations also
Fentanyl		7–12		Can be administered as a continuous intravenous or subcutaneous infusion 100 μg/h is roughly equi-analgesic to morphine 4 mg/h
Transdermal fentanyl		16–24	48–72	100 μg/h is roughly equi-analgesic to morphine 4 mg/h. A ratio of oral morphine to transdermal fentanyl of 70:1 may also be used clinically

* Oral dose equivalent to 10 mg morphine (intramuscular).

Several studies have however found no peripheral effects of opioids. New peripherally restricted opioids that have recently entered human trials include new slow release morphine analogues, M-6-G drug, a synthetic opioid (propiram) and opioids that have reduced dependency.

Intranasal opioids

The intranasal route of absorption has been examined for many opioids as a quick and relatively non-invasive means of providing analgesia. Reliable absorption depends on lipid solubility. The nasal mucosa is richly vascularized and the subepithelial cells are lined by fenestrated epithelium. There is a large surface area, uniform temperature and high permeability. The vascular drainage is the facial and sphenopalatine veins so drugs avoid the first pass metabolism. Many of the opioids have been used in this way. They can be administered as a dry powder or dissolved in water or saline. A spray produces a wider distribution than drops. The intranasal route has been used either to provide preoperative sedation or for postoperative pain control.

INTRANASAL DIAMORPHINE

Diamorphine is rapidly and well absorbed because it is lipophilic and has a high aqueous solubility which allows administration in a small volume.

The relative potency compared to an intramuscular dose is 50 per cent. It has been used for management of trauma in children and provides as rapid an effect as an intramuscular dose but with better parent acceptability.

Doses for children

The dose is approximately 0.1 mg/kg in 0.2 mL saline.

1. Assess the weight of the child to the nearest 5 kg.
2. Add saline in amount shown in Table 3.5 to 10 mg diamorphine.

Table 3.5 *Intranasal diamorphine for children: calculation of the volume of saline added to the opioid*

Weight of child to nearest 5 kg	Volume saline (mL) added to 10 mg diamorphine
15	1.3
20	1.0
25	0.8
30	0.7
35	0.6
40	0.5
50	0.4
60	0.3

3 Draw up 0.2 mL.
4 Administer via a 1 mL syringe or metered spray.

Inhalational opioids

The drug is administered by nebulizer in a 2–6 mL volume. Factors affecting bioavailability (17–5.5 per cent) are the design of the nebulizer, amount of drug swallowed and inspiratory/expiratory ratio of the respiratory cycle.

DOSES

- Morphine 10–25 mg
- Fentanyl 100–300 μg

BENEFITS

- Non-invasive.
- Rapid absorption.
- May be useful in palliative care for relieving breathlessness.

CLONIDINE

Clonidine is an α adrenergic agonist and the only such drug to be in common clinical use. Its properties include:

- Analgesia – clonidine reduces the postoperative requirement for pain relief and can be as effective as opioids. It reduces opioid requirements when both drugs are used together.
- Sedation in the intensive care unit.
- Treatment of withdrawal to control autonomic symptoms.
- Transdermally it relieves hyperalgesia in sympathetically mediated pain.
- It prolongs analgesia produced by local anaesthetics.
- It may be useful in noradrenaline-sensitive neuromata.
- Antihypertensive.
- Antisialagogue.
- It can be reversed by naloxone.

The sedative, antihypertensive and antisialagogue effects may limit its usefulness. It can be given orally, intravenously, epidurally or caudally. There appears to be no clinical advantage of giving it via the extradural route over the intravenous route.

Mechanism of action

Clonidine stimulates the central descending noradrenergic inhibitory system acting on the spinal dorsal horn neurones of laminae IV and V. There is recruitment of other neuromediators that can modulate pain perception (adenosine, acetylcholine and endorphins) and inhibition of substance P release. Clonidine has a centrally mediated direct effect on spinal pre- and postsynaptic α2 adrenergic receptors in the dorsal horn. It also has supraspinal effects and inhibits acetylcholinesterase. The resultant analgesia is related to cerebrospinal fluid (not plasma) concentration.

Side effects

- Hypotension
- Bradycardia
- Sedation
- Anxiolysis
- Dizziness
- Dry mouth
- Decreased bowel motility
- Diuresis

Clonidine should not be given to patients who are haemodynamically unstable because of the possibility of hypotension.

Dose

ORAL

- (Half-life = 6–20 hours.)
- 50–150 μg three times daily produces peak plasma levels in three to five hours.
- 4 μg/kg given 105 minutes before induction reduces postoperative analgesic requirements, particularly in children.

CAUDAL

A dose of 2 μg/kg via the caudal approach may prolong analgesia but may cause respiratory depression.

Indications for intrathecal/epidural/peripheral clonidine with local anaesthetic

- Opioid-sparing effect
- Epidural clonidine has been used for spasms in multiple sclerosis
- Malignant pain
- Spinal cord injury
- Multiple sclerosis
- Diabetic neuropathy
- Complex regional pain syndrome (CRPS)

ENTONOX®

Historical background

Nitrous oxide was discovered by Joseph Priestly, a Yorkshire chemist. In 1799 the scientist Humphry Davy inhaled the gas and found it gave him rapid pain relief from an infected tooth. On one occasion he reported momentarily losing consciousness, waking up laughing about the pleasurable feelings he had experienced, hence the term 'laughing gas'. It was some time before the analgesic properties were recognized as useful.

The mixture of gases containing equal parts of nitrous oxide and oxygen is known as Entonox.

Indications

- Situations where pain is predictable and of a short duration.
- Wound dressing changes.
- Debridement of wounds.
- Removal of drains or sutures.
- Turning a patient with a fracture or a pressure ulcer.

Administration

The gas is administered using a facemask or mouthpiece. Gas flow is controlled by a sensitive demand-valve activated by the patient's inspired breath. Pressurized gas from the cylinder flows through a pressure regulator into the lungs at a steady rate. Longer and deeper breaths allow greater volumes of gas to be taken into the lungs if necessary.

The gas is rapidly absorbed on inhalation, providing analgesia within minutes. It is excreted, largely unchanged, by the lungs and is rapidly eliminated from the body on cessation of inhalation. There is no risk of overdose as the patient's level of consciousness governs their ability to maintain the flow of gas.

Use in children

Entonox is safe for any age group. It is an excellent analgesic for children, providing pain relief, distraction and relaxation.

Contraindications

Entonox causes an enclosed air-pocket in the body to expand rapidly in volume as the gas mixture is absorbed from the blood into the space, resulting in a build-up of pressure. It must therefore never be used if the patient has any condition where air is trapped in the body and expansion would be dangerous.

- Where there is artificial, spontaneous or traumatic pneumothorax.
- Air embolism.
- Decompression sickness.
- Abdominal distension or suspected bowel obstruction.
- Maxillofacial injuries.
- Following a head injury where consciousness is impaired.

Entonox may also expand and cause pain in other cavities, such as the sinuses, middle ear and gut.

Side effects

Repeated exposure may result in **megaloblastic anaemia** owing to interference with the action of vitamin B_{12}. It interferes with methionine synthetase activity causing impaired DNA synthesis and folate metabolism leading to bone marrow depression. If a procedure is to be carried out more frequently than every four days, the patient should be monitored and a routine blood cell count carried out. Exposure should be limited to one hour per day.

Protocol for administration

Entonox should be administered according to a locally agreed protocol following a period of instruction or training. The patient should be instructed on how to hold the mask over the nose and mouth, or in the case of the mouthpiece, between the teeth sealing around it with the lips, and to then breathe normally. The patient should breathe the gas for around two minutes before commencing the procedure. The mask should never be held on the patient's face by another person as his or her active involvement is crucial to the safety of the system. At all times the patient should be able to obey commands, but if a momentary loss of consciousness does occur, the seal around the mask or mouthpiece will be lost as it falls away and the demand valve will fail to operate, causing the flow of gas to stop. On breathing normal air these effects will quickly wear off.

Although Entonox is rapidly eliminated from the body, the British Oxygen Company (BOC) advises that patients should not drive or operate machinery for at least 12 hours.

CROSS-INFECTION

The Blood Borne Viruses Advisory Panel of the Association of Anaesthetists of Great Britain (AAGBI) produced an advisory report in 1996 following cases of cross-infection with hepatitis C (HCV). Its recommendations included the need for an appropriate filter to be placed between the breathing system and the patient.

OPERATIONAL PROTOCOLS

In the UK, Entonox is not classed as a prescription-only medicine but is designated as a pharmacy product. This means that it does not require a doctor's prescription, but must be issued by a pharmacist, who may be unwilling to do so without confirmation from a doctor.

BISPHOSPHONATES

Bisphosphonates are analogues of endogenous pyrophosphates, which inhibit osteoclastic bone resorption. They bind tightly to the surface of trabecular bone and inhibit its resorption. They are effective for osteoporotic pain (alendronate), Paget's disease of the bone (disodium etidronate), cancer-induced hypercalcaemia and bone pain in myeloma (pamidronate and clodronate). Pamidronate and clodronate may reduce malignant bone pain. Etidronate and alendronate reduce the incidence of fractures and relieve bone pain in osteoporosis. They should be used for two to three years only because they are toxic and remain in bone for a long time.

Doses

- Alendronate: 10 mg at least 30 minutes before breakfast.
- Etidronate: 5 mg/kg as a single daily dose for at least six months.
- New drugs include zelodronate and ibandronate.
- For doses of pamidronate and clodronate see Chapter 16.

KETAMINE

Ketamine is a phencyclidine derivative and is the most potent NMDA receptor channel blocker available for use. It binds to the phencyclidine-binding site when the channels are open in the active state.

Ketamine is a racemic mixture (i.e. as an equal mixture of the two enantiomers) of two isomers, S-(+)-ketamine and R-(−)-ketamine, but the S-enantiomer is more potent.

Metabolism

Ketamine is metabolized in the liver to nor-ketamine. Nor-ketamine has 30 per cent of the activity of ketamine. The distribution half-life $(T1/2\alpha)$ is rapid (minutes) and the elimination half-life $(T1/2\beta)$ is two to three hours.

Mechanism of action

Ketamine depresses neurones in the cortex and thalamus and simultaneously increases activity in the limbic system. This is known as 'functional disorganization'. Non-competitive action at NMDA receptors reduces 'wind-up' and central sensitization. It has an effect on γ-aminobutyric acid (GABA) receptors and inhibits synaptic uptake of serotonin and noradrenaline. With regard to opioid receptor binding, it has μ, δ and κ opioid-like effects and reduces opioid requirements. It acts on non-NMDA glutamate receptors, on muscarinic receptors and cholinergic transmission and voltage gated Na^+, K^+, Ca^{2+} channels. It also has anti-depressant effects.

Dose

Ketamine can be given orally, intravenously, intramuscularly, subcutaneously, sublingually and intranasally. The preservative-free form can be used epidurally.

ORAL DOSE FOR NEUROPATHIC PAIN

The parenteral drug can be given orally starting with 10–50 mg and increasing the dose as necessary. The taste is unpleasant and the bioavailability is only 17 per cent but it does work in some patients with neuropathic pain. It is also used orally in palliative care. A new oral preparation of ketamine is now available (5 mg/5 mL) which is more palatable. The same dose given sublingually has better absorption and an improved effect.

For procedures

Give 4–10 mg/kg orally, usually with 0.4 mg/kg oral midazolam.

INTRAVENOUS DOSE FOR ANALGESIA

- 0.3–0.5 mg/kg produces analgesia.
- A 0.15–0.2 mg/kg bolus dose preoperatively reduces postoperative pain for up to four hours and reduces opioid requirements by 25–50 per cent. It has a pre-emptive effect by reducing the sensitization of second order neurones in the spinal cord. It has a better effect if given before surgery.
- 1 mg/kg ketamine preoperatively has eliminated phantom breast pain in 25 per cent of patients.
- 10 mg intravenously produces a 40 per cent reduction in opioid consumption during the first five hours after cholecystectomy.

Infusion rate

A ketamine infusion postoperatively ($2.5\,\mu g/kg$) lowers morphine requirements (50 per cent over 48 hours). The aim is to achieve a theoretical plasma concentration of $100\,ng/mL$ to produce analgesia without important side effects. Analgesia occurs at $100–150\,ng/mL$ plasma concentration ($3–4\,\mu g/kg$ per minute after loading dose). Give:

- $10\,\mu g/kg$ per minute for five minutes
- $7.5\,\mu g/kg$ for 30 minutes
- $5\,\mu g/kg$ per minute for 45 minutes
- $2.5\,\mu g/kg$ per minute thereafter

INTRAVENOUS DOSE FOR NEUROPATHIC PAIN

The starting dose of ketamine is usually $15–25\,mg$ intravenously over 30 minutes but this is variable depending on effect. It is usually given with intravenous midazolam $2–5\,mg$ to prevent hallucinations occurring. Reduction in pain and dysaesthesia may last up to six weeks following a single dose.

Side effects

There is a very small therapeutic range between analgesia and side effects, which include:

- 20–30 per cent psychomimetic effects (bizarre dreams or hallucinations)
- Nystagmus
- Sedation
- Euphoria
- Neurobehavioural and cognitive depression
- Tolerance.

Ketamine may have greater efficacy in the very young because there are larger numbers of receptors and a wider distribution. The receptors may also have different functions.

Ketamine patient controlled analgesia

- Morphine $1\,mg/mL$ and ketamine $1\,mg/mL$
- Fewer opioid side effects, e.g. nausea, pruritus and urinary retention.

Epidural ketamine

The preservative-free form of the drug must be used in the epidural space. Analgesia is produced with a dose of $20–30\,mg$ but it is not as good as with $2\,mg$ diamorphine. It produces better analgesia when combined with local anaesthetic agents. Caudal bupivacaine and ketamine $0.5\,mg/kg$ gives 12.5 hours of analgesia in children but not in adults. It is probably not superior to parenteral administration.

Intranasal ketamine

The intranasal route produces rapid and effective relief of pain within 10 minutes, lasting up to 60 minutes. Adverse effects are dose related. The dose is $10–50\,mg$ using a $10\,mg/0.1\,mL$ spray also containing 10 per cent aqueous solution with 0.002 per cent benzacromium chloride (vehicle) in the pump.

AMANTADINE

Amantadine is an antiparkinsonian drug and an antiviral agent used to treat influenza. It also causes NMDA receptor antagonism and occasionally reduces nerve injury type of pain.

Dose

- $50–100\,mg$ daily orally
- $200\,mg$ in $500\,mL$ saline over three hours intravenously on three consecutive days may have a prolonged effect.

TRICYCLIC ANTIDEPRESSANTS

Despite the accepted and widespread use of antidepressants in pain management we know little about how tricyclic antidepressants produce analgesia. The older ones such as amitriptyline are better for the relief of pain than the newer selective agents.

Amitriptyline

METABOLISM

Amitriptyline is converted in the liver to nortriptyline.

USES

- Control of neuropathic pain.
- Normalizing disturbed sleep patterns.
- Elevation of mood in depression.
- The effect of antidepressants in pain occurs within a week whereas the antidepressant effect may take more than 10 days.

THEORIES ABOUT MECHANISM OF ACTION

Mood altering effects

Studies suggest drugs exert a central analgesic effect independent of the anti-depressant effect.

Monoamine hypothesis

Noradrenaline reuptake inhibition is thought to be a key mechanism as the noradrenergic system is involved in almost all aspects of brain function that affect pain from sensory perception to motor attention, memory and motivation. One theory suggests that chronic pain can result from a deficiency in endogenous pain inhibition which is in turn mediated by noradrenaline, serotonin and endogenous opioids. By blocking the reuptake of noradrenaline and serotonin and activating opioid receptors, antidepressants may restore the endogenous pain system to a normal state. The problem with this explanation is that there is little evidence for either the cause or the treatment.

Neurodegenerative changes, altered synaptic function, endocrine dysfunction

Tricyclic drugs also:

- have neurotrophic effects and regulate synaptic plasticity
- have antagonistic effects at $\alpha 1$ adrenoceptor
- produce H_1 histaminergic receptor block
- have anticholinergic effects
- lead to increased neurogenesis
- enhance endocrine function.

The tricyclics normalize sleep cycles and patients who sleep well complain of less pain than those who have disrupted sleep.

SIDE EFFECTS

- Dryness of mouth (inhibits saliva production)
- Sedation
- Constipation
- Hallucinations
- Disturbed cardiac rhythm in patients with ischaemic heart disease (slowed atrioventricular and intraventricular conduction producing slowing of the heart)

Other tricyclic drugs such as nortriptyline and dosulepin may have a similar effect without the side effects.

DOSE

- Initial dose – amitriptyline or nortriptyline 10 mg one hour before bedtime.

Table 3.6 *Number needed to treat (NNT) for antidepressants in various conditions*

Disease	NNT with antidepressants
Diabetic neuropathy	3.0 (2.4–4.0)
Post-herpetic neuralgia	2.3 (1.7–3.3)
Atypical facial pain	2.8 (2.0–4.7)
Central pain	1.7 (1.1–3.0)*

* Small trials only.

- This can be increased in 10 mg increments every three days to a maximum of 50 mg nocte.
- Doses higher than this do not usually have any greater benefit for chronic pain.
- Dosulepin – 25–50 mg nocte.

Antidepressants and neuropathic pain

Antidepressants are not licensed for use in neuropathic pain in the UK. It is not known which one is most effective. It is also not known how they compare with anticonvulsants. Their effect on reaction time is not clear and there appears to be a variable disease effect (Table 3.6).

Only one trial has shown a greater benefit with lower risk than anticonvulsants.

- NNH Minor = 3.7 (2.9–5.2)
- NNH Major = 22 (14–58)

SELECTIVE SEROTONIN REUPTAKE INHIBITORS

Selective serotonin reuptake inhibitors are antidepressants. There is limited experience of their use for pain management and consistent results are hard to achieve. More research is needed but they do not appear to be as useful as the tricyclic drugs so far. They elevate 5-HT.

Venlafaxine is an example that has been shown to have an effect in chronic pain, otherwise generally they have poor outcomes in chronic pain.

ANTICONVULSANTS

Anticonvulsants have been used for chronic pain since the 1960s. They were initially used mainly for trigeminal neuralgia but are now used in the management of many different neuropathic pain states with variable success. They are also useful in the management of acute neuropathic pain such as that seen in nerve trauma. It is not possible to predict which drug will be effective.

Carbamazepine

Carbamazepine suppresses spontaneous activity and pain produced by inflammatory mediators. It remains the first line treatment for trigeminal neuralgia but it is used less commonly now because of the availability of newer agents that have fewer side effects. See Table 3.7 for NNTs with carbamazepine and Table 3.8 for NNTs for other drugs.

Gabapentin

ACTION

The action of gabapentin is still unclear, but it has an inhibitory action at the voltage-gated calcium channels where it blocks the $\alpha2\beta$ subunit.

SIDE EFFECTS

- Sedation
- Dizziness
- Headaches

DOSE

- May range from 100 mg three times daily to a maximum of 5200 mg in divided doses (occasionally used in the USA for postherpetic neuralgia).
- Maximum recommended dose is 1800 mg/day.
- Beginning treatment with low doses reduces the incidence of side effects. Some patients may benefit from low doses.
- It accumulates in renal impairment and the dose interval should be increased for example from three times a day to twice a day.

Pregabalin

Pregabalin (S(+)-3-isobutyl GABA) is a new drug licensed for use in epilepsy, neuropathic pain and anxiety states. The pharmacology is similar but not identical to gabapentin.

MECHANISM OF ACTION

Pregabalin blocks specific calcium channels within the nerves. It has a rapid onset and shortened period of titration than gabapentin. It is potentiated by alcohol and oxycodone. Ninety eight per cent is excreted in the urine. It improves sleep, pain and global impression of change.

SIDE EFFECTS

- Dizziness
- Drowsiness
- Water retention

DOSE

- 75 mg twice daily up to 200 mg three times daily.
- If creatinine clearance is under 60 mL/min the daily dose should not exceed 300 mg.

Table 3.8 *Number needed to treat (NNT) for other drugs in various conditions*

Drug	Disease	NNT	NNH
Tricyclics	Post-herpetic neuralgia	2.1	2.7 (minor)
	Diabetes	3.4	
Anticonvulsants	Diabetes	2.7	2.7 (minor)
	Post-herpetic neuralgia	3.2	
	Trigeminal neuralgia	2.6	
Carbamazepine		2.7	3.7
Gabapentin		3.7	2.5
Dihydrocodeine		9	

Table 3.7 *Number needed to treat (NNT) for carbamazepine in various conditions*

Disease	Treatment	NNT	NNH
Trigeminal neuralgia	Carbamazepine 400 mg to 2.4 g/day Better than tizanidine No different from tocainide Less effective than pimozide	2.6 (2.2–3.3)	Minor = 3.4 (2.5–5.2)
Diabetic neuropathy	Carbamazepine Very few trials	2.5 (1.8–4.0)	Minor = 3.1 (2.3–4.8)
Migraine prophylaxis (also sodium valproate)	Carbamazepine	1.6 (1.3–2.0)	2.4 (1.9–3.3)

Lamotrigine

Lamotrigine is an anticonvulsant that acts by stabilizing presynaptic membranes via blockade of voltage-dependent Na^+ channels, so preventing pathological release of excitatory neurotransmitters, principally glutamate in the spinal cord (i.e. it prolongs inactivation of Na^+ channels). It prevents the activation of secondary spinal nociceptive neurones via AMPA (α-amino-3-hydroxy-5-methyl-4-isoxazolepropionic acid) and NMDA receptors.

Occasionally lamotrigine can be helpful when other drugs have failed. It has been used in conjunction with carbamazepine for the treatment of resistant trigeminal neuralgia. It may cause skin rashes and, rarely, Stevens-Johnson syndrome.

DOSE

- Initially 25 mg once daily for two weeks.
- Increase to 50 mg for two weeks then increase by 50–100 mg every 7–14 days to a maximum of 500 mg/day.
- The usual dose is 100–200 mg/day in two divided doses.
- The dose should be reduced when prescribed with carbamazepine.

Oxcarbazepine

Oxcarbazepine is a 10-ketoanalogue of carbamazepine. It has a longer half-life so it can be administered twice a day. It has less enzyme induction than carbamazepine. It has been used for the treatment of resistant trigeminal neuralgia.

DOSE

- 300 mg twice daily up to 2.4 gm/day maximum in two divided doses.

Phenytoin

Phenytoin is rarely used for treatment of neuropathic pain because of side effects but it is licensed for use in trigeminal neuralgia and can be useful in patients with resistant symptoms.

Sodium valproate

DOSE

- 200 mg twice daily.

SIDE EFFECTS

- Altered liver enzymes

- Increased prothrombin ratio
- Pancreatitis

Topiramate

MECHANISM OF ACTION

Topiramate modulates voltage gated Na^+ and Ca^{2+} ion channels. It potentiates GABA inhibition and blocks excitatory glutamate neurotransmission. It inhibits carbonic anhydrase.

So far there is little experience with this drug but trials show it is effective in some neuropathic pain states.

DOSE

- 25 mg nocte for one week increasing by 25–50 mg every two weeks to a maximum of 400 mg in two divided doses.

LOCAL ANAESTHETICS

Lidocaine

MECHANISM OF ACTION

Lidocaine is a local anaesthetic of the amide type. It produces a reversible blockade of impulse propagation along the nerve fibres by preventing the inward movement of sodium ions through the nerves. When the membranes are repeatedly depolarized by an increased frequency of stimulation, more sodium channels open and more local anaesthetic can enter the nerve and increase the block.

The free base of the local anaesthetic drug, which is highly lipid soluble, interacts with sodium channels in a manner that is exquisitely sensitive to the voltage-dependent conformational state of the ion channel. When depolarized in the presence of lidocaine, sodium channels assume a longlived quiescent state. The lidocaine receptor has been localized to the inner aspect of the aqueous pore but the actual mechanism of action remains uncertain.

Lidocaine is absorbed from injection sites including muscle and its rate of absorption is determined by factors such as the site of administration and the tissue vascularity. Except for intravenous administration, the highest blood levels occur following intercostal nerve block and the lowest after subcutaneous administration. Temperature sensation is lost first followed by sharp pain and then light touch.

INTRAVENOUS USE

When used intravenously for management of neuropathic pain lidocaine suppresses the discharge of neurones or reduces their sensitivity to stimulation. It stabilizes the neuronal membrane and prevents initiation of nerve impulses.

METABOLISM

Lidocaine is metabolized in the liver and about 90 per cent of a given dose undergoes *N*-dealkylation to form monoethylglycinexylidide and glycinexylidide, both of which may contribute to the therapeutic and toxic effects. The elimination half-life of lidocaine following an intravenous bolus injection is one to two hours, but this may be prolonged in patients with hepatic dysfunction.

DOSE

First treatment

The usual adult intravenous bolus dose is 50–100 mg administered at a rate of approximately 25–50 mg per minute. If the desired response is not achieved, a second dose may be administered five minutes after completion of the first injection. Not more than 200–300 mg should be administered during a 1-hour period but this should produce a response by the end of the infusion. Elderly patients may require smaller bolus doses.

Further treatment

Recurrent treatments can be given on a daily or weekly basis until the desired effect has been achieved. A trial of mexiletine orally can be undertaken. Doses of up to 600 mg mexiletine may be necessary but it is rarely possible to achieve this without unacceptable side effects such as indigestion, nausea, dizziness and palpitations. Other oral local anaesthetics include flecainide and tocainide but these are rarely used because of the incidence of side effects.

CONTRAINDICATIONS

Local anaesthetics should be used with caution in patients with:

- epilepsy
- ischaemic heart disease
- cardiac conduction disturbances
- congestive heart failure
- bradycardia
- impaired respiratory function
- impaired hepatic function.

There is a risk of cardiac dysrhythmias with intravenous lidocaine so the patient should be monitored with an electrocardiogram and resuscitation facilities must be available.

SIDE EFFECTS

Adverse reactions to local anaesthetics are rare and are usually the result of raised plasma concentrations due to accidental intravascular injection, excessive dosage or rapid absorption from highly vascular areas, or may result from a hypersensitivity, idiosyncrasy or diminished tolerance on the part of the patient (Table 3.9). Toxicity mainly involves the CNS and/or the cardiovascular system.

CNS reactions

- Excitatory and/or depressant
- Nervousness
- Tremor
- Blurred vision
- Nausea and vomiting
- Drowsiness
- Coma
- Respiratory arrest

Cardiovascular reactions

- Hypotension
- Bradycardia
- Myocardial depression
- Cardiac arrest

The excitatory CNS reactions may be brief or may not occur at all, so that the first signs of toxicity may be drowsiness, followed by coma and respiratory failure.

Allergic reactions

These are rare and include:

- Cutaneous lesions
- Urticaria
- Oedema
- Anaphylactoid reactions.

Table 3.9 *Side effects of lidocaine at various plasma concentrations*

Plasma concentration (μg/mL)	Side effect profile
4–6	Light-headed, numb tongue, metallic taste, ↑BP, dizzy
8	Visual and auditory disturbances, disassociation, muscle twitching, ↓BP
12	Convulsions (treat with benzodiazepines)
16	Coma
>20	Respiratory arrest and CVS collapse

BP, blood pressure; CVS, cardiovascular system.

Skin testing for allergy to lidocaine is not considered to be reliable.

LIDOCAINE PATCH (LIDODERM®)

Lidocaine 5 per cent is impregnated into a patch. Each patch contains 700 mg of lidocaine. Up to three patches can be worn together for a maximum of 12 hours per day.

Mechanism of action

Lidocaine infiltrates subcutaneous tissues to the damaged nerve and also protects the sensitive area. There may also be some systemic absorption. Sodium channel blockade leads to suppression of spontaneous ectopic activity and hyperalgesia. Blood concentrations remain very low even when using four patches twice a day. It produces only analgesia and no local anaesthesia.

Evidence of efficacy

Fifty-three of 100 patients with post-herpetic neuralgia were shown to have moderate relief and 29 patients a lot or complete pain relief. The lidocaine patch is effective in reducing ongoing pain and allodynia in the first hour after application and over seven days. The NNT is 4.4.

The effect only lasts while the patches are being used and there is no prolonged period of pain relief after treatment.

Advantages of topical treatment

- Few and mild side effects
- Easy to handle
- Once daily application

Bupivacaine

The advantage of bupivacaine over lidocaine for local anaesthesia is its longer duration of action which makes it more suitable for spinal and epidural anaesthesia. It is not indicated for intravenous use.

Levobupivacaine

Levobupivacaine appears to be equivalent in potency to the racemic bupivacaine mixture used for years, but does have the decreased potential for arrhythmogenicity expected of the pure L-isomer. It may be the drug of choice when large doses of long-acting local anaesthetic must be injected with little chance for dose fractionation, such as in upper or some lower extremity nerve blocks for surgery. Unless evidence suggests some advantage (less motor block or some subjective advantage for the patient) of levobupivacaine over bupivacaine, it is unclear whether there is a role for levobupivacaine.

Ropivacaine

Ropivacaine is synthesized and sold as the pure L-isomer to take advantage of the fact that the D-isomer of local anaesthetics possesses more of the arrhythmogenic potential. Ropivacaine causes less motor block than equivalent doses of bupivacaine.

Emla® 5 per cent cream

Lidocaine 2.5 per cent plus prilocaine 2.5 per cent are mixed together to produce a soft white cream. Emla also contains polyoxyethylene hydrogenated castor oil, carbomer 974P, sodium hydroxide and purified water. Application provides dermal analgesia, and the depth of analgesia depends on the application time, the dose and the thickness of the skin. It causes transient vasoconstriction or vasodilation of the area.

For venepuncture about 2 gm should be applied to the skin for a minimum of one hour and a maximum of five hours and covered with an occlusive dressing. The procedure should be started soon after the dressing is removed; the duration of action should be about two hours. For larger areas and other applications about 1.5–2 gm/10 cm^2 should be applied.

SYSTEMIC ABSORPTION

Systemic absorption is low. For example, following an application of 60 g cream over 400 cm^2 for three hours on the thigh about 5 per cent is absorbed, giving maximum blood concentrations of 0.12 µg/mL lidocaine and 0.07 µg/mL prilocaine after two to six hours.

METHAEMOGLOBINAEMIA AND PRILOCAINE

Systemic absorption of prilocaine is low but care must be taken in the following:

- patients with glucose-6-phosphate dehydrogenase deficiency
- congenital idiopathic methaemoglobinaemia
- anaemia
- patients taking additional therapy known to cause methaemoglobinaemia such as sulphonamides.

Amethocaine

Amethocaine 4 per cent (Ametop®) is formulated as a free base to allow the tetracaine to diffuse across the skin to the pain receptors just below the corneum stratum. It has a shorter onset time than Emla (20–30 minutes) and a longer duration of action (four to six hours). It may cause erythema, oedema and blistering, and it is contraindicated in neonates.

Phenol and alcohol

Both phenol and alcohol cause protein coagulation and necrosis of the axon without disruption of the Schwann cell tube so axonal regeneration can occur. Recovery is faster with phenol than alcohol. Destruction is not selective – both motor and sensory nerves are destroyed.

PHENOL

Aqueous phenol 6 per cent is for peripheral use and 5 per cent in glycerol for intrathecal use. Contact with somatic nerves may lead to neuritis.

Dose

- Maximum dose in a 70 kg man = 600 mg (50 mg/mL = 12 mL).

ALCOHOL

Alcohol also produces a non-selective destruction of nerves but has a very high incidence of neuritis. Alcohol is more likely than phenol to destroy the cell bodies as well as causing a permanent block. It is usually only used for coeliac plexus blocks where the large volumes required preclude the use of phenol. The large volumes may cause alcohol overdose especially in small or elderly people.

RECENT ADVANCES IN THE PHARMACOLOGICAL MANAGEMENT OF PAIN

New NSAIDs

Dexketoprofen trometamol is a dextrorotatory enantiomer of ketoprofen, which is an NSAID that has been used for about 20 years. Arylpropionic acids (APAs) are a group of NSAIDs currently produced in racemic form. The pharmacological effect resides with the S(+) enantiomer and production of single isomer drugs is underway.

BENEFITS

- Production of the new isomer
- Better analgesia
- Faster onset
- Increased therapeutic index

- Simplified pharmacokinetic profile
- 50 per cent dosage reduction

The tromethamine salt also increases solubility and so leads to faster absorption. A recent study demonstrated similar pain relief using rofecoxib 50 mg and dexketoprofen trometamol 25 mg and there were also similar side effects.

Sites of action of potential analgesic drugs

Pharmacotherapy for neuropathic pain is generally disappointing. There is no treatment to prevent the development of neuropathic pain, or to adequately, predictably and specifically control established neuropathic pain. Research is continuing into the causes and management of neuropathic pain and a few of the possible treatments are mentioned here.

NITRIC OXIDE SYNTHETASE INHIBITORS

A COX-2 drug that donates nitric oxide at sites of inflammation is being investigated. Nitric oxide should reduce inflammation.

B1 AND B2 RECEPTOR ANTAGONISTS

Both antagonists show analgesic activity and may prove useful, but probably only when potent non-peptide compounds are discovered.

LTB4 RECEPTOR ANTAGONIST

In trials these drugs reduced general clinical symptoms and histological changes of arthritis but there was no evidence of analgesic activity.

CYTOKINE SUPPRESSIVE ANTI-INFLAMMATORY DRUGS (CSAIDS)

Cytokine (interleukin-1 and tumour necrosis factor (TNF)-α) production is regulated at transcriptional and translational level. CSAIDs can inhibit their production and antagonists can block inflammatory hyperalgesia, but no compounds are available for clinical use yet.

TUMOUR NECROSIS FACTOR-α ANTIBODIES FOR THE TREATMENT OF RHEUMATOID ARTHRITIS

Tumour necrosis factor-α antibodies decrease hyperalgesia in inflammatory models, e.g. anti-TNF therapy in rheumatoid arthritis reduces pain (e.g. infliximab, see Chapter 13).

SLOW TETRODOTOXIN-RESISTANT CHANNELS

These offer an attractive drug target, blocking transmission in the polymodal neurones. It would be a highly specific therapeutic strategy.

CHANNEL BLOCKERS

Potassium ion channel

Opening the K^+ channels leads to membrane hyperpolarization and inhibition of membrane excitability. There are two types of K^+ channel:

- Large conductance Ca^{2+} dependent channel (maxi-K channel)
- ATP-sensitive K^+ channel.

Sodium ion channel

Na_v 1.8 and Na_v 1.9 channels are specific to neurones and central pain regulation. Drugs specific for these channels could be produced. (Phenytoin and carbamazepine act at these sites.)

Calcium ion channel blockers

Pregabalin is an example of a selective calcium channel blocker. Following nerve injury, there is an up-regulation of the $\alpha2\beta$ subunit of calcium channels, suggesting a greater number of channels are active at any one time. These findings have relevance to the mode of action of the drug, gabapentin, used in neuropathic pain, since gabapentin binds to this component of calcium channels, where it can he presumed to act as an antagonist.

NERVE GROWTH FACTOR

Primary afferent neurones can regenerate. If there is an injury to the peripheral nerve, then there is selective death of nociceptive cells and non-nociceptive cells sprout to fill the void. This can be prevented by using nerve growth factor (NGF) because it stops the degeneration of the small fibres so there is no void for the cells to sprout into.

ADENOSINE

Anti-nociceptive action results from activation of A1 receptors, which exert pre- and postsynaptic inhibitory effects in the dorsal horn. Central and peripheral A1 receptors mediate anti-nociceptive effects and A2 receptor agonists have the opposite effect. Selective A1 receptor agonists might prove useful analgesic agents and trials are about to begin. Adenosine itself given as an intravenous infusion has been shown to reduce some types of neuropathic pain, in particular, reduced hyperaesthesia to tactile stimuli.

Dose

- Test dose 10 μg/kg/min over 10 minutes
- Followed by 50–70 μg/kg per minute over 60 minutes if there are no side effects

- Pain relief occurs gradually (over several days)
- Repeat weekly

There is no tolerance, and there are no side effects.

EPIBATIDINE

This is produced from the skin of the Ecuadorian frog. It has a very potent anti-nociceptive effect in rats and mice. It is a potent nicotinic agonist and produces analgesia but has motor and autonomic effects at doses very close the anti-nociceptive doses. It is roughly 100 times more potent than morphine.

CHOLECYSTOKININ (CCK)

Cholecystokinin (CCK) differs from the other nociceptive neuropeptides by acting indirectly rather than directly. It antagonizes the effect of μ-opioid agonists at the receptor, but CCK does not produce hyperalgesia when applied alone. It is normally located in laminae I and II of the dorsal horn. The amount of CCK is increased in neuropathic pain and decreased in inflammatory pain. This may explain the relative opioid resistance and sensitivity respectively of these two pain syndromes. Antagonists to CCK are unlikely to be useful as analgesics on their own but could enhance the effects of opioids. They may also be useful in tolerance and addiction.

The CCK antagonists devazepide and lorglumide are currently under investigation. They also appear to be anxiolytic.

NMDA RECEPTOR ANTAGONISTS

NMDA receptor antagonists available so far are ketamine, amantidine and dextromethorphan. They have major unwanted side effects but drugs continue to be developed. The therapeutic window for NMDA receptor antagonists maybe improved by use of subtype-specific drugs as there are four subunits of the receptor. The NR2B subtype of the receptor, for example is an interesting target since it has a restricted distribution yet antagonists appear to be effective in reducing nociception.

GLYCINE RECEPTORS

Drug companies are looking at drugs that would block glycine reuptake into nerve cells.

CANNABINOIDS

Cannabis was withdrawn from the *British Pharmacopoeia* in 1976 (in 1942 in the USA). The major active constituent of *Cannabis sativa* is delta-9-tetrahydrocannabinol (Δ^9 THC). It was isolated in 1964.

CB1 and CB2 receptors were cloned in the 1990s. CB1 receptors are found in the brain and spinal cord in high concentrations, especially in the olfactory areas, cortex, hippocampus, cerebellum, and basal ganglia. Activation of CB1 receptors inhibits voltage sensitive Ca^{2+} channels and augments K^+ channels, producing increased membrane hyperpolarization and inhibition of adenylcyclase. CB2 receptors are found in the spleen, macrophages, lymphocytes and mast cells, peripheral nerve terminals, vas deferens and the myenteric plexus.

Δ^9 THC content varies tremendously among different sources and preparations, complicating the interpretation of previous reports of analgesic benefit. When smoked, 50 per cent Δ^9 THC is absorbed rapidly through the lungs. When taken orally it undergoes first pass metabolism producing a delayed and reduced effect. Sprays are being developed containing THC and cannabidiol. Trial results show some positive outcomes but the potential of cannabinoids has not yet been fully recognized.

Mechanism of action

The first natural cannabinoid (anandamide) was discovered in 1992. All cannabinoids appear to play a part in memory, appetite, control of movement and modulation of pain. Animal studies show cannabinoids lower the response of pain neurones in the spinal cord and thalamus. The sites of cannabinoid action in the CNS are confined to specific areas especially the dorsal horn of the spinal cord. There are more cannabinoid receptors than opioid receptors in the brain. Cannabinoid and opioid receptors may interact and even operate synergistically but at the moment our knowledge is still limited. They may attenuate the NGF-mediated inflammatory response and may help both visceral and neuropathic pain.

Δ^9 THC possesses anti-nociceptive properties and is mediated by CB1 receptors. A double blind comparison with placebo in chronic pain shows an opioid sparing effect. It probably acts at brain and spinal cord sites producing opioid receptor agonism and cannabinoid receptor antagonism. It also reduces arachidonic acid induced inflammation. Intrathecal cannabinoids may help pain without the central effects.

$$20 \, mg \, THC \equiv 120 \, mg \, codeine.$$

Studies and effectiveness

The main therapeutic use of cannabis currently is as an antiemetic. There are numerous anecdotal reports of the benefit of cannabis but the attitude towards it as being a drug of abuse has limited proper studies into its use. Animal studies indicate that cannabinoids will be useful and human studies are currently underway. It may be useful in cancer pain.

LEVONANTRADOL

Levonantradol 1.5–3 mg may be good in postoperative pain.

Δ^9 THC

Δ^9 THC 2.5–15 mg relieved spasticity in multiple sclerosis, but some patients became dysphoric. A recent study looking at 5 mg Δ^9 THC in postoperative pain for abdominal hysterectomy showed no difference between drug and placebo. This dose was chosen because 10 mg caused an unacceptably high number of side effects.

NABILONE

One patient with multiple sclerosis has been reported to have improved with nabilone but some have reported dysphoria. Nabilone 1 mg is probably too much for most pain patients. Its half-life is two to four hours but the half-life of the metabolite is 20 hours. Of a single dose, 84 per cent is eliminated in seven days. The initial dose should be 1 mg every three days up to 1 mg three times daily. The dose should be tapered gradually if used for more than a few weeks.

All patients who have tried cannabis as well as nabilone have preferred the former because of increased effectiveness, less dysphoria and ease of titration.

DRONABINOL

In a dose of 10 mg per day dronabinol has been shown to reduce central pain in multiple sclerosis by an average of 21 per cent. The NNT is 3.45.

COMMONEST SIDE EFFECTS OF CANNABINOIDS

- Dizziness – 58 per cent
- Sedation and drowsiness – 42 per cent
- Headache – 25 per cent
- Myalgia – 25 per cent
- Tachycardia and palpitations – 17 per cent
- Euphoria – 13 per cent
- Dry mouth – 13 per cent

SUBSTANCE P ANTAGONISTS

These agents act at the NK-1 receptor and are potent for reducing hyperalgesia but not baseline nociceptor reflexes so they may be useful in chronic pain states. Although NK-1 receptors are widely distributed, side effects do not seem to be a problem. So far these drugs have not proved useful clinically.

NEUROKININ-1 RECEPTOR ANTAGONISTS

Neurokinin-1 receptor antagonists inhibit enhanced spinal excitability and should be available soon. Neurokinin-2 receptor antagonists are potent for nociception. Calcitonin gene-related peptide (CGRP) is released from nociceptive afferents and causes slow depolarization of the dorsal horn cells. It also potentiates the spread of substance P (non-synaptic volume transmission) by competing for the same breakdown peptidase. There are no useful receptor antagonists available yet, but antibodies to CGRP are analgesic.

ANTI-NOCICEPTIVE NEUROPEPTIDES

Somatostatin analogues

Somatostatin content in the dorsal horn is increased after noxious thermal stimuli. Application of somatostatin or its stable peptide analogues (octreotide and vapreotide) is analgesic in animal and human models. The major disadvantage of somatostatin in clinical use is its short half-life, requiring administration by continuous infusion. To date these drugs have been used effectively to treat cancer pain either intrathecally or epidurally. The dose of octreotide is 5–20 μg/h.

GALANIN AGONISTS

Galanin is co-localized with substance P and CGRP and is thought to exert a tonic inhibitory effect on spinal cord nociceptive transmission. Unlike the other two transmitters, its production is up-regulated in nerve damage. Agonists would be analgesic.

Novel drug delivery methods

IONTOPHORESIS

Iontophoresis is being developed to allow rapid delivery of a transdermal drug for acute pain. Iontophoresis is the transdermal administration of drugs in an ionized state by electric current. It was first described by Veratti in 1747 and Leduc at the beginning of the twentieth century. If a drug is applied to the skin in an electrode of the same charge as the drug (e.g. lidocaine/anode) and an electric current is applied, the drug will pass with the current and be deposited superficially and in deeper tissue. The circuit is completed by the drug-free electrode of opposite charge placed close to the active electrode. Emla applied for 60 minutes under an occlusive dressing has been compared to iontophorectically applied lidocaine (5 per cent 0.5 mL with 0.1–0.2 mAcm^2) for 10 minutes. Both methods produced skin analgesia but the iontophoretic technique abolished pain on injection. This technique also reduces pain associated with intravenous propofol.

Other drugs used with iontophoresis are:

- fentanyl – iontophoresis improves drug delivery, leads to a rapidly steady state, with the ability to vary the delivery rate and is therefore better for acute pain

- sufentanil
- morphine.

The delivery is affected by the physicochemical nature of the drug, the solution and the voltage (duration and nature).

Botulinum toxin (Botox®)

Clostridium botulinum is a Gram-positive anaerobic bacterium that produces seven types of toxin. It was first isolated in 1895 from food of victims with food poisoning.

Botulinum A binds irreversibly to the presynaptic membrane of the motor end plate and blocks acetylcholine release. The toxin enters the presynaptic cholinergic nerve terminals and causes localized destruction so preventing release of acetylcholine. It inhibits muscle contraction and so acts as a muscle relaxant.

The end plate shrivels but then re-grows after about three months and the collateral sprouting of axons restores the initial situation within three to six months. Tachyphylaxis has been shown but injections into the affected muscles can be repeated. The onset of action is about three days with maximum effect at one to two weeks. Accompanied by physiotherapy it can improve muscle function.

MECHANISM OF ACTION

Treatment of tender points and trigger points causes relaxation of the muscle which in turn leads to decompression of afferent nociceptive neurones, decompression of muscular blood vessels, reduction in the elevated concentration of excitatory metabolites because of improved blood supply and normalization of excessive muscle spindle activity.

SIDE EFFECTS

- 'Flu-like' symptoms (2.6 per cent)
- Numbness of the surrounding area (6.5 per cent)
- Muscle weakness
- Difficulty swallowing if used around the neck

USES

- Blepharospasm – 90 per cent improve
- Spasmodic dystonia – 90 per cent improve
- Spasmodic torticollis – 80 per cent improve
- Cervical dystonia
- Cervicogenic headache
- Myofascial pains – neck, shoulder, low back, painful muscle spasms
- Painful contractures (cerebrovascular accidents, CRPS)
- Postural pains

- Migraine
- Cluster headache
- Tension headaches

DOSE

See Table 3.10. Inject at the site of pain or trigger points. Pain relief is usually obtained before muscle spasm and is more marked. Tolerability and safety are high, and efficacy builds stepwise. The improvement may last up to 90 days.

Table 3.10 *Dose chart for botulinum toxin*

Muscle	Dose (IU)
Scalenus anterior	50
Trapezius	100
Rhomboid	100
Supraspinatus	50
Brachioradialis	25
Iliopsoas	50
Quadratus lumborum	50
Piriformis	100

Capsaicin

Capsaicin is the active ingredient in chili pepper and when applied to the skin causes a severe burning feeling. It is used in:

- post-herpetic neuralgia (licensed)
- osteoarthritis (licensed)
- post-mastectomy pain
- diabetic neuropathy
- post-amputation pain.

An adequate trial should last eight weeks. The burning sensation can be relieved with 5 per cent lidocaine ointment. The cream is absorbed through the skin and depletes substance P from primary afferent C fibre endings in the periphery and dorsal horn. Axon transport is blocked and synthesis of substance P is decreased. It thereby inhibits central transmission of pain. It is transported in neurotubules and neurofilaments from the periphery to the dorsal horn. Cream 0.075 per cent is applied liberally to the painful area three to four times per day but contact with hands and mucous membranes should be avoided.

Intracellular messengers

Protein kinase C (PKC) is activated in conjunction with the NMDA receptor and is a critical step in long-term increases in neuronal excitability. Gangliosides significantly reduce hyperalgesia in neuropathic pain models. The mechanism may involve blockade of PKC translocation and activation.

FURTHER READING

Moore JE, Barden J, McQuay H. *Bandolier's Little Book of Pain*. Oxford: Oxford University Press, 2003.

Section Two

4 Management of Acute Pain: Principles and Practice

ACUTE PAIN

An explosion of research into the management of acute pain occurred in the 1980s and 1990s. Prior to this there were no pain management specialists, no training in pain management, no research or funding and no journals. The lessons that have been learnt are gradually improving the management of patients in pain.

Acute pain is pain of recent onset and probable limited duration. It usually has an identifiable and causal relationship to injury or disease. There are not only wide variations from patient to patient in the amount of pain experienced, but also great differences in responsiveness to particular therapeutic approaches. This is partly genetic and partly due to physiological modulating factors such as anxiety, fear, sense of control, ethno-cultural status and the meaning to the patient of the pain state.

In September 1990 the Royal College of Surgeons of England and the Royal College of Anaesthetists produced the *Report of the Working Party on Pain after Surgery*. It identified the very poor quality of pain relief at that time and recommended that improvements be made (Box 4.1). It is now a condition for accreditation for training by the Royal College of Anaesthetists that an acute hospital has a pain team.

Seventy five per cent of adult patients believe postoperative pain is to be expected and 60 per cent regard this as their primary fear before surgery. In a questionnaire, 515 patients indicated that among the general public there is little or no understanding of the nature of postoperative pain or of the methods currently available to treat it.

The extent of satisfaction with the provision of analgesia depends on the knowledge and expectations of the patient and should not provide grounds for complacency when such knowledge is poor. Postoperative pain does not confer any benefit on a patient. Although we believe good pain relief speeds recovery there is no evidence this is so but some reports indicate that effective analgesia leads to early restoration of oral feeding and aggressive regimens reduce hospital stay. In the past, up to 50 per cent of patients have had inadequately

relieved pain (Box 4.2), but there is now a clear directive that clinicians have a moral obligation to treat pain more effectively.

How much pain and how much pain relief?

Anyone, expert or not, observing someone who is injured, almost inevitably assigns an appropriate amount of pain to the injury. Staff of an emergency room thought 40 per cent of patients made a terrible fuss, 40 per cent were 'denying pain' and 20 per cent gave an appropriate answer. A further area that hinders research into acute pain and its management is the problem of assessing how much pain relief is enough. How much pain relief do patients require before they are comfortable, and how variable is this among patients? Significant pain relief for one person may be insufficient pain relief for another. Current studies suggest that a reduction of 3 in the visual analogue scale score, or a reported 30 per cent reduction in pain, is clinically significant in terms of studies, but is

---

BOX 4.1 UK working party recommendations to improve the management of pain after surgery

- Need for education and training in changing antiquated staff attitudes and practice together with adequate resources
- Systematic recording of patient's pain, as with blood pressure/heart rate
- A named member of staff to be responsible for a hospital policy towards postoperative analgesia, subject to continuous audit and appraisal
- All major hospitals performing surgery should introduce an acute pain service using a multidisciplinary team approach with input of medical, nursing, pharmaceutical and psychological expertise. The anaesthetist has a primary role to play
- There is a need for powerful, well-tolerated analgesics and long-acting non-toxic local anaesthetics

---

BOX 4.2 Reasons for ineffective analgesia

- Pain is subjective and difficult to quantify
- The common idea that pain is merely a symptom and not harmful in itself
- The belief that a certain degree of injury justifies an appropriate amount of pain
- Concerns about respiratory depression, nausea and vomiting associated with opioids
- Lack of understanding of the pharmacology of the agents used
- Lack of appreciation of the variability in analgesic response to opioids
- Prescriptions for opioids that include the use of inappropriate doses and/or dose intervals
- Misinterpretation of doctors' orders by nursing staff, including the use of lower doses and delaying administration
- Patients' difficulties in communicating their need for analgesia
- A nursing culture that believe opioid drugs are only for the dying
- Poor supervision of pain relief by physicians

See also Table 4.1.

Table 4.1 *Some myths and truths about analgesia*

Myth	Truth
Analgesia makes accurate diagnosis difficult or impossible	Good analgesia may improve diagnosis because an adequate examination can be made
Patients will become addicted to opioids	In 10 000 patients with burns requiring opioid therapy there were no cases of drug addiction
The patient's weight is the best predictor of opioid requirement	The amount of opioid required can vary eight-fold between patients. Age is a better predictor of requirement. 100 − age = mg morphine required in 24 hours
Opioids should only be given four hourly	Opioids should be titrated to full effect. Intravenous doses can be given every 10 minutes as required
If the patient is pain free at the scheduled time of dosing, the analgesic drug should be missed	Pain is controlled because analgesia has been given. If a dose is missed pain may return and it is then more difficult to treat. Constant blood levels of the drug provide better analgesia

---

this enough for the patient? Assessment of outcome of treatment is therefore not straightforward.

Most patients do not seek complete pain relief. They often weigh up the benefits of analgesia against the side effects caused by the drugs. Physicians and relatives may have differing perspectives regarding the relative importance of the outcomes. To optimize patient care it is necessary for physicians to understand better how patients value outcomes and they may have different relative preferences for different types of side effect.

Incidence of pain on a general medical ward

The Joint Royal Colleges of Surgeons and Anaesthetists report in 1992 that was the precursor to the development of the Acute Pain Service in the UK was primarily concerned with postoperative pain. It did not look at pain management in other areas of the hospital setting or in the community. A recent survey revealed that 20–25 per cent of patients admitted to medical wards had pain scores of 6 out of 10 or greater and 12 per cent had unbearable pain. The reasons for this were given as:

- inadequate information
- poor assessment
- poor prescribing and administration
- poor patient reporting
- 16 per cent of those patients would like better pain control
- 29 per cent would like fewer side effects
- 39 per cent would like more information on pain relief
- 16 per cent would like more involvement with their pain management.

Ethnic differences in pain perception and pain response

Laboratory studies show psychological pain thresholds do not vary considerably among different groups. However, clinical studies do show ethnic differences and minorities remain at risk for inadequate pain control.

In patients undergoing internal fixation of a femur, of American patients given an average of 30.2 mg morphine 80 per cent reported inadequate pain control, yet among Vietnamese patients who received on average 0.9 mg morphine, only 8 per cent reported inadequate pain control. The Vietnamese patients had a more accurate impression of how much a femoral fracture should hurt prior to the injury than the Americans. African Americans in the USA are less likely to be given analgesia. Asian patients receive 24 per cent lower postoperative analgesic agents than Europeans if given by nurses. If the two groups are given patient controlled analgesia (PCA) they use the same amounts of opioids. Among patients who had had an open reduction and fixation of a fractured limb, white patients had an average of 22 mg morphine per day, Hispanics 13 mg morphine per day and black patients just 6 mg of morphine per day.

The most important variable in the under-treatment of minority pain is the staff perception of pain intensity. The ethnicity of the clinician is also important. A patient will have better analgesia if they share a language. Gender, age, generation, socioeconomic status, level of ties to the mother country, primary language spoken at home and the degree of isolation of the individual all affect how closely an individual identifies with an ethnic group. Beliefs about pain influence treatment compliance, outcome and how patients manage their pain.

Physiological changes associated with pain

Injury not only produces pain, but it is also associated with stress. Surgical trauma, psychological factors, environmental factors and other factors (e.g. drugs) combine to produce several physiological responses. Substances released from injured tissue also evoke stress hormone responses. The body tries to achieve homoeostasis using neural, hormonal and behavioural activities leading to the following physiological changes:

- sympathetic activation
- hypercoagulability due to platelet aggregation
- immunosuppression

- nausea
- ileus
- hypertension
- tachycardia
- increased cardiac work
- vasoconstriction with impaired wound healing
- inability to cough
- substantial reductions in respiratory parameters
  - low oxygen tension
  - poor perfusion
  - reduced deposition of collagen in tissue undergoing repair
  - restricted breathing and low-grade hypoxia
- psychological effects.

Those patients at greater risk of adverse outcomes from unrelieved pain are those with concomitant medical illness, major surgery, and the very young or very old. It is particularly important in these patients to modify these changes by providing effective analgesia to minimize this increased risk.

Metabolic and endocrine responses to surgery

See Table 4.2.

The acute pain team

The first acute pain service started at the University of Seattle in 1986. By the late 1990s, 88 per cent of British hospitals had an acute pain team.

Table 4.2 *Metabolic and endocrine responses to surgery*

Endocrine	Metabolic			Water and electrolyte flux
	Carbohydrate	Protein	Fat	
↑catabolic hormones: ↑ACTH, cortisol, ADH, growth hormone catecholamines, angiotensin II, aldosterone, Glucagon, IL-1, TNF and IL-6	Hyperglycaemia: ↑hepatic glycogenolysis, gluconeogenesis	Muscle protein catabolism, ↑synthesis acute phase proteins Leads to protein breakdown	↑lipolysis and oxidation: ↑catecholamines, cortisol, glucagon and growth hormone	Retention of water and sodium, ↑excretion of potassium and ↓functional ECF with shifts to ICF
↓anabolic steroid: ↓insulin and testosterone	Insulin resistance and glucose intolerance: ↓insulin secretion/action			

ACTH, adrenocorticotropic hormone; ADH, antidiuretic hormone, IL, interleukin, TNF, tumour necrosis factor, ECF, extracellular fluid, ICF, intra cellular fluid.

OBJECTIVES

1 To improve the quality of postoperative analgesia, and minimize discomfort.
2 To expand the range of techniques used.
3 To increase the safety and efficacy of analgesia.
4 To facilitate the recovery process.
5 To avoid or effectively manage side effects of treatment.
6 To increase awareness among healthcare staff of the importance of postoperative pain and the availability of new analgesic techniques.
7 To improve pain management in all patients including medical admissions.
8 Audit.
9 Research.
10 To make therapy cost effective.

It seems likely that, for most patients, better postoperative pain control will require application of existing knowledge rather than the introduction of new analgesic agents or expensive equipment.

Factors to consider when choosing treatment

- The underlying problem – some procedures are more painful than others.
- Coexisting illness.
- Institutional factors:
  - available staff
  - available equipment
  - cost.
- Risk and unwanted effects of various options.
- Appropriateness of chosen intervention for that pain.
- Evidence of efficacy for the chosen intervention.
- Patient factors:
  - what would they like
  - mental capacity
  - control.
- Surgical factors:
  - type of operation
  - likes and dislikes.

Steps to successful management

- Guidelines to follow to act on reported pain scores.
- Relieving anxiety decreases pain – psychologist or explanation and understanding of patient's fears.
- Involve patient directly in management of pain especially with self-administered drugs.
- Improved monitoring of side effects may decrease tendency to under-prescribe opioids such as the use of pulse oximetry.

- Treatment should be individualized.
- Where pain can be prevented efforts should be made to achieve this.
- Keep side effects to a minimum.
- Balanced analgesia may be used to improve efficacy and reduce side effects. This means using a combination of analgesic agents such as paracetamol, a non-steroidal anti-inflammatory drug (NSAID) and an opioid.
- Restoration of function should be a clear goal.
- Adverse physiological and psychological effects result from unrelieved severe pain.
- Regular assessment of pain and adverse effects – proper assessment and control of pain require patient involvement, frequent assessment and reassessment of pain intensity and charting of analgesia.
- Prevention is better than treatment – pain that is established and severe is difficult to control.
- Protocols for monitoring and treating pain – effective pain relief requires flexibility and tailoring of treatment to an individual rather than rigid application of formulae and prescriptions. Allow patient control – ordering the same analgesic doses and administering intervals for all patients while failing to regularly reassess efficacy will provide suboptimal results. Patients under 40 years have twice the amount of incident pain as those over 70 years. They also have a three times higher use of opioids.
- Postoperative analgesia should be planned preoperatively with consideration given to the type of surgery, medical condition of the patient, perioperative use of analgesics and regional anaesthetic techniques.
- Postoperative requirements for early mobilization should be discussed with the patient and the timing of appropriate and adequate analgesia considered.
- Protocols for monitoring and treating adverse effects.
- Titration of doses at short intervals until the pain is relieved.
- Use more than one approach when necessary.
- Appropriate back-up by identified personnel.
- Continuing in-service training and education of staff and patients.
- Opt for safety and simplicity.
- Choose evidence-based interventions.
- While it is not possible or always desirable to alleviate completely all pain in the postoperative period, it should be possible to reduce pain to a tolerable or comfortable level.
- A multidisciplinary approach to the management of acute pain, particularly in a formal acute pain service, leads to improved pain relief and better patient outcomes. When patients are managed with PCA in hospitals with acute pain teams they have the same pain scores but a lower incidence of side effects compared with hospitals without acute pain teams.

- Effective pain management is fundamental to the quality of care. The key to successful pain management is education and training of all staff and patients. The introduction of simple methods of pain assessment, recording of pain on movement and at rest and the treatment of pain using simple algorithms can significantly reduce postoperative pain.
- Ultimate responsibility for pain management should be assigned to those most experienced in its administration and not to the most junior staff members.

Estimates of economic benefit of acute pain teams

Estimates suggest that the development of an acute pain team may be cost effective and the team provides improved quality of service for patients undergoing surgery. A reliable and rapid response from the acute pain service is the best way to gain the cooperation of nursing staff and confidence of surgical colleagues.

Standards

The Welsh Office set a target in acute pain that was to be reached by 2002. It states that <5 per cent of patients should be suffering severe pain postoperatively by this time. Evidence for best practice in pain management remains fairly limited, and at present we have little guidance on which to base best practice. The National Health and Medical Research Council (NHMRC) in Australia, through the Health Care Advisory Committee, has produced a document entitled *Acute Pain Management – The Scientific Evidence*. This document has assessed all available evidence and provides some best practice guidelines for pain management. McQuay and colleagues in Oxford have done similar meta-analyses of studies to produce guidelines on effective and ineffective treatments.

Effectiveness of acute postoperative pain management – the evidence

LEVEL 1 EVIDENCE

See Table 4.3 for definition of levels of evidence.

- Postoperative epidurals can significantly reduce the incidence of pulmonary morbidity.
- Epidural opioids are more effective when used with local anaesthesia.
- Currently available NSAIDs do not reduce severe pain when used alone for major surgery, but they are useful when used as a component of multimodal analgesia as they reduce

Table 4.3 *Levels of evidence*

Level 1	Randomized controlled trial, systematic review and/or meta-analysis
Level 2	One or more well-designed randomized controlled trials
Level 3	Well designed, non-controlled studies, cohort or case controlled studies
Level 4	Opinions from recognized authorities, descriptive studies or reports of expert committees

Table 4.4 *Relief of pain: current levels of achievement*

	Intramuscular (%)	Patient controlled analgesia (%)	Epidural (%)
Moderate to severe pain at rest	66	36	21
Moderate to severe pain on movement	78	25	38
Severe pain on movement	29	10	8
Poor pain relief	2	4	5
Poor or fair pain relief	21	16	19

opioid requirements. Multimodal analgesia improves the effectiveness of pain relief with a reduced dose of each drug and the intensity of the side effects.

- Paracetamol is an effective postoperative analgesic and codeine 60 mg produces additional analgesia.
- In 15 of 17 studies that used transcutaneous electrical nerve stimulation (TENS) postoperatively there was no benefit.

LEVEL 2 EVIDENCE

- More aggressive approaches to management of early postoperative pain may reduce the transition to chronic postoperative pain.
- Multimodal analgesia improves the effectiveness of analgesia after surgery.
- Patient controlled analgesia provides greater patient satisfaction and improved ventilation compared with conventional routes.

A review of studies published up to this time demonstrated the present situation. They show that over the period 1973–99 there has been a highly significant reduction in the incidence of moderate-severe postoperative pain. The mean incidence of catheter dislodgement was 5.7 per cent. The figures in Table 4.4 show that one in five patients reported poor or fair pain relief (21 per cent), which far exceeds the level we should be achieving.

Assessment of pain

Pain should be assessed regularly throughout treatment, using self-reporting techniques as described in Chapter 2. As pain varies so markedly among individuals, patient involvement in the initial and continuing assessment of their pain is essential. Pain should be assessed both at rest and during activity, and before and after treatment is administered to assess the effect of the intervention. Pain relief must be assessed with regard to its adequacy to allow appropriate function.

Unexpected levels of pain or pain that suddenly increases, especially when associated with changes in other vital signs, may signal the development of a new surgical or medical diagnosis (e.g. postoperative complication, neuropathic pain). Although not specific, an important indicator of neuropathic pain is the inability to relieve pain with opioids, or no apparent relief of pain with a rapidly increasing opioid dose.

The role of acute pain in the development of chronic pain

The severity of postoperative pain is a predictor of the development of chronic pain. In a study looking at postoperative hernia pain, 28.7 per cent of patients had persistent pain after surgery with 11 per cent having pain severe enough to interfere with work or leisure activities. At one year 20 per cent of patients undergoing inguinal hernia repair had pain and 6 per cent of these patients felt their pain was moderate or severe. Trauma is responsible for approximately 19 per cent of long-term pain. In general the pain scores were higher or the pain persisted longer in these patients than in patients without persistent pain. It is unknown whether good pain control can alter these outcomes, but until we know more about this, optimum pain control should be the aim in all patients.

Psychology in acute pain

Many pain conditions, whether acute, chronic or secondary to malignancy, are only treatable up to a point. All pain problems can be partially maintained or exacerbated by psychological, psychosocial and behavioural factors.

Acute pain associated with strong negative emotions such as fear, grief or anger can persist long after a precipitating physical injury. Situations that trigger strong negative emotions, feelings of lack of control or conflicting feelings (e.g. guilt or anger) can impair a patient's recovery from pain.

The pain of relatively minor physical injuries sustained in a psychologically traumatic event (e.g. road traffic accident, physical assault) may have a prolonged course compared with the pain of comparably greater physical injuries from a less traumatic incident. A patient's appraisal of the impact of pain on his or her life and their ability to control the pain influence whether or not the patient becomes depressed. Depression, anxiety, anger and hostility complicate and often impede pain rehabilitation and recovery.

Behavioural and psychological intervention at this time may prevent pain from becoming a long-term problem, Focused psychological intervention can improve pain management outcomes by helping pain patients learn self-management techniques and build coping skills.

Risk factors creating barriers to recovery from acute pain

- Multiple invasive procedures, for example patients with burns.
- The perception of how an injury will affect the future particularly in patients with amputations and scarring from burns.
- A history of prolonged recovery from previous similar types of pain.
- Job dissatisfaction – this is particularly relevant in the context of work-related injuries.
- A history of emotional or physical trauma.
- A history of physical, emotional or sexual abuse.
- Low levels of activity.

Psycho-educational interventions to improve postoperative pain

Education about the aims and risks of pain therapy is an essential part of pain control and can lead to an improvement of postoperative analgesia. Preoperative education to help reduce postoperative pain should include:

- Information on:
  - Preparation for surgery
  - Timing of procedures
  - Functions and roles of healthcare providers
  - Self-care actions
  - Management of pain/discomfort
- Behavioural instructions
- Cognitive interventions
- Relaxation
- Emotion-focused coping
- Skills teaching:
  - Coughing
  - Breathing and bed exercises
  - Relaxation exercises
  - Hypnosis

- Psychosocial support
  - Identifying/alleviating concerns
  - Reassurance
  - Problem solving with patient
  - Encouraging questions

Small to moderate sized beneficial effects on recovery, postoperative pain and psychological distress are found in patients who have received this information. Length of hospital stay is also decreased compared with patients who do not receive this information.

Preoperative interventions which combine sensory and procedural information significantly reduce postoperative pain and distress and negative affect. Preoperatively patients should be offered information-giving interventions that include explanations of what will happen to them (**procedural**) and how they can expect to feel (**sensory**). Combined information is significantly better than procedural or sensory information alone.

GENERAL PRINCIPLES OF PAIN MANAGEMENT (BOX 4.3)

- Remove the cause of pain – surgery or splinting
- Medication
  - The analgesic ladder
- Regional analgesia
  - Epidural
  - Spinal
  - Nerve blocks
- Physical methods
  - Physiotherapy
  - Manipulation
  - TENS
- Psychological
  - Relaxation
  - Hypnosis
  - Psycho-prophylaxis
  - Other methods

BOX 4.3 The American Pain Society key strategies to improve pain management

- Recognition and prompt treatment of pain
- Making information about analgesics available
- Defining policies for use of advanced analgesic technologies
- Examining the process and outcomes of pain management with the goal of continuous improvement

---

PRE-EMPTIVE ANALGESIA

Background

The rationale behind pre-emptive analgesia is to stop pain from starting by blocking the usual response to pain. The pain of surgery begins during the incision with tissue damage producing primary hyperalgesia. We have also seen that the noxious stimulus produces 'wind-up' and receptive field expansion within the dorsal horn of the spinal cord causing secondary hyperalgesia (Chapter 1). Experimentally, analgesia commenced before surgery in animals can depress central sensitization to pain signals and enhance central inhibition mechanisms. This finding has led to studies using NSAIDs, opioids, ketamine and local anaesthetic preoperatively, with the aim of reducing postoperative pain.

Problems

- Animal models used have not provided sufficient information on what we are trying to modify. This raises several questions:
  - What time frame do we need to use?
  - What mechanisms are we trying to prevent (i.e. inflammation or nerve damage)?
  - Which type of pain will respond best (somatic, visceral, acute, chronic)?
- What type of pain are we trying to prevent?
  - Are we trying to reduce postoperative nociceptive pain or are we aiming to prevent the central sensitization that produces hyperalgesia and pain in non-injured tissues?
  - Or are we trying to reduce the incidence of chronic pain?
- Surgical nociception is much more longlasting, multimodal and intense than its experimental counterparts.
- Most clinical studies use only short-term analgesia, e.g. preoperative NSAID versus postoperative NSAID when the stimulus is longlasting. Pre-emption must correspond to the duration and extent of the nociception involved if it is to be effective. Postoperative surgical inflammation can still induce sensitization.
- The mechanism of action of epidural or peripheral nerve block in the role of postoperative pain is unclear. Is it due to a decrease in peripheral or central hypersensitivity?

Evidence

- NSAIDs/paracetamol should reduce peripheral sensitization secondary to prostaglandin release. Overall, studies show no measurable difference in pain scores if given before or after surgical incision.

- Spinal opioids – one study showed reduced pain for six hours postoperatively.
- Intravenous opioids – one study produced better pain relief if given prior to incision but methodology was poor.
- Epidural for abdominal hysterectomy – no difference.
- Inguinal field block – no difference.
- Intravenous ketamine during renal transplant led to reduced hyperalgesia around the wound, but when used for aortic aneurysm repair there were no benefits. Ketamine is thought to reduce the excitability of the spinal cord and reduce central sensitization. The dose is 0.15 mg/kg 10 minutes before incision and 3 μg/kg/min until the end of surgery.
- Combined intravenous ketamine and epidural morphine in gastrectomy have led to reduced postoperative pain scores.
- Pre-emptive epidural bupivacaine or fentanyl versus postoperative epidural in 100 patients undergoing radical prostatectomy led to 33 per cent less pain while the patients remained in hospital. However, at 9 weeks 86 per cent of the pre-emptive group had no pain compared with 47 per cent of the control group and they also had higher activity levels.

Summary

Limiting treatment to the preoperative period alone may be insufficient because the tissue damage produces an inflammatory reaction that outlasts the block and can cause central sensitization. To be maximally effective, treatment should start before surgical incision, continue though the surgery and into the postoperative period until surgical inflammation has subsided as a result of natural healing. This should be achieved using balanced analgesia, i.e. a mixture of NSAIDs, opioids, local anaesthesia and possibly ketamine to provide optimum pain management throughout.

THE WORLD HEALTH ORGANIZATION ANALGESIC LADDER

The principle of the analgesic ladder (Fig. 4.1) provides a simple way of prescribing drugs for pain relief.

1   The first step: Patients should be prescribed a non-opioid analgesic drug such as paracetamol, regularly. If this provides inadequate pain relief, an NSAID should be introduced, also prescribed regularly. Only about 80 per cent of individuals will respond to the first NSAID prescribed and if no benefit is obtained it is worth changing to a different NSAID. In those over 65 years, a cyclo-oxygenase

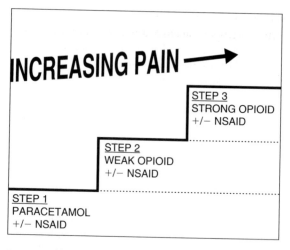

Figure 4.1 *WHO analgesic ladder*

(COX)-2 NSAID should be used as directed by the National Institute for Clinical Excellence (NICE).

2   The second step: If the first step fails to provide adequate relief, a weak opioid should be introduced with the paracetamol and NSAID. The addition of codeine to paracetamol may improve pain relief provided both drugs are administered at the same time.

3   The third step: When the patient is experiencing severe pain it is usually necessary to give a strong opioid such as morphine. If the patient is allowed oral intake this can be given orally. If the patient is nil by mouth, the opioid can be given intramuscularly but is best delivered intravenously, usually as PCA. If more than three doses of intramuscular drug are required it is better to provide PCA. Where possible and if not contraindicated the patient should always be prescribed paracetamol and an NSAID at the same time as they both have opioid-sparing effects and allow a smaller dose of opioid to be used, thus reducing the risk of side effects from the opioid.

The analgesic ladder and postoperative pain relief

Any patient who requires an opioid drug should also be prescribed paracetamol and an NSAID as well if there are no contraindications.

Role of benzodiazepines

Acute pain causes intense distress and anxiety, which then leads to increased pain levels. Research shows there is a linear relationship between anxiety and pain. Insomnia is also a serious and distressing problem. Benzodiazepines are very useful in controlling anxiety associated with acute pain. The anxiolytic properties are similar and are a result of potentiation of neural inhibition mediated by γ-aminobutyric acid (GABA). Lorazepam at bedtime has a slow onset and prolonged action.

SIDE EFFECTS

- Weakness
- Headache
- Blurred vision
- Vertigo
- Nausea
- Vomiting
- Diarrhoea

Benzodiazepines may augment respiratory depression therefore one should be careful with morphine infusion or PCA.

REGIONAL ANALGESIA

Spinal anaesthesia and epidural analgesia are excellent ways of providing both analgesia for surgery and postoperative pain relief. About 92 per cent of hospitals are using epidural analgesia for postoperative patients. In some hospitals these patients are cared for on general wards, but in others all patients with epidurals are kept in a high-dependency setting.

There is no doubt that the best results from epidural analgesia are achieved in intensive care units, high-dependency units and recovery areas. However it is not possible in most British hospitals for all patients with epidurals to be nursed in these areas and postoperative management of the epidural falls to the acute pain service. This management must follow a strictly defined routine with clear guidelines on how to manage complications. It has been recommended that a minimum of 80 per cent of the ward nurses receive education in the management of epidurals and be assessed as competent.

Epidural analgesia with local anaesthetics, opioids, or α agonists alone, or in combination, can provide superior analgesia over conventional systemic routes (intravenous or oral) with minimal systemic side effects (nausea, sedation, constipation). Drugs administered epidurally are distributed by three main pathways:

- diffusion through the dura into the cerebrospinal fluid (CSF), then to the spinal cord or nerve roots
- vascular uptake by the vessels in the epidural space into systemic circulation
- uptake by the fat in the epidural space; creating a drug depot from which the drug can eventually enter the CSF or the systemic circulation.

EPIDURAL ANALGESIA

Aims

Epidural analgesia aims to block the sensory nerves to provide pain relief but allow the motor nerves to continue to function so the patient can move his or her limbs. The smaller the nerve the easier it is to block the function because the local anaesthetic does not have so far to travel. The autonomic nerves are the smallest and the motor nerves are the largest. Thus if sensory blockade is achieved it is inevitable that the autonomic nerves are blocked as well, but it is usually possible to maintain motor function.

The aim of a continuous infusion is to produce a band of analgesia around the area of the wound. The epidural tip should be as close to the nerve supply of that region as possible. For example, if the incision covers T4–T10 (upper abdominal surgery) the catheter should be inserted at T7–T8 and approximately 6 cm of catheter left in the space. For a low abdominal incision the catheter may be inserted at a lower thoracic level and lumbar for lower limb surgery.

Benefits and indications

DOES EPIDURAL ANALGESIA IMPROVE SURGICAL OUTCOME?

Some studies have shown improved outcome with the use of epidural anaesthesia and others have shown there is no difference between regional techniques and other methods of pain relief. The Veterans Affairs Hospital study in 2001 in 1021 high-risk patients showed the only significant difference was in patients undergoing aortic aneurysm repair where those with epidurals had a lower mortality, fewer myocardial infarctions and strokes and less respiratory failure. The Yeager study also showed that patients undergoing aortic aneurysm repair or lower extremity vascular surgery fared better with epidural analgesia. In the MASTER trial in Australia (2002) which looked at 915 high-risk patients the only significant difference was a lower rate of respiratory failure in the epidural group.

When epidurals are used for hip and knee surgery there is reduced blood loss, faster surgery, reduced morbidity and faster rehabilitation. Epidural opioids are associated with a lower incidence of atelectasis, and epidural local anaesthetic use leads to a higher PaO_2, fewer pulmonary infections and pulmonary complications compared with systemic opioids even though there is no difference in forced expiratory volume in one second (FEV_1), forced vital capacity (FVC) and peak expiratory flow rate (PEFR). Local anaesthetic and opioid in the epidural solution is better than epidural local anaesthetic and systemic opioid.

Previous meta-analyses showed reduced mortality up to 30 per cent but there may have been differences in patients and treatment in the groups; however, there have been recent changes in anaesthetic and surgical practices that have radically altered perioperative morbidity. The changes are regarding drugs, anti-embolism treatment, preoperative optimization, monitoring, etc. Moreover, since positive trials are published preferentially the overall outcome of meta-analyses is altered.

IF THERE ARE NO MAJOR BENEFITS ARE THERE ANY BENEFITS?

- The results of the PIRAT study show general anaesthesia with regional blockade significantly reduces the re-operation rates for graft occlusion in vascular surgery compared with general anaesthesia alone. It is recommended that an epidural is used for 48 hours.
- Allows more effective physiotherapy.
- Fewer cardiac ischaemic events.
- Improved cough.
- Reduced atelectasis and hypoxaemia possibly because of better analgesia.
- Earlier recovery of gut function in gastrointestinal surgery. It may be because a block from T5 to T12 antagonizes the sympathetically mediated peristaltic inhibition and preserves vagal and sacral parasympathetic outflow.
- Better analgesia.
- Reduced blood loss.
- Improved bowel motility.
- Improved activity levels.
- Improved quality of life.

All the above are important for patient satisfaction.

INDICATIONS

- Thoracic, abdominal, pelvic and lower limb surgery
- Pancreatitis
- Labour
- High risk patients, i.e. cardiovascular or respiratory disease
- Obese patients
- To improve lower limb perfusion and graft survival
- To improve gastrointestinal motility
- Deep vein thrombosis (DVT) prophylaxis
- To encourage earlier mobility
- To minimize side effects of drugs

CONTRAINDICATIONS

- Untrained nursing and medical staff
- The patient does not consent, or informed consent cannot be obtained
- Patient anticoagulated
- Infection near the site of injection
- Bacteraemia
- Bleeding disorders
- Low platelets
- Allergy to local anaesthetics
- Site of surgery – motor block may hinder mobilization, e.g. knee surgery
- Coexisting neurological disease

Epidurals are rarely essential!

Epidurals provide far superior analgesia to opioids given by the intramuscular or intravenous route when they work well. Unfortunately only about 35 per cent of epidural infusions work well throughout their use. Another 35 per cent will work after they have been modified in some way but 30 per cent do not provide especially good analgesia. An overall comparison of intramuscular analgesia, PCA and epidural found that PCA and epidural were significantly better than intramuscular analgesia but there was little difference between PCA and epidural within a group.

Epidural level and site of surgery

See Table 4.5.

Major complications

RESPIRATORY SYSTEM

Epidurals can produce respiratory depression in two ways: spread of diamorphine in the CSF and absorption into the blood stream. The opioid in the infusion has a direct effect on the respiratory and chemoreceptor centres in the brain. Predisposing factors are opioid naivety, co-administration of opioids by different routes, impaired respiratory function and immaturity (neonates and infants). If respiratory depression occurs for this reason, the epidural should be switched off and naloxone 4 μg/kg given intravenously.

Table 4.5 *Epidural level and site of surgery*

Surgery site	Dermatomes	Puncture level for epidural insertion
Neck	C2–C4	C6–C7
Shoulder	C4–T2	T1–T2
Arm	C5–T2	T1–T2
Cardiac surgery	T1–T8	T3–T4
Thorax	T2–T10	T6–T7
Abdomen above the umbilicus	T6–T10	T8–T9
Abdomen below the umbilicus	T9–L1	T11–T12
Hip/knee	L2–L5	L3–L4

If the epidural block is very extensive the bupivacaine may cause paralysis of the intercostal muscles and diaphragm. Respiratory depression from this cause requires the epidural to be switched off and the patient's breathing supported by intubation and ventilation. Increasing sedation is a warning sign. The risk is greater in the old and sick. **For this reason, patients receiving epidural opioids should not be given opioids by any other route except on the advice of an anaesthetist.**

CARDIOVASCULAR SYSTEM

Cardiovascular changes may occur depending on the level of the block. Extensive epidural blocks might result in a sympathetic blockade causing reduced peripheral resistance leading to hypotension. Intravenous fluids are given to counteract this. If hypotension does not respond to volume loading then ephedrine should be given intravenously.

Hypotension

Hypotension occurs in 14 per cent. Sympathetic blockade leads to peripheral vasodilation. Venous dilation reduces venous return and therefore cardiac output. Mean arterial pressure decreases in proportion to the decrease in cardiac output and, less importantly, due to the venous dilation. This produces hypotension.

In patients with ischaemic heart disease the systolic pressure and the heart rate should be kept within 20 per cent of the normal angina-free limits. There is increased risk of myocardial infarction if systolic blood pressure is >30 per cent less than normal for >10 minutes.

Management
- Raise legs (do not put head down).
- An infusion of 500–1000 mL saline or 500 mL Gelofusine® (succinylated gelatin) over 15 minutes is often sufficient to restore blood pressure.
- If hypotension is severe give ephedrine 3–6 mg/min until systolic blood pressure >90 mm Hg.

Factors increasing the risk of hypotension

Hypovolaemia increases the risk of hypotension. Adequate fluid replacement is important postoperatively because vasoconstriction is not possible to compensate for the inadequate circulating volume and so the patient is more susceptible to hypotension. Once the block is established the circulation should remain stable with good management, which includes adequate fluid replacement, but continued bleeding may lead to hypotension *without* a tachycardia. Hypotension may develop on the ward because of ongoing hypovolaemia with no compensatory mechanisms available (i.e. vasoconstriction).

Urine output should be maintained at a minimum of 0.5 mL/kg per hour but preferably at 1 mL/kg per hour. Also a block at T1–5 may block the cardio-accelerator fibres so the patient cannot respond to hypotension with a tachycardia.

Left ventricular failure

When the epidural wears off, vasoconstriction can occur. The capacity of the blood vessels will fall and fluid will be squeezed back into the tissues. In some vulnerable patients this may precipitate heart failure and a diuretic may be required.

Pulse

Tachycardia may indicate hypovolaemia or sepsis. Bradycardia may indicate very high epidural block (cardio-accelerator fibres to the heart blocked).

NEUROLOGICAL COMPLICATIONS

Depending on the drugs used and the concentrations given, each patient may experience some type of motor or sensory loss. Permanent neurological complications such as paraplegia and arachnoiditis are very rare and are caused mainly by damage to the spinal cord or spinal nerve roots.

Peripheral nerve damage

The nerves can be traumatized directly by the needle. They may be damaged by preservative-containing local anaesthetic solution. Often damage pre-exists (usually an underlying polyneuropathy) and is simply uncovered by the epidural infusion. One in 500 patients with nerve damage may have prolonged numbness with ultimate recovery. One in 5–10 000 patients have a permanent deficit of some kind. Surgery and positioning can also be the cause of neural damage.

The problem may be limited by performing the epidural with the patient awake. If a nerve root is touched the patient will experience pain and the needle can be re-sited.

Epidural haematoma

Epidural haematomas occur rarely. Coagulopathy is the most significant risk factor but the incidence is increased by the use of low-molecular weight heparin therapy, concomitant anticoagulant and antiplatelet drug use or clotting abnormalities. The incidence is greater using the epidural approach and with the insertion of a catheter. Haematomas can present up to a week after removal of the catheter. Up to 60 per cent of clinically important spinal haematomas occur after the removal of the catheter.

Diagnosis

- Back pain possibly localized to the side of the haematoma.
- Motor and sensory deficits. Weakness from the epidural alone is unlikely so onset of pain and or loss of function and sensation, particularly in the perineal area, should always be regarded with suspicion.
- Bladder dysfunction.

The diagnosis can be difficult and the patient should have an urgent magnetic resonance imaging (MRI) scan if there is any suspicion of a haematoma.

Outcome

It is important that patients are monitored for signs of neurological dysfunction for a minimum of 48 hours after removal of the catheter. If the diagnosis is made promptly then outcome is usually good. Sixty per cent of patients operated on within eight hours of diagnosis of epidural haematoma will make a complete recovery. Unfortunately the chance of a full recovery after this time is small.

INFECTION

Meningitis

Meningitis following an epidural is very rare. Epidurals should never be used in patients with septicaemia or bacteraemia where infection is blood borne. Local sepsis is also a contraindication where the catheter and needle would be inserted through infected tissue.

Epidural abscess

This is rare but may be devastating. The infection occurs:

- during insertion of needle
- along the catheter
- endogenous source – bacteraemia
- haematoma with secondary infection
- multiple attempts.

Diagnosis

- Pyrexia, raised white cell count, always raised C-reactive protein.
- The onset of symptoms is often three to four days after the block is established but it can be anywhere from one to 60 days.
- There is nearly always localized spinal or paraspinal tenderness and back pain.
- The presence of both erythema and local discharge is a good indicator of infection. There is rarely a positive culture in patients with erythema alone or when there are no local signs.

The risk of abscess formation is increased in:

- diabetes
- intravenous drug abuse
- alcohol abuse
- coexistent infection.

Abscess formation generally occurs secondary to a respiratory or urinary tract infection.

Treatment

Staphylococcus aureus is the commonest bacterium found in epidural abscess formation (73 per cent). Treatment should be with antibiotics and drainage of the abscess. The symptoms of haematoma and abscess are similar in that they both can present with the sudden onset of any abnormal neurological signs although infection is often a later event.

Minor complications

Epidural air – although rare, injection of air into the epidural space during the insertion of an epidural catheter can cause a variety of problems.

- Pneumoencephalos
- Venous embolism
- Unblocked segments and incomplete analgesia
- Subcutaneous emphysema
- Venous embolism
- Multiradicular syndrome
- Lumbar root compression
- Paraplegia

MOTOR NERVE BLOCK

Motor block is common in the first few postoperative hours because the patient will often have been given 0.5 per cent bupivacaine. The block usually wears off as the weaker local anaesthetic solution is used. Motor nerve block is more likely with a lumbar epidural because it will block the nerves to the legs. Patients do not like the sensation of numbness and it may distress them more than the pain itself.

UNILATERAL BLOCK

The epidural space may contain fibrous strands that prevent local anaesthetic spreading to both sides of the space. The catheter may also lie more to one side than another or pass out of a foramen. Loss of sensation or unilateral motor block may develop. This is just as bad as no block at all because unrelieved pain is still present on the other side. Sometimes withdrawing the catheter and giving a bolus dose may overcome this but the epidural may need to be re-sited or discontinued.

NAUSEA AND VOMITING

Nausea and vomiting is worse with morphine than fentanyl. Nausea and vomiting is due to opioid action on the chemoreceptor trigger zone of the brain and is common in surgery involving the viscera. Hypovolaemia and pain can also produce nausea and vomiting. Any opioid absorbed into the CSF can travel upwards to the brain. Ambulant patients can have more problems as vestibular stimulation enhances the emetic effect. It is worse when opioids are used but it is less common than with intravenous opioids. The administration of oxygen by facemask may reduce nausea and vomiting. Patients having epidural analgesia should be prescribed antiemetics – conventional antiemetics or 0.04 mg naloxone. It may be necessary to use plain bupivacaine.

PRURITUS

There is a higher incidence of itching when opioids are given by the epidural route as opposed to the intravenous route, especially in the facial area. It is commoner with diamorphine and morphine than with fentanyl. Histamine release is thought to play a role in the production of spinal-induced pruritus. Antihistamines are not always effective for treating this and naloxone given intravenously by infusion can be more effective. Patients on epidurals are prescribed chlorphenamine to relieve itching. If not effective a small dose of naloxone can be given (0.04 mg naloxone subcutaneously) or infuse continuously in the intravenous fluids. The opioid dose may need to be reduced or omitted, but the bupivacaine concentration will often need to be increased to 0.25 per cent to produce adequate analgesia.

URINARY RETENTION

Opioids given by any route can cause urinary retention. If a patient with an epidural has not passed urine for over 15 hours postoperatively they should be catheterized. Retention may respond to naloxone. Most patients have a urinary catheter sited during surgery. This also allows measurement of urine output to ensure adequate fluid replacement. Urine output should be greater than 0.5 mL/kg per hour. Sufficient fluids should be given to maintain urine output. Patients sometimes require large volumes. If the urine output tails off 500 mL of Gelofusine STAT should be given. The patient should be re-examined in one hour. If there is no response a senior member of the medical team should be alerted.

CONSTIPATION

Opioids may also cause constipation. Morphine may reduce gut motility postoperatively and prolong paralytic ileus following abdominal surgery.

CATHETER FALLEN OUT

It is difficult to stop this problem, but tunnelling the catheter a few centimetres is probably the best way of ensuring that it stays in place. Many devices are available to anchor the catheter but none are without problems.

PAIN DESPITE INFUSION

Supplementary medication may be required to treat symptoms beyond the scope of the epidural block, e.g. generalized discomfort, shoulder tip pain, etc. Often this can be managed with an NSAID or a small dose of opioid (ask the acute pain team).

MACHINE NOT WORKING

Sometimes after changing the syringe some air gets trapped in the filter and the pump does not work properly. The syringe needs to be removed from the pump and a small bolus given (2 mL).

SEDATION

Sedation may be respiratory depression from opioids and the score should be recorded as for PCA/intravenous infusion. Sedation may develop over a number of hours.

See Table 4.6 for a summary of management of complications.

Incidence of complications of epidural analgesia

The occurrence of neurological complications (Table 4.7) and the development of haematomas has led many to discuss the way in which epidurals are given. Severe neurological injury is one of the greatest tragedies for the patient. Following two instances of neurological complications in Germany, the following guidelines were produced:

- No epidural should be inserted above L1–2 in anaesthetized patients.
- There should be careful consideration of the risk:benefit ratio.
- Lumbar epidurals or spinals should only be inserted in anaesthetized patients in exceptional circumstances.
- Difficulty in catheter insertion or needle placement should be considered a warning for possible adverse outcome.

The risk can be reduced by:

- Any complaint of lancinating pain during insertion of the needle is taken as a sign of root or cord trauma and the procedure is abandoned.
- The needle is inserted below the termination of the spinal cord wherever practical and medically appropriate.
- The patient should be awake in all but rare circumstances.

Table 4.6 *Epidural analgesia: management of complications*

Nausea and vomiting	Prochlorperazine 12.5 mg/cyclizine 50 mg
	Ondansetron 4 mg
Itching	Chlorphenamine 4 mg or naloxone 0.1 mg subcutaneously up to four doses
Urinary retention	0.1 mg naloxone subcutaneously. If fails catheterize
Respiratory depression	<8 breaths per minute – stop PCA/epidural
	Give O_2
	Call physician
	Draw up 0.4 mg (1 mL) naloxone and mix with 3 mL saline (total 4 mL)
	Give 1 mL every 30 s to one minute until respiratory rate >10/min
	Respiratory depression may reoccur after 20 minutes
	It may be necessary to give further doses of naloxone or to set up an infusion
Oversedation	Sedation score >2 call physician
	Patient will require intravenous naloxone
	Stop infusion
	Draw up 0.4 mg (1 mL) naloxone and mix with 3 mL saline
Hypotension	Systolic BP <90 mmHg
	Stop infusion
	Lie flat
	Give 500 mL Gelofusine STAT. Consider other causes of hypotension
	Call physician
Urine output	This should be at least 0.5 mL/kg per hour. If the volume falls below this give 500 mL Gelofusine and increase rate of fluid administration
	If urine output falls below this for >2 hours consecutively contact either pain service or senior member of firm

PCA, patient controlled analgesia.

Table 4.7 *Epidural analgesia: risk of complications*

Complication	Risk
The overall incidence of severe complications	0.01–0.001%
Minor and reversible lesions	0.01%
Puncture of epidural vessels	3–12%
Dural puncture	0.16–1.3%
Headache from dural puncture	16–86%
Pruritus	29–44% especially on the face
Urinary retention	11%
Nausea and vomiting	54–78% (severe in 12.5–47%)
Intrathecal migration	0.15–0.18%
Intravascular migration	0.18%
Epidural haematoma	Possible 1:200 000
Epidural abscess	1:7000–1:500 000

Dermatomal level of block

Even if not charted, nurses caring for patients with an epidural infusion should be aware of the expected level of block. Ideally the block should extend from just below the wound to just above it. The level can be tested using a pin or a cold spray.

Management of the failed epidural

The epidural catheter should be left in place as it may be possible to alter the catheter position and get the epidural working. Either intramuscular morphine can be used or PCA started but remember the patient will require a bolus of intravenous morphine first to re-establish good pain control.

Drugs used for epidural infusion

LOCAL ANAESTHETICS

Bupivacaine/ropivacaine

Local anaesthetics block transmission of messages along the nerves. The ability of local anaesthetic to penetrate the myelin sheath of the nerve fibres depends on the concentration used. A low concentration will block the small C and Aδ fibres, but a higher concentration will block the larger motor fibres. The longer the infusion is continued, the more likely there will be a block of the motor nerves, regardless of the concentration of the local anaesthetic. It is important to use the most dilute local anaesthetic agent possible while still providing analgesia.

OPIOIDS

Opioid drugs alone in the epidural space will provide analgesia but the doses required would result in significant side effects. The opioid is therefore usually given mixed with a local anaesthetic. Using a combination of local anaesthetic and opioid, both in minimal doses, allows good analgesia while minimizing the risks associated with larger doses of either of the other drugs.

Any drug injected into the epidural space can spread up to the brain and cause unwanted effects such as respiratory depression so the infusion rate should also remain at a reasonable level. Opioids are lipophilic so they are rapidly absorbed into the tissues.

Diamorphine

Diamorphine is more lipophilic than morphine and is less likely to spread through the CSF to the brain. It is more rapidly absorbed and therefore safer. The dose ranges from $50\,\mu g/mL$ to $200\,\mu g/mL$. It may be excluded if the patient is elderly or there are pre-existing respiratory difficulties. The strength of the bupivacaine may then need to be increased, e.g. to 0.25 per cent.

Fentanyl

Fentanyl is commonly added to a local anaesthetic epidural infusion. The concentration of the infusion is usually $2\,\mu g/mL$ for adults. It is thought that the main mechanism of action is via absorption into the bloodstream rather than a direct epidural effect. Using a combination of local anaesthetic and opioid, both in minimal doses, allows good analgesia while minimizing the risks associated with larger doses of either drug.

Rate of epidural infusion

The rate of infusion is usually between 5 mL/h and 10 mL/hr. Once adequate analgesia has been established at a particular infusion rate, there is no need to alter this rate. There is a tendency for the rate to be progressively reduced to a minimal level. This results in the level of the block falling and analgesia then becomes inadequate. If the patient is sleepy it is better to reduce the amount of opioid present rather than to reduce the rate of infusion.

Changing the infusion

Syringes must be changed immediately when they run out because the block will regress. It takes too long for the infusion to reach the required level once that level has fallen. For the same reason it should not be discontinued when the patient goes to X-ray! The block will subside to nothing over about two hours.

Duration

The acute pain of thoracic or upper abdominal surgery lasts for three to five days. The infusion is therefore usually continued for up to six days. The patient can be mobilized at the same time. Prolonging the infusion longer than this is usually unnecessary and increases the risk of infection. Some examples are:

- Vascular patients, e.g. femoropopliteal bypass – usually two days. Used for the beneficial effects of vasodilatation on the blood flow through the graft.
- Scoliosis – three days.
- Abdominal/pelvic surgery – three to five days.
- Amputation – variable. Five days or more postoperatively may reduce the incidence of phantom limb pain.

Checking the epidural site

The site should be checked regularly for signs of leakage, redness and infection. If the catheter comes apart at any site it can be reassembled after wiping with an alcohol wipe. Bupivacaine is bacteriostatic and the catheter so long that infection is unlikely to enter via this route. Most infections arise from contamination around the entrance site.

Figure 4.2 gives an algorithm for the use of epidural infusion.

Anti-coagulation and epidural infusions

Guidelines for epidurals with anticoagulation include:

- Aspirin/NSAID – no contraindication.
- Clopidogrel – stop seven days preoperatively.
- Subcutaneous unfractionated heparin – give four hours before or one hour after epidural/spinal block.
- Intravenous unfractionated heparin – stop two to four hours before the block and restart not less than one hour after the block.
- Low molecular weight heparin (LMWH) – ideally an epidural catheter should not be inserted for a minimum 12 hours following a dose of LMWH and 12 hours should

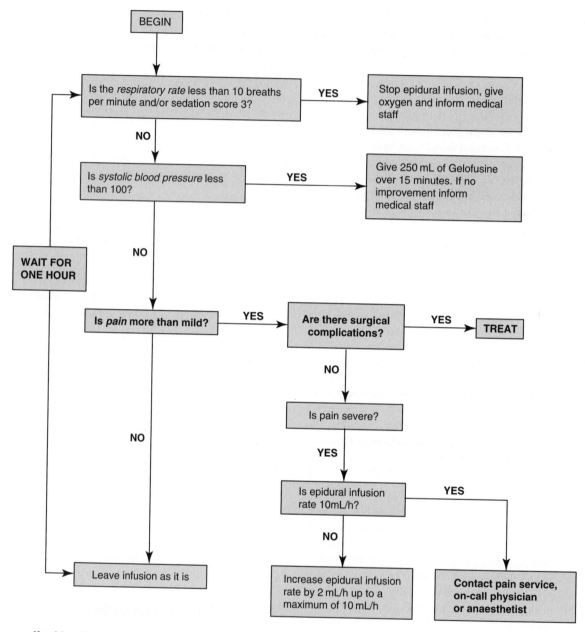

If epidural is not providing analgesia and an anaesthetist is not available – STOP (DO NOT REMOVE CATHETER) EPIDURAL and consider patient controlled or intramuscular analgesia as algorithm (Fig. 4.3). Contact the pain service as soon as possible

Figure 4.2 *Algorithm for use of epidural infusion*

elapse prior to removal of the catheter. Low molecular weight heparin can be given two hours after the block. The addition of antiplatelet drugs to LMWH should be avoided. Providing there are no contraindications, aspirin should be stopped one week before surgery.

PERIOPERATIVE INTRAVENOUS HEPARIN

If a bloody tap occurs during catheter insertion prior to surgery there is no need to delay surgery if the intravenous dose of heparin will be 3000–5000 IU as in vascular surgery. However, if the epidural is inserted for cardiac surgery when doses of 300 IU/kg are used, it is sensible to delay surgery as the risk of epidural haematoma is very high.

The catheter should not be removed if there are any concerns about the clotting status of the patient. The international normalized ratio (INR) or activated partial thromboplastin time (APTT) should be measured in any patient where there may be a risk of bleeding. The APTT should be normal and the INR should be below 1.5. Monitor daily for the symptoms listed below and for 24 hours after removal of the epidural catheter. Contact the pain service urgently if any of these symptoms are discovered:

- tenderness or redness of the epidural site
- backache – this may be the only symptom
- leg weakness. Lower limb weakness is probably the most important sign
- loss of leg/perineal sensation
- loss of bladder control
- leaking catheter
- blood under dressing/in catheter.

The patient MUST have a patent intravenous cannula at all times until the epidural catheter is removed. The epidural should run at a rate within the prescribed range to keep the patient comfortable. Other forms of analgesia, e.g. NSAIDs may be administered concurrently. There is no benefit in trying to reduce the rate of the infusion if the patient is stable and comfortable.

Monitoring

It is recommended that a minimum of 80 per cent of the nurses on the ward are trained in managing epidurals. All staff involved with managing epidurals should:

- be familiar with the operation of the pump
- check regularly according to hospital guidelines that the pump is delivering the correct volume
- check blood pressure, pulse, respiratory rate, urine output regularly as per guidelines
- check the catheter
- check for leaks
- check the insertion site
- know what side effects may occur and how to manage them
- be aware of the guidelines for removal of the catheter
- know when to call for help.

Heart rate, blood pressure, respiratory rate, pain, sedation, nausea/vomiting score and the volume of the infusion that has been given should be recorded:

- quarter-hourly for 2 hours then half-hourly for 2 hours
- hourly on return to the ward for ... hours

The frequency of heart rate and blood pressure observations may be reduced to four hourly after 12 hours if the patient remains haemodynamically stable. If a bolus of any drug is given into the epidural, blood pressure should be recorded at 5-minute intervals for 30 minutes. If the rate of infusion is increased all observations must be recorded half-hourly for two hours.

PATIENT CONTROLLED EPIDURAL ANALGESIA

Patient controlled epidural analgesia (PCEA) is another new progressive, patient-centred approach. The basic idea is simple and analogous to intravenous patient-controlled postoperative analgesia: if we let the patient decide how much they need, they will usually use less medication and will feel more in control. Some controversy exists about whether to provide a basal infusion to which the patient adds their own doses, or to allow the patient to control all doses.

Advantages

- Increased efficiency
- Higher patient satisfaction
- Decreased opioid use
- Reduced risk of sedation
- Reduced sedation
- Reduced anxiety
- Adjustment of medication by patient
- Anticipatory dosing

Patient controlled epidural analgesia is often used to supplement a basal rate to allow a patient to manage breakthrough pain in order to meet their individual analgesic requirements. Like intravenous PCA, PCEA can provide more timely pain relief, more control for the patient, and convenience for both the patient and nurse to reduce the time required to obtain and administer required supplemental boluses. Unlike intravenous PCA, the lockout interval of PCEA varies widely based on the lipid solubility of the opioid administered – from 10 minutes with fentanyl to 60–90 minutes when morphine is used. If local anaesthetic is used, the lockout interval should be at least 15 minutes to allow for peak effect of the supplemental local anaesthetic dose.

Pain is the most common cause of night-time sleep disturbance and the use of analgesics is the effective method of restoring sleep in most patients. Analgesics are given most often during two time intervals: between 08:00 and 12:00, and between 20:00 and 00:00. When PCEA alone is compared with an infusion plus PCEA, the number of requests for supplemental analgesia is lower for PCEA plus night-time infusion than for PCEA alone. The infusion decreases the incidence of postoperative pain, provides a better sleep pattern, and reduces the degree of the pain associated with coughing during the night.

Set-up

The PCEA pump contains an opioid and local anaesthetic of choice. The infusion rate is 2–4 mL/h with 4–5 mL bolus on demand and a lockout interval of 15–20 minutes. The incidence of side effects does not differ from other epidural analgesia techniques and it does not appear to reduce the incidence of itching.

PCEA in thoracic surgery

Epidural local anaesthetics improve the postoperative diaphragmatic function and chest wall compliance and reduce postoperative pulmonary morbidity by improving analgesia. There is a significant decrease, both in the incidence of atelectasis in association with epidural opioid therapy, and in the incidence of pulmonary infections and pulmonary complications overall in association with epidural local anaesthetics. It has been suggested that PCEA potentially reduces postoperative pulmonary morbidity and minimizes drugs given. In view of the quality of analgesia reached, the absence of unwanted effects and the overall degree of patient satisfaction, PCEA is the technique of choice to provide adequate pain treatment following thoracic surgery.

SPINAL AND COMBINED SPINAL/EPIDURAL TECHNIQUES

Advantages

- Rapid onset
- Reliable procedure – more objective endpoint (CSF) than traditional epidural
- Ambulation easily and reliably achieved
- Simple modification of existing technique
- Lower total local anaesthetic doses
- Decreased inadvertent dural puncture rate
- Improved patient satisfaction
- Improved subsequent epidural analgesia

Disadvantages

- More complex procedure
- Dural puncture
- Increased risk of unintended dural puncture, with epidural needle during manipulation
- Catheter placement not really 'tested' until later use
- Increased risk of infection/meningitis (*very* small risk, if any)

Start the epidural infusion immediately (within 5 minutes) after the spinal dose is given to avoid the loss of analgesia at the end of the spinal effect (one to two hours). By the time the spinal is wearing off, sufficient epidural medication has been administered so that there is usually a smooth transition between the two modes of drug delivery without the need for a rescue dose.

Regional blocks

GENERAL POINTS

Whenever a surgical procedure is planned it is worth considering whether there are any nerve blocks that can help reduce postoperative pain. This is particularly the case for day-case patients but anything that can reduce the need for postoperative pain relief should be used in all patients. Many local blocks can be performed quickly before or after induction of analgesia and wherever possible can be continued into the postoperative period.

INFILTRATION

The use of local anaesthetic agents can reduce the requirement for postoperative analgesia. Infiltration of the surgical area prior to incision has been shown to reduce the amount of morphine required postoperatively. Infiltration after surgery does not have a similar effect.

PREPARATION OF PATIENT – PREOPERATIVE CONSIDERATIONS

- Visit the patient.
- Take a full history and examine the patient as necessary.
- Check for any problems that prevent local anaesthesia – infection, clotting problems, drugs, allergy to local anaesthesia, refusal by patient, neurological condition, obesity.
- Explain the procedure to the patient.
- Prescribe premedication where necessary.

PROCEDURE

- Insert an intravenous cannula.
- Position the patient correctly for the procedure.

- Check the drugs and equipment required for procedure, including needles, catheters, syringes and nerve stimulators.
- Check other equipment required such as the resuscitation facilities.
- It is important the procedure is carried out under aseptic conditions.

Specific nerve blocks

Detailed descriptions of how to perform specific nerve blocks can be found in several textbooks on regional analgesia and will not be described here. These blocks should be considered for all patients undergoing surgery to reduce postoperative pain. Many of the blocks can be continued into the postoperative period by using an infusion of local anaesthetic. See Table 4.8 for a summary of specific nerve blocks.

PATIENT CONTROLLED ANALGESIA

Patient controlled analgesia simply means allowing the patient to administer their own analgesia whether it is oral, intramuscular or intravenous. The term, however, has become synonymous with the pump that allows a patient to self-administer intravenous opioids. The term should not be specific to the machine but to the patient. It usually represents intravenous opioid but it could be oral, subcutaneous, nasal, etc. All analgesia should be patient controlled. In the UK, 99 per cent of hospitals are now using PCA.

Sechzer first described the PCA machine in 1968. The first commercially pumps were available in 1970 but they were expensive compared with intramuscular injections. The use of PCAs became commoner after the report of the Joint Colleges of Surgery and Anaesthesia, which showed that pain management in all hospitals was generally very poor. It was seen as a way of improving pain control, by giving control to the patient and not relying on nursing staff to administer the drugs.

Patient controlled analgesia – management protocol

When the PCA is to be used for postoperative pain management the anaesthetist should assess the suitability of the patient for a PCA preoperatively. The doctor must ensure the patient understands the use of the PCA and is able to manage to activate the machine, using either the handset or an appropriate adaptation. Ideally the handset should be shown to the patient before surgery if possible.

Table 4.8 *Summary of specific nerve blocks*

Region	Block	Indication
Head	Scalp block	Craniotomy
		Bat ears
Thorax	Intercostal nerve block	Fractured ribs
	Interpleural nerve block	Thoracotomy
	Paravertebral nerve block	Scoliosis
	Epidural	
Abdomen	Intercostal nerve block	Cholecystectomy
	Inguinal nerve block	Inguinal hernia repair
	Penile block	Circumcision
	Epidural	Circumcision, hernia
	Spinal	Haemorrhoids
Upper limb	Brachial plexus:	
	interscalene	Shoulder
	subclavian	Upper arm
	axillary	Arm/hand
	Peripheral:	
	Intercostobrachial	
	Lateral cutaneous nerve of	
	forearm	Hand and fingers
	Ulnar nerve	
	Median nerve	
	Radial nerve	
	Digital nerves	Fingers
	Intravenous regional analgesia	
Lower limb	Lumbosacral plexus:	Fractured neck of femur
	Femoral nerve (L2–4)	
	Lateral cutaneous nerve	Arthroscopy, fractured
	of thigh (L2–3)	neck and shaft of
	Obturator (L2–4)	femur
	Three in one block (femoral,	Leg
	lateral cutaneous nerve,	
	obturator)	
	Sciatic nerve block	Foot
	Blocks at knee:	
	Sciatic nerve block	
	(popliteal fossa)	Foot, toes
	Saphenous nerve block	
	Blocks at ankle:	
	Ankle block	
	Digital nerve block	
	Intravenous regional analgesia	
	For arthroscopy:	
	Spinal	
	Epidural	
	Three in one block + sciatic	
	(but get tourniquet pain)	
	Infiltration	

A loading dose of a long-acting opioid should be administered if the patient is in pain, and the patient should be comfortable before starting the PCA. Intravenous PCA usually consists of 50 mL syringe connected either via tubing directly to an indwelling cannula or to the long end of a Y-connector. If an intravenous infusion is used it should be connected to the one-way valve on the Y-connector to prevent any of the opioid drug entering the intravenous infusion line and the patient inadvertently receiving an extra bolus dose of the opioid. The PCA can be connected to a central line. The intravenous infusion can be:

- normal saline
- Hartmann's solution
- dextrose saline
- 5 per cent dextrose
- Gelofusine
- any pre-prepared bags, e.g. normal saline +20 mmoL potassium chloride.

Blood should not be given through the same line as the PCA as it is not known if the opioid drug remains stable in blood.

'Locus of control'

Effectiveness of self-administered analgesia depends on the patient's appropriate response to the pain perceived. For the majority of patients, having control over their pain confers positive effects both for analgesia and recovery. The potential for control to confer positive benefits is closely linked with provision of information. The provision of information, instruction and continuing supervision represents a major contributing factor to improved analgesia – probably of more importance than the analgesic method *per se*.

The efficacy of an analgesic technique lies not intrinsically in that technique but in the quality of its implementation. The proper use of PCA often decreases morphine requirement because a sense of control over the pain decreases the need for analgesia. It has also recently been shown that patients mainly like PCAs because they do not have to disturb the nursing staff to ask for analgesia.

The advantages of PCA can be negated by failure to address deficiencies in knowledge and pain management by both ward staff and patients. The limitations of currently available analgesics with inadequate education of ward nurses and medical staff regarding acute pain may be the main factors contributing to inappropriate use of and consequent suboptimal efficacy of PCA rather than the technique itself.

Age and patient controlled analgesia

Younger patients (<60 years) use significantly more morphine in PCAs.

Advantages of patient controlled analgesia

- Postoperatively, patients are often cold and perfusion to the buttock or thigh may be poor. A drug given intramuscularly may not be absorbed and stays in the tissue. The patient is still in pain so more morphine is given. Gradually the patient warms up and the morphine is absorbed all at once leading to an overdose. Patient controlled analgesia allows patients better control of their analgesia and is safer than intramuscular injection.
- The dose of morphine is varies among patients and in the same patient at different times. Patient controlled analgesia allows a variable dose to be given for each individual.
- The intensity of acute pain is rarely constant and with the PCA the amount of opioid delivered can be titrated according to increases and decreases in pain stimulus.
- Patients often do not request analgesia until pain is severe and then they must wait until the drug is delivered. The small and frequent intravenous doses of opioid given when required by PCA are more likely to maintain a reasonably constant blood concentration of the drug, improve pain control and lower drug consumption.
- Side effects do occur with opioids but PCA allows the patient to titrate the amount of opioid delivered against both pain and side effects.
- Patients are more comfortable when using PCA and patient satisfaction is better than with intramuscular injection.
- Intramuscular injections may lead to nerve damage and this risk is removed when using PCA.
- The incidence of chest infection is lower than with intramuscular opioid.
- Patients mobilize and eat sooner with PCA than with intramuscular opioid and they have a shorter stay in hospital.

Safety features of the patient controlled analgesia machine

Standardized concentrations of opioid are used. There are guidelines for use of PCA which include regular monitoring of the patient by the nursing staff. The machine is tamperproof because a key is required to open the pump. The patient is also monitored by the acute pain team, which has also been associated with improved safety. Preoperative instruction to the patient should include discussion of the use of the technique with the patient, parents and nursing staff. Every nurse must understand the technique. Children over the age of six years should be able to understand:

- the technique
- the rationale for PCA
- the use of the machine
- an explanation of the safety features
- an explanation of the monitoring, e.g. pain scores and sedation scores
- the likely duration of pain therapy.

Problems with patient controlled analgesia

MEDICATION RELATED

About 22 per cent of patients fear addiction and 30 per cent of patients fear overdose. This may prevent them from using the PCA machine as well as they should and improved explanation should help to overcome this problem.

EQUIPMENT RELATED

These include equipment malfunction, operator error, incorrect programming, cracked syringes and defective one-way valves.

PATIENT RELATED

Persisting pain:

- Is the patient activating the machine?
- Is the patient receiving the drug?
- Are the settings correct?
- Check the history – attempts versus successes
- Is the patient anxious?
- Opioid naive – increase bolus
- Opioid tolerance – start infusion

Some pumps default to the previous setting when they are turned off and then on again. If the pump has previously been set up for a different drug dose, e.g. pethidine, an overdose of morphine may be given by mistake. To improve safety, the pump should default to zero and would therefore require reprogramming every time. Some of the newer pumps do this but every machine should be checked prior to use.

RESPIRATORY DEPRESSION

- Incidence
  - PCA: 0.1–0.8 per cent
  - intramuscular: 0.2–0.9 per cent
  - Infusion: 1.7 per cent
  - Infusion +PCA: 1.1–3.9 per cent

Acute pain stimulates respiration and antagonizes the effects of opioids. Systemically administered opioids reduce the respiratory rate and the tidal volume.

The most serious complication is respiratory depression. The incidence is between 0.07 and 1.2 per cent. This includes a respiratory rate <10, $PaCO_2 >7\,kPa$ and $SpO_2 <90$ per cent for >1 minute. Opioids alter respiratory regulation by decreasing the slope of the carbon dioxide response curve and shifting it to the right. This may precede respiratory depression. The risk is higher in those aged >65 years, smokers, those with an American Society of Anethesiologists score (ASA) $\geqslant 3$ and preoperative $PaO_2 <10\,kPa$.

Monitoring the respiratory rate alone is inadequate – a falling respiratory rate is a late and unreliable indicator of respiratory depression. The sedation score is a much more reliable means of detection. The use of multiple modalities further improves detection rate. Respiratory depression can occur, but it is commoner in the first 48 hours. Tolerance to the respiratory effects develops very quickly. Provided the patient is monitored according to hospital guidelines, respiratory depression should be detected and treated early.

The causes of respiratory depression include:

- wrong dose put in machine
- patient especially sensitive to opioids
- someone else presses trigger
- mechanical fault.

Respiratory depression is increased by:

- infusion
- bolus $>1\,mg$
- respiratory disease
- hypovolaemia
- proxy control
- concomitant sedatives/opioids
- operator error
- equipment failure
- wrong drug
- wrong programming
- obesity and Pickwickian syndrome – no background, lower bolus. There is a 10-fold difference in opioid requirement among obese patients using a PCA
- spina bifida.

Management: if respiratory rate <10 or sedation $= 2$, stop pump, give oxygen and contact the physician. Draw up 0.4 mg naloxone (1 mL) in a 10 mL syringe and add 9 mL saline $= 40\,\mu g/mL$. Give 1 mL every two minutes.

SEDATION

Sedation is the **best** clinical indicator of early respiratory depression.

- Sedation is due to a mixture of the opioid and increase PCO_2.
- Sedation score should be <2.
- All opioids in equianalgesic doses cause the same degree of respiratory depression.
- If the dose of opioid is titrated to the need the risk is small.

Confusion

- PCA – 2.3 per cent
- intramuscular – 18 per cent
- therapeutic doses of opioids are not usually the cause
- more likely to be:
  - hypoxia
  - sleep deprivation
  - drugs
  - sepsis
  - unusual environment.

NAUSEA, VOMITING AND PCA

- Nausea – 28.8 per cent
- Vomiting – 15 per cent

Despite the common clinical opinion that PCA should be renamed 'patient controlled nausea', there is little evidence in support of the notion that postoperative nausea and vomiting are exacerbated by the method. It is often more a complication of the surgery than of the opioid, e.g. gynaecology and breast surgery.

Patients with more extensive surgery often use PCA and are therefore more likely to have nausea and vomiting also. The PCA is frequently discontinued because of this. If nausea and vomiting is not related to the opioid dose it cannot be opioid dependent. Reduction in opioid usage using NSAIDs does not reduce incidence of nausea and vomiting neither does a reduction of opioid dose on second day. It seems therefore that the nausea and vomiting is not related to the dose of opioid received. The problem is sometimes solved by changing the opioid or giving a regular antiemetic.

Postoperative nausea and vomiting adversely affect the analgesic perception and it stops the patient using the PCA leading to an increase in pain. Occasionally if the patient is very nauseated within a short space of time after receiving a bolus of opioid, increasing the dose delivery time may reduce the nausea and vomiting. The opioid can be delivered over two to three minutes. Nausea and vomiting are more common in:

- women
- age ≤65 years

- PCA > epidural
- gynaecological procedures.

Antiemetics in PCA

Adding antiemetics to the syringe may be beneficial for the first 24 hours but because the side effects increase with time and dose, the risk of sedation and dystonic reactions also increase after this time. Regular antiemetic doses are probably at least as good.

The cost effectiveness of treating everyone with antiemetics must be considered as most patients only have one episode, and only a few have prolonged problems.

ITCHING

- 7.3 per cent
- Due to morphine
- Treatment:
  - chlorphenamine 4 mg oral/intramuscular or 0.1 mg naloxone subcutaneously.

URINARY RETENTION

- Can be caused either by pain or by morphine.
- Treat with 0.1 mg naloxone subcutaneously or catheterize.

CONSTIPATION

See Table 4.9.

HYPOTENSION

- Usually only occurs with opioids if there is hypovolaemia.
- Give 500 mL Gelofusine.

Patient controlled analgesia machine

CONCENTRATION

Morphine 50 mg in 50 mL, 60 mg in 60 mL or 100 mg in 50 mL saline are standard mixtures. The initial bolus is 1 mg but this can be altered depending on the analgesic response.

THE SYRINGE AND GIVING SET

A disposable PCA or 50/60 mL syringe is most commonly used. The PCA giving set has a syringe connected to thin tubing, and an intravenous infusion connected to a Y end. This contains a Cardiff antireflux valve, which prevents the drug in the syringe travelling back up the intravenous infusion giving set instead of into the patient.

Table 4.9 *Management of constipation*

Drug	Dose*	Action
Lactulose	20–60 mL PO twice to four times daily	A semisynthetic disaccharide that is not absorbed from the digestive tract It produces osmotic diarrhoea of low faecal pH
Senna Movicol	Two tablets at night, twice or thrice daily Two to three sachets per day in divided doses dissolved in 125 mL water. Start with one sachet per day in elderly people	Osmotic laxative containing macrogol '3350' (polyethylene glycol '3350') 13.125 g, sodium bicarbonate 178.5 mg, sodium chloride 350.7 mg, potassium chloride 46.6 mg Osmotic laxatives work by retaining fluid in the bowel by osmosis
Bisacodyl suppositories (Dulcolax two tablets) Milk of magnesia Phosphate enema	One to two If no bowel movement in 24 hours repeat 15–30 mL with mineral oil twice daily 1 PR	

* It normally takes two to three days before any treatment will have any effect. Laxatives should always be prescribed if opioids are being used.

LOADING DOSE

This setting on the PCA is not used routinely especially on the wards. A bolus dose of the opioid to be used should be given intravenously prior to starting the PCA to achieve blood levels that produce analgesia either in theatre or recovery.

BOLUS DOSE

Microprocessor-driven syringe pumps deliver a preset bolus of a drug when the patient presses a demand button connected to the pump. Access to the pump is only possible using a key and infused over several seconds. Morphine 0.5 mg is not enough, 2 mg increases respiratory depression. The pump is usually set at 1 mg STAT. Fentanyl = 40 μg over 10 minutes.

If the patient has had sufficient analgesia they will be sedated and therefore unlikely to press the demand button. It is important nurses and relatives (particularly parents) do not press the button (except in exceptional circumstances).

DOSE DURATION

If a subcutaneous dose is used, rapid delivery may cause stinging. The main advantage in giving the bolus dose more slowly intravenously is if the patient experiences nausea with a rapid infusion. Slower delivery of the opioid may prevent the nausea and vomiting associated with pressing the button of the PCA.

BACKGROUND INFUSION

A background infusion increases the risk of overdose of opioid in opioid-naive patients in particular. In adults a background infusion of morphine along with the PCA function tends to increase the consumption of morphine without improving pain relief. It may be that a sense of control over pain relief decreases the requirement. It also removes the safety features of the patient control. Circumstances where an infusion may be used include:

- patient already taking long-term opioid drugs and nil by mouth
- long-term PCA use with poor pain control
- children
- patients unable to use the PCA, who require morphine for pain control
- use for opioid tolerance
- opioid naive with high opioid requirements
- severe pain causing waking at night.

FOUR HOUR LIMIT

It is possible to set a limit on how much opioid the patient can receive in a 4-hour period. This is not usually set because it contravenes the philosophy of a PCA – one is making a pre-judgement about the patient's four hourly requirement.

LOCKOUT TIME

The lockout time should take into account the time taken to achieve the full effect of the opioid to minimize the side effects. The full effect may not be seen for 15 minutes. Ginsberg suggests 7–11 minutes with morphine and five to eight minutes for fentanyl. There is no difference in analgesia, side effects or anxiety with these times. The lockout time is still five minutes in the majority of hospitals. When the patient has pressed the demand button the pump will not deliver another bolus until the preset time has been reached.

Within five minutes 90 per cent of the action of morphine has occurred. Having a lockout period helps to prevent overdose but still allows the patient to receive a reasonable dose of analgesia in a reasonable time. Studies have shown that increasing the lockout period up to 10 minutes increases safety without compromising pain relief.

HISTORY

This setting tells you how much morphine the patient has used since the PCA was reset. It also tells you how many attempts were unsuccessful. The PCA settings should be altered if there have been many unsuccessful attempts. The patient needs a higher dose of morphine so the bolus dose should be increased.

OTHER DRUGS

Paracetamol and an NSAID (e.g. ibuprofen) should be given at the same time because they have morphine-sparing effects – i.e. they lower the dose of morphine required. Other drugs that are prescribed for the relief of pain preoperatively, e.g. amitriptyline and gabapentin, should be given while the PCA is running.

Any other opioid-containing drugs should not be given while the patient has a PCA, including co-proxamol, tramadol, cocodamol, co-dydramol and dihydrocodeine. It takes 20–30 minutes for these oral drugs to work. During those 30 minutes the patient could have administered 6 mg morphine. The extra opioid dose may be too much and lead to respiratory depression.

Sedatives

Giving sedative drugs to a patient with a PCA does increase the risk of respiratory depression but sedation is not contraindicated. Some patients are especially anxious postoperatively causing increased distress from pain. A sedative drug rather than more painkillers is more likely to improve that patient's pain. Similarly night sedation, e.g. 20 mg temazepam, is unlikely to cause major problems especially if the patient is monitored properly. If a patient is taking oral sedative drugs consider whether oral analgesia could be prescribed instead of the PCA.

Patients who will benefit from patient controlled analgesia

- Major surgery
- Not permitted oral fluids (i.e. cannot take oral analgesia)
- Those with marked incident pain, e.g. physiotherapy or dressing changes
- Those who are not allowed intramuscular injections

Contraindications

- Current or past history of addiction to opioid drugs (debatable)
- Untrained staff
- Patient rejection (some patients do not wish to be in control of their analgesia)
- Inability to comprehend technique
- Extremes of age
- Inability to use the demand button

Changing to oral analgesia

Do not discontinue PCA to mobilize patient, use it to provide analgesia during mobilization. Convert to Oramorph® (morphine sulphate) initially, and then to cocodamol or paracetamol as the pain subsides. Do not stop PCA without ensuring further analgesia is prescribed. The PCA should be maintained until oral agents are sufficient to control pain.

There should be no nausea or vomiting, pain mild to moderate only and no further interventions should have been planned. If the patient is allowed oral fluids then oral analgesia can be given. The PCA should be maintained until oral agents are sufficient to control pain and there should be some overlap of therapies so oral analgesia has time to work.

If opioid use has been prolonged it may be necessary to continue with opioids orally. Twenty-four hours after resumption of gastric emptying change to low-dose long-acting oral opioids to maintain a continuous plasma concentration of drug to produce analgesia but less than the dose which will cause serious side effects. The oral dose required can be calculated from the preceding 24-hour PCA consumption. Prescribe about twice the previous 24-hour PCA dose as an oral agent in two divided doses. A short-acting opioid such as Oramorph should also be prescribed two hourly for breakthrough pain. If the daily PCA dose is less than 30 mg the pain may be controlled with a less potent agent, e.g. cocodamol or an NSAID. Always combine the opioid with paracetamol and NSAIDs as long as these are not contraindicated.

Adapting patient controlled analgesia for no hands

There are times when a patient would benefit from a PCA but is unable to use his or her hands, e.g. burns, rheumatoid arthritis, etc. Another method may be more suitable, for example, some patients are able to use their toes to activate the machine. In some machines the handpiece can be removed from the machine and replaced with green bubble tubing and the patient can blow into the tube and activate the machine.

Diamorphine subcutaneous patient controlled analgesia

With diamorphine subcutaneous PCA there is less local irritation and erythema, and improved sleep pattern on first and second nights because of fewer peaks and troughs. Nausea and vomiting is the same as above but is not associated with pressing the button.

SET-UP

- 50 mg diamorphine in 20 mL water
- 2.5 mg bolus (1 mL)
- 20 minute lockout
- Y-can into deltoid

Patient controlled analgesia for children

Children as young as 4 years can use a PCA with adequate instruction. Add 1 mg morphine/kg to 50 mL saline. For example, if the child weighs 35 kg add 35 mg morphine to 50 mL saline; 1 mL of the solution is equivalent to 20 μg/kg morphine. The bolus dose is 1 mL with a 5-minute lockout as for adults.

The success or otherwise of the PCA depends on how well the PCA is used.

Summary: patient controlled analgesia guidelines (Fig. 4.3)

1 50 mg morphine made up to 50 mL with normal saline.
2 Bolus dose is 1 mg/mL.
3 Duration of injection – STAT (30 seconds).
4 5-minute lockout.
5 No background infusion of morphine (unless discussed with acute pain team).
6 An antisiphon device must be used.
7 Prescription for antiemetics.
8 Check drug chart has no other opioids prescribed.
9 Prescribe naloxone 100–400 mg intravenously slowly (or 400 mg intramuscularly) if respiratory rate <8/min.
10 Oxygen via nasal prongs at 2–3 L/min while PCA in progress to be prescribed on front of drug chart. Higher rates may mask significant hypoventilation.

Monitoring the patient

It is a nursing responsibility to monitor the vital signs of the patient throughout the time the PCA is in use. Respiratory depression, hypoxia and increased sedation will then be detected and treated early. This should minimize the occurrence of more serious side effects. Postoperatively record the following:

- Observations:
  - heart rate
  - blood pressure
  - respiratory rate
  - sedation scores
  - pain scores
  - nausea score.
- Amount (mg) opioid used.
- Infusion rate.
- Changes of settings.
- Syringe changes.
- Blood pressure/pulse/respiratory rate/SaO$_2$
  - quarter hourly for one hour or while patient remains unstable
  - half hourly for two hours
  - one hourly for 12 hours
  - four hourly for 24 hours.
- Pain/sedation/nausea scores:
  - hourly for 12 hours
  - two hourly for 12–24 hours
  - then four hourly.
- Record respiratory rate, sedation score and amount (mg) opioid used, hourly **until the infusion is discontinued**.
- Two hourly observations of heart rate, blood pressure, pain and nausea should continue but the frequency of heart rate and blood pressure may be reduced to four hourly after 12 hours if the patient remains haemodynamically stable.
- Scoring systems should be used to record:
  - pain score
  - sedation score
  - nausea score.

See Table 4.10 for management of problems with PCA in the postoperative period.

Morphine infusions

INDICATIONS

- Continuous infusions of morphine should generally not be used in opioid-naive patients.
- Patients who normally take opioids but are nil by mouth.
- Patients who have used a PCA or who have had intramuscular/intravenous opioids for a while and pain relief is inadequate.
- Intensive care setting.

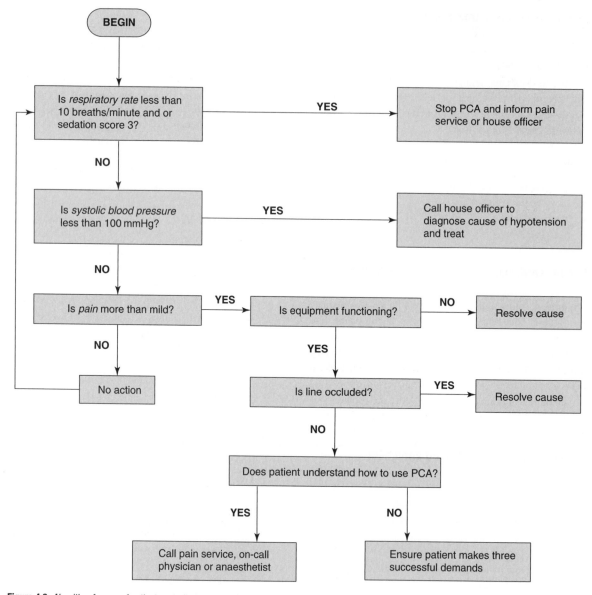

Figure 4.3 *Algorithm for use of patient controlled analgesia (PCA)*

■ Children especially postoperatively in a high-dependency area.

COMPLICATIONS

■ Accumulation:
  – renal failure
  – hypovolaemia, e.g. with active bleeding. There may be reduced liver blood flow and therefore a reduced rate of drug elimination.
■ Mechanical failure.

DISADVANTAGES

■ Not flexible and pain is rarely constant.
■ Requires careful monitoring and training.

Gastrointestinal prophylaxis and NSAIDs

There is no justification for the routine prescribing of drugs for the prophylaxis of peptic ulcer disease in all patients receiving NSAIDs. NSAID-induced erosions are found more commonly

Table 4.10 *Management of problems with patient controlled analgesia*

Problems	Action
Respiratory rate (adults) <8 breaths per minute	**STOP PCA** Naloxone* 0.4 mg (1 mL) in 9 mL saline. Give 1 mL at a time until respiratory rate increases

Respiratory rate (children)
  <1 year <25 breaths
    per minute
  2–5 years <20 breaths
    per minute
  6–12 years <15 breaths
    per minute
  >12 years <10 breaths
    per minute
	STOP PCA
	Naloxone* 4 μg/kg repeated as
	necessary

Sedation score of 2 or more	**STOP PCA – Call physician** – may require naloxone*

* Naloxone effects may be short lived and respiratory depression may re-occur after 20 minutes.

in the stomach than the duodenum, but the incidence of bleeding and perforation from the two sites is similar. lbuprofen is associated with the lowest risk of peptic ulcers.

Patients at high risk of peptic ulcer disease include frail, elderly people, those with a previous history of peptic ulceration or of gastric intolerance to NSAIDs, those on systemic steroids, anticoagulants (excluding low-molecular weight heparin) or high-dose NSAIDs.

WHICH PROPHYLACTIC AGENT SHOULD BE USED?

For frail/elderly people, those on NSAID + anticoagulant or NSAID + systemic steroid, those with previous gastric or duodenal ulcer, the recommended prophylactic regimen is: lansoprazole 30 mg daily orally or omeprazole 20 mg daily (if a suspension is required).

Lansoprazole (30 mg daily orally)/omeprazole (20 mg daily) are licensed for the prophylaxis of NSAID-induced ulcers occurring in the stomach or duodenum. Lansoprazole is the first choice for oral treatment on the basis of cost.

Use of NSAIDs in surgical patients

In all patients the usual medical contraindications to NSAIDs apply. In 'low-risk' surgery (e.g. microdiscectomy, general surgery, etc.) they can be introduced immediately. NSAIDS can be used orally when the patient is nil by mouth if this is only a short-term situation.

Neurosurgery

There is no evidence that the earlier introduction of NSAIDs is dangerous. Indeed some neurosurgical centres use them immediately postcraniotomy *if* there are no problems with clotting. The vast majority of postoperative intracranial haematomas develop in the first six hours postoperatively – perhaps NSAIDs should be started six hours postoperatively.

Guidelines for management of postoperative nausea and vomiting

Identify at-risk patients with two or more of the following:

- Patient factors:
  - History of motion sickness or postoperative nausea and vomiting
  - Female
  - Obese
  - Delayed gastric emptying
- Anaesthetic and surgical factors:
  - Use of opioids especially with PCA
  - Hypotension
  - Nitrous oxide
- Specifically in neurosurgery:
  - Raised intracranial pressure
  - Foramen magnum decompression
  - Low pressure headache
- External factors:
  - Movement, e.g. transfer from trolley to bed
  - Give prophylaxis for at-risk patients:
    - ☐ Regular cyclizine 50 mg orally or intravenously slowly eight hourly for 36 hours
    - ☐ Ondansetron 4 mg orally/intramuscularly/ intravenously 12 hourly
    - ☐ Dexamethasone 4–8 mg intravenously

Postoperatively:

- Prescribe an antiemetic in all patients:
  - Cyclizine 50 mg oral/intramuscularly/slow intravenous (six hourly) up to 150 mg/24 h.
  - Prochlorperazine 12.5 mg intramuscularly eight hourly (or 10 mg oral eight hourly).
  - Ondansetron 4 mg orally/intramuscularly/ intravenously 12 hourly as required, or regularly if nausea continues. Ondansetron maximum dose = 16 mg in 24 hours
  - Prescribe a 'rescue' antiemetic in all patients (to be given after one hour if no response to first line antiemetic).
  - Consider regular cyclizine if nausea remains problematic (this has not caused problems with sedation).

- Metoclopramide has been shown in many studies to be ineffective for most forms of postoperative nausea and vomiting.

Non-invasive methods for patient controlled analgesia in pain management

New modes of drug administration or new delivery systems are being developed with the aim of improving pain control. Patient controlled analgesia with an intravenous opioid has become one of the most effective techniques for acute post-operative pain relief. Prerequisites for intravenous PCA are an intravenous cannula and an appropriate pump for drug administration. Because intravenous cannulae are often painful and restrict the patient's mobility, and because the number of PCA pumps are limited in most hospitals, alternative routes for opioid administration have been investigated with respect to their suitability for PCA.

TRANSDERMAL PCA

Transdermal opioid delivery is non-invasive, is not subject to hepatic first pass metabolism and offers convenient, comfortable and consistent analgesia to the patient. However, diffusion of fentanyl through the skin is slow. Peak plasma concentrations are reached only within 14 hours. The penetration of the skin by fentanyl is enhanced by iontophoresis. Iontophoresis is a physicochemical method by which ionizable drugs can be forced into the skin under the influence of an external electrical field. In the case of fentanyl only the positively charged molecule can be propelled into the skin from the anode along the electrical field. By introducing fentanyl into an acidic medium, the amount of positively charged drug can be increased and therefore more opioid is available for iontophoresis. Application of direct current (1–2 mA) for a 2-hour period has been shown to deliver clinically significant doses of fentanyl. The amount of drug delivered within a certain time period depends on the drug concentration in the device applied to the skin, the duration of current application and the current intensity.

Fentanyl has been incorporated into an electro-transport therapeutic system (ETS) with an internal electrical power source. Activation of this system delivers a fentanyl bolus of 40 µg over a 10-minute period. The electro-transport therapeutic system has been reported to result in consistent transdermal fentanyl delivery independent of frequency of demand. The safety is reported to be high, with the majority of subjects having very little erythema at the application site 24 hours after patch removal. Transdermal iontophoretic delivery of fentanyl could be a useful non-invasive method for PCA if further studies confirm its effectiveness.

PATIENT CONTROLLED INTRANASAL ANALGESIA

Opioids are absorbed well by the nasal mucosa. The nasal mode of opioid administration has the following advantages:

- perfusion of the nasal mucosa is excellent
- rapid absorption
- rapid rise in plasma concentration
- venous outflow of the nasal mucosa bypasses the liver and therefore the hepatic first pass effect
- high bioavailability of nasally administered drugs
- most people are familiar with nasal administration of drugs
- nasal spray bottles are common, handy and easy to use.

Fentanyl has a high affinity for the µ-opioid receptor subtype, good lipid solubility and high potency, and is good for nasal PCA since even a small number of molecules diffusing through the nasal mucosa can produce good analgesia. The maximum serum concentration can be detected five minutes after a total dose of fentanyl sprayed into both nostrils. Intranasal boluses of fentanyl have proved to be as effective as intravenous treatment with the same doses for postoperative pain. Nasal application of fentanyl has turned out to be a highly effective method of analgesia with a short onset time and is very well accepted by all patients. No local problems in the nasal mucosa of any patient have been reported. Respiratory depression or clinically significant haemodynamic side effects could not be observed. The overall incidence of side effects has been reported as:

- euphoria in 3.6 per cent
- dizziness in 1.4 per cent
- nausea in 1.4 per cent
- vomiting in 0.7 per cent
- itching in 0.7 per cent.

These are typical opioid-related side effects, and there was no difference in their incidence between the intranasally and the intravenously treated patients. An electronically controlled intranasal PCA device with safety features comparable to an intravenous PCA pump and of similar size as a common nasal spray bottle is currently under consideration for marketing approval with the health authorities. The small size, ease of use, and the comparably low production costs will make opioid PCA therapy available for great numbers of hospitalized patients as well as outpatients.

PATIENT CONTROLLED ORAL ANALGESIA

Since oral administration is the most convenient form of drug administration, it should be the route of first choice. A device for oral PCA should have the same safety features as an electronic pump for intravenous PCA. To compensate for the delay in intestinal absorption and for oral bioavailability of morphine, the initial oral PCA dose is 40 mg, and all subsequent doses are 20 mg (lockout interval of one hour). Analgesia is of the same quality as intravenous PCA. An electronically controlled, small and handy device for patient controlled oral analgesia will probably be available in the near future.

SUMMARY

Non-invasive PCA can be achieved by different routes of drug administration. The intranasal route has been investigated most thoroughly so far. Nasal PCA seems to be especially indicated for the treatment of breakthrough cancer pain, but it may also be greatly advantageous in the postoperative period. Electronically controlled devices for nasal and oral PCA will be commercially available in the near future and are currently under clinical investigation. Oral PCA seems to be especially promising in the postoperative period following extra-abdominal surgery. Transdermal PCA has been shown to be effective in volunteers; however, this has still to be proved in clinical studies.

TRANSCUTANEOUS ELECTRICAL NERVE STIMULATION IN ACUTE PAIN

There is no good evidence that TENS offers pain relief in acute pain, partly because blinding is difficult. Of 17 studies, 15 showed no benefit. However, it may have an effect in decreasing opioid requirements in gynaecological or haemorrhoids surgery and it may reduce pain in rib fractures and some hand infections, and improve ventilatory function in rib fractures.

It is cheap and safe and may be worth trying because some patients may benefit, but evidence remains inconclusive. If it is to be used, education and information and adequate demonstration are essential.

LOCAL ANAESTHETIC INFILTRATION

Local anaesthetic infiltrated along the incision is effective in reducing pain for hernia repair up to seven hours when given prior to surgery. Wound infiltration at the end of surgery has not been shown to improve postoperative pain relief.

ACUTE NEUROPATHIC PAIN

Neuropathic pain is commonly described as burning, stabbing, stinging, shooting, aching or electric shock-like in quality. It may be felt superficially or in deep tissues, may be present intermittently or constantly and can occur spontaneously or be triggered by various stimuli. It may have been present preoperatively and is sometimes temporarily worse following surgery. Therefore any preoperative treatment should be continued in the postoperative period and discontinued (slowly) when the neuropathic pain goes. Acute neuropathic pain is sometimes seen for the first time postoperatively and is usually temporary. It presumably results from inflammation around nerve roots following surgery. Severe, persistent neuropathic pain postoperatively needs to be investigated to exclude compression of nerve roots for example by haematoma or infection.

Suggested treatments

DEXAMETHASONE

Typically neuropathic pain responds poorly to simple analgesics and opioids. Most patients require centrally acting drugs. If inflammation around a nerve root is thought to be the cause of the neuropathic pain dexamethasone 4 mg four times daily orally or intravenously for two days can be very effective.

CENTRALLY ACTING DRUGS

Amitriptyline

Start at 10 mg nocte and increase the dose every two days if there are no troublesome side effects, up to a maximum of 50 mg.

Gabapentin

Some patients show a response to gabapentin within hours. There are many different ways to prescribe gabapentin but the aim is to start with a low dose and gradually increase it as required. In this way side effects are kept to a minimum and the lowest effective dose can be used. In acute pain the initial dose is 300 mg once daily, if tolerated. Increase dose until pain improves, as follows:

- day 2 – 300 mg twice daily
- day 3 – 300 mg three times daily
- day 4 – 400 mg three times daily.

The maximum dose is 2.4 g/day in three divided doses.

Acute pain as a cause of chronic pain

Neuropathic pain can occur years after the initial insult and 17 per cent of patients attending a pain clinic attribute their symptoms to surgery. The incidence of chronic pain after surgery may depend on the type of procedure performed and this is discussed in more detail in Chapter 13. Surgery can also be responsible for different types of postoperative pain, for example breast surgery has an incidence of postoperative pain of 11–49 per cent. These pains consist of phantom pains (13 per cent), scar pain (30 per cent), and also chest wall and arm pain. Chronic pain also follows thoracotomy (5–67 per cent), cholecystectomy (3–56 per cent), hernia repair (0–63 per cent) and vasectomy (0–37 per cent). The symptoms do have a tendency to decrease with time but can lead to prolonged and distressing symptoms for many.

Prevention

Good perioperative pain management is the key to reducing the severity of as many of the long-term symptoms as possible, but it may not be possible to prevent their occurrence altogether. The use of regional techniques, pre-incisional local anaesthesia and optimum drug therapy should all be considered. Any patient experiencing pain for a prolonged period should be seen and treated aggressively as soon as possible.

Treatment

Several studies have failed to show any effect from the interventions below, but other studies show a benefit.

- Preoperative gabapentin may decrease postoperative morphine requirements and also decrease movement pain.
- Regional anaesthesia may reduce the incidence of phantom limb pain.
- Ketamine may reduce the incidence of phantom limb pain.
- Optimal perioperative pain relief may reduce phantom limb pain.
- Early treatment for neuropathic pain may reduce intensity or duration.

Evidence that any treatment can alter long-term outcome is still needed, but as the symptoms can be so distressing, it is still worth optimizing perioperative pain relief in the hope that this will reduce postoperative problems as much as possible.

CASE SCENARIO

You are called to see a morbidly obese patient at 10 pm on the ward. He has been prescribed intramuscular morphine for pain relief after a laparotomy but he is in a great deal of pain despite frequent injections. He is not moving or coughing well and he is nil by mouth. How would you deal with the situation?

Problems

- Poor intramuscular absorption
- Dose of morphine required
- Sleep apnoea
- Coughing and movement
- Physiotherapy
- Difficulty of procedures, e.g. epidural/cannulation

Check whether adjuvant analgesia has been prescribed

PARACETAMOL

Paracetamol should be prescribed to be given six hourly. If he is unable to take it orally then it should be given intravenously.

NSAIDS

It is safe to give NSAIDs even when the patient is nil by mouth for a short time. NSAIDs given by any route have the same incidence of gastrointestinal problems but if he has just had bowel surgery he may not absorb oral drugs so it is best to administer them rectally or intravenously.

OPIOIDS

In the large majority of people, especially the obese, drugs given intramuscularly are often subcutaneous. The blood supply to the tissues postoperatively may be poor and absorption from the fat may be slow and lead to poor analgesia. If recurrent doses are given the patient could receive an overdose of the drug when blood supply to the area has improved.

It is better to give morphine intravenously to overcome this problem, particularly in the obese patient. It is difficult to know at first what the optimum dose of morphine is going to be in each patient and the use of PCA with small doses of intravenous opioid is normally the easiest and most effective way of delivering the drug.

The bolus should always start at 1 mg with a minimum of a 5 minute lockout time in the opioid-naive patient. If this is insufficient the bolus can be increased in 0.5 mg increments.

A background infusion is rarely required in the postoperative opioid-naive patient. Once he is taking fluids orally he could be put on oral morphine instead. The dose of oral morphine prescribed should be based on the previous daily intravenous use. For example if the patient has had 60 mg morphine from the PCA, the oral dose is between two and three times the intravenous dose, i.e. 120–180 mg morphine orally. This could be prescribed as 20 mg two hourly prn but altered as required.

As the patient recovers and requires less morphine he can be put onto paracetamol and codeine orally. Oxygen should be prescribed while the patient is receiving intravenous morphine.

EPIDURAL

Surgery in the morbidly obese patient is associated with a significant risk of respiratory problems. Poor gas exchange and hypoxia are exacerbated by morphine. There is increased risk of infection because of poor cough. There may be sleep apnoea and Pickwickian syndrome.

If the patient demonstrates any of these problems an epidural infusion should be considered to improve lung function and gas exchange. It ought to be placed at the time of surgery as it will be a difficult procedure in a large patient who is in pain and unable to move well. However, if gas exchange is a significant problem, it may be necessary. Also remember that the patient may now be having low-molecular weight heparin and timing of the siting of the epidural will be important.

There is no doubt that when an epidural infusion works well it provides the best available analgesia but about a third of epidurals fail to provide adequate analgesia.

FURTHER READING

Wildsmith JAW, Armitage EN. *Principles and Practice of Regional Anaesthesia.* 3rd edn. Edinburgh: Churchill Livingstone, 2002.

5 Acute Pain: Special Situations

INTRODUCTION

The basic principles of pain assessment and management are universal and frequent reassessment of the patient should be made to treat any pain that rapidly waxes and wanes. This chapter deals with specific situations within the management of acute pain.

PAIN DURING PREGNANCY

The issue of fetal pain was first raised in 1996, when the Royal College of Obstetricians and Gynaecologists set up a working party in response to parliamentary questions relating to fetal pain and awareness. The research areas highlighted were:

- developmental pathways for transmission of noxious stimuli in the fetus and neonate, i.e. how the ability to experience pain develops during fetal life
- placental transfer of analgesic drugs in the second trimester, i.e. the effect of analgesic drugs administered to the mother which pass through the placenta to the fetus
- effects of analgesic drugs on stress responses in animal and human fetuses/neonates
- potential long-term effects of intrauterine procedures, with or without analgesics
- animal research on the effects of analgesics on the development of the fetal brain.

Can the fetus feel pain? It is generally accepted that awareness of pain requires the involvement of the cerebral cortex. Connections to the cortex begin to develop at about 20 weeks' gestation. In the early stages of pregnancy, the experience of pain is not physiologically possible. The process develops over many pre- and postnatal months and there is no time when pain is suddenly 'switched on'. The neural 'wiring' continues to develop during childhood and into adolescence. Awareness of pain is subject to many factors including consciousness, anxiety, memory and individual experience, which develop in early life and change over time.

What are the effects of analgesic drugs that pass through the placenta to the fetus? Harmful effects on the fetus of analgesic drugs given to the mother during delivery are rare. The time of exposure is short and drug levels very low. Little is known about the effects of drugs on fetal development in the second trimester (fourth, fifth and sixth months of pregnancy). There is a need for more research but ethical and practical considerations mean this is difficult in pregnancy.

What are the potential long-term effects of intrauterine procedures, with or without analgesics? In the UK, surgical procedures are rarely carried out in the womb, with only about 250 performed per year. Of more practical importance is the effect both of pain and of powerful analgesics on infants born prematurely, and whose stage of brain development is similar to that of a fetus in the third trimester of pregnancy. Premature babies may require many such interventions.

It is thought that painful procedures experienced by premature babies may affect them later in life in a variety of ways. These may include an increased prevalence of behavioural disorders and psychosocial problems. It is difficult to know if these result from the procedures or from other disadvantages that premature babies may suffer but there is some evidence that behavioural problems may be correlated with the number of procedures that had to be performed, rather than with clinical factors such as how premature the baby was. It is important to determine how severe the behavioural problems are and whether or not they persist in the longer term.

Teratogens

Teratogens are substances that can cause congenital malformations, spontaneous abortion, or other structural or functional abnormalities in the fetus or the child after birth. In the pre-embryonic period (up to 17 days post-conception) a toxic insult is believed to lead to either death of the embryo or replacement of damaged cells and intact survival (the 'all or nothing' principle). From 18 days to 10 weeks post-conception the fetus is most vulnerable to toxins affecting organogenesis. After this period teratogens may interfere with fetal growth and development. Teratogens are not toxic in all cases of exposure.

Prescribing in pregnancy

Most drugs are unlicensed for use during pregnancy because there is no evidence from clinical trials about their use in pregnant women. However, extensive circumstantial evidence of the safe use of several drugs during pregnancy enables many conditions to be treated appropriately.

GENERAL PRINCIPLES OF PRESCRIBING

- Almost all drugs cross the placenta except high molecular weight drugs such as heparin.
- Prescribe drugs only when necessary.
- Consider topical treatment before systemic treatment.
- Use the lowest effective dose for the shortest possible time, but remember that under-treatment poses risks to maternal wellbeing and may also affect the fetus.
- Use the minimum number of drugs.
- Prescribe older, more established drugs in preference to newer drugs. For instance, use antacids rather than proton pump inhibitors, and older rather than more recently introduced antidepressants.
- Teratogenic risk should be considered when prescribing for **any** woman who may become pregnant.

PARACETAMOL

Paracetamol products can normally be used at recommended dosages during pregnancy, and mothers who are breastfeeding may use paracetamol products. One report has shown that daily or almost daily use of paracetamol by the mother during the later stages of pregnancy almost doubles the risk of wheezing in children at 30–42 months of age. This did not occur with normal occasional use at recommended dosages. The association was strongest when the symptoms appeared before the child was 6 months old. Use of paracetamol before 20 weeks was not associated with an increased risk. However, the risk still remains small (1 per cent) and paracetamol remains the analgesic drug of choice if used infrequently.

There may also be an increased risk of hypertension in the mother with paracetamol and non-steroidal anti-inflammatory drugs (NSAIDs, but not aspirin).

NSAIDs

There are only a few reports of the use of opioids, NSAIDs, antidepressants and anticonvulsants in the treatment of pain in pregnancy. Controlled trials in humans of the use of aspirin have not shown evidence of teratogenic effects. However, studies in animals have shown that salicylates can cause birth defects including fissure of the spine and skull, facial clefts and malformations of the central nervous system, viscera and skeleton. Ingestion of aspirin during the last two weeks of pregnancy may increase the risk of fetal or neonatal haemorrhage.

Regular or high dose use of salicylates late in pregnancy may result in:

- constriction or premature closing of the fetal ductus arteriosus, if taken after 30 weeks
- transient risk of wheezing before the age of 6 months
- increased risk of stillbirth or neonatal death
- decreased birthweight
- prolonged labour
- complicated deliveries
- increased risk of maternal or fetal haemorrhage
- possibly persistent pulmonary hypertension of the newborn or kernicterus in jaundiced neonates.

Pregnant women should be advised not to take aspirin in the last three months of pregnancy unless under medical supervision. Aspirin is distributed in breast milk and should be avoided while breastfeeding.

OPIOIDS

Most of the work so far has concentrated on the effects of maternal drug abuse on the fetus. Opioids can cross the placenta and enter the fetal blood stream. The use of opioids in pregnancy can lead to an increased risk of medical and obstetric complications affecting both mother and fetus. None of the opioid drugs has been shown to produce physical birth defects in babies.

Alternating between intoxication and withdrawal can result in an unstable uterine environment that can be fatal to the fetus. The most consistently reported effect on neonates is intrauterine growth retardation, resulting in smaller-than-normal head size and low birthweight. Other effects include:

- abnormal fetal electroencephalogram
- abnormal fetal breathing activity
- abnormal glucose regulation
- increased risk of stillbirth
- increased risk of fetal distress
- increased risk of aspiration pneumonia in the neonate
- may be a higher than usual rate of visual defects (i.e. strabismus)
- withdrawal syndrome in the neonate in 60–70 per cent (especially with opioid use in the last three months of pregnancy). Neonatal abstinence syndrome primarily affects an infant's central nervous system and gastrointestinal tract.

In mice codeine can lead to delayed ossification and in rats to increased bone resorption. Generally the use of opioids in pregnancy in the short term and in recommended doses appears to be safe, but further studies are needed.

It appears that infants born to women on methadone maintenance, who receive good prenatal care, have relatively higher birthweights than do babies born to women who abuse heroin during pregnancy and have no prenatal care. The effects of *in utero* exposure to prescribed methadone are relatively benign.

Effects during breastfeeding

Opioids are transmitted to the baby via breast milk although research shows that exposure levels are lower than prenatal exposure levels. Opioids should be avoided where possible in women who are breastfeeding.

Long-term effects

Although research on animals suggests that exposure to any drug *in utero* has long-term physiological effects across the entire lifespan, there has been very little research on the long-term effects of intrauterine opioid exposure in humans and results have been inconclusive. So if there are long-term effects they may be quite subtle or may take years to appear.

ANTIDEPRESSANTS

Tricyclic antidepressants have a long history of use without increasing teratogenic risk in pregnant women. Doses of tricyclic antidepressants may need to be higher during pregnancy because of physiological changes such as increased hepatic metabolism. Where appropriate, to avoid withdrawal symptoms in the neonate, antidepressants should be slowly withdrawn or reduced to the minimum dose prior to delivery.

ANTICONVULSANTS

Reported incidences of congenital deformities in pregnant women taking one or more antiepileptic drugs vary from 0.5–1 per cent with a single drug to 20–30 per cent with four drugs. The risk is greater with polypharmacy and higher doses of drugs. Less information is available about the newer agents such as gabapentin or lamotrigine but they have not been found to be teratogenic in experimental animals and are used at some centres. With sodium valproate, peak plasma concentrations should be reduced by changing dosing from twice daily to three times daily or to the modified-release preparation (before conception if possible). About 1 per cent of women taking carbamazepine during pregnancy will have a child with a congenital malformation but this may be mild.

SUPPLEMENTATION WITH ANTICONVULSANTS

Folic acid deficiency has been implicated in teratogenicity caused by antiepileptic drugs. Therefore, supplementation with folic acid at a dose of 5 mg daily is recommended, ideally starting three months before conception. Vitamin K deficiency may occur more frequently in neonates who were prenatally exposed to antiepileptic drugs that induce liver enzymes. This can be prevented by giving oral vitamin K (as phytomenadione, 10–20 mg daily) to the mother during the last month of pregnancy.

PAIN IN CHILDREN

Long-term consequences of pain in infancy

There is considerable controversy around the short- and long-term consequences of pain in early infancy. Until recent years, infants received inadequate or no analgesia for a range of medical procedures and even major surgery. Some people believe that neonates do not experience pain, that they do not remember pain, or that if pain is experienced as suffering, it produces no lasting consequences. Others believe that untreated pain in early infancy can have profound and lasting consequences, particularly longlasting emotional consequences.

Animal studies

Adult rats that have undergone repetitive neonatal injury show an increased preference for alcohol, increased latency in exploratory and defensive withdrawal behaviour, and a prolonged chemosensory memory in the social discrimination test. Newborn animals exposed to morphine when not in pain need higher doses of morphine later in life to achieve pain control.

Clinical studies

The model for neonatal analgesic studies is circumcision. Boys having circumcision without analgesia have a lowered pain threshold to vaccination at six months. Twin studies show behavioural differences between those who experienced pain and those who did not.

Developmental plasticity in the neonatal pain system and developing brain suggest that early painful experiences may have long-term neurobiological effects. This leads to altered behaviour during childhood – increased behavioural and physiological responses, including vulnerability to stress disorders, addictive behaviour and anxiety states. Preterm

BOX 5.1 Physiological differences in neonates

- Organs mature during the first three months of life; adult physiology by three months.
- There is no evidence that neonates feel less pain.
- Side effects of opioids are greater – the prolonged elimination time means they should be given in smaller doses.
- Ventilatory differences in neonates: babies <1 month are sensitive to opioids and should be monitored in high-dependency units or intensive care units (ITUs) and apnoea alarms used; reduced response to hypoxia and hypercarbia; reduced ability to breathe against restrictive loads; chest wall instability; increased tendency to alveolar collapse; fatigue of diaphragm; and apnoea attacks.
- A higher percentage of bodyweight of neonates is water and there is less fat, so water-soluble drugs have a larger volume of distribution and so need larger doses than expected.
- Brain and viscera form a greater amount of body mass so increased passage into brain of drugs such as morphine.
- Most drugs are conjugated in the liver. Neonates have delayed maturation of these systems leading to a delay in conjugation of opioids, paracetamol, NSAIDs and local anaesthetics.
- The glomerular filtration rate is lower in the first week so most analgesics have a significantly longer half-life. Neonates can clear most medications by two weeks.
- The number and distribution of μ receptors is different in the newborn causing a greater propensity toward respiratory depression and higher analgesic requirements with an increased risk of respiratory depression at opioid doses necessary for analgesia.
- Neonates have less albumin and α1 acid glycoprotein, greater availability of drug and increased risk of acute toxicity.

- An understanding of infant neurobiology and pharmacology is essential.
- Parenteral opioids and other potent drugs should only be used in a specialist environment.
- Dangerous complications should be anticipated and treated without delay.
- Cyclo-oxygenase (COX)-2 drugs have not yet been evaluated in children.
- Morphine in neonates undergoes prolonged elimination so the maintenance dose should be reduced and the dose interval should be increased. Up to 14 per cent of spontaneously breathing infants receiving opioids have an apnoea attack or respiratory failure.

Pain assessment in children

Assessment of pain in infants and children remains a challenge. Behavioural pain measures for neonates are better than for 2–4-year-olds, partly because measurement at this age is confounded with fear and anxiety. Some children cannot separate the unpleasantness of a needle stick from the pain of the needle stick even up to the age of 12 years.

PAIN SCORING SYSTEMS FOR YOUNG CHILDREN AND BABIES

Many scoring systems have been developed for use in this age group and all have advantages and disadvantages, however, they generally include changes in behaviour. See Table 5.1 for the FLACC (Face, Legs, Activity, Crying and Consolability) pain assessment tool.

Other methods include:

- CHEOPS (McGrath,1985) which includes assessing the cry and observing the facial response, torso movement, wound touching and movement of the legs.
- Facial action coding for neonates. This method involves making a video of the baby and assessing it later. It requires training and is better for research purposes than for bedside assessment of pain.

Faces scale: Many different scales have been produced for pain measurement in children as well. Some are based on pictures such as the faces scale (Fig. 5.1) and some use physiological assessment. All of them have advantages and disadvantages, but the faces scale is simple to use. It can be used from about 4 years up to about 10 years.

Unlike adults, children tend to go for extremes and when tears are used on the diagram this often makes children use the more severe diagram. It may be better to have a series of faces without tears.

neonates seem to display a lower pain threshold, which tends to decrease even further after exposure to repeated painful stimuli (see Box 5.1). These children do react differently to pictures of painful events, but it is not clear whether it is the pain that produces these changes as they have other altered behaviour as well.

Principles of pain management in children

- Effective pain management depends on accurate pain assessment.
- Multimodal analgesia should be used where possible.

Table 5.1 *FLACC (Face, Legs, Activity, Crying and Consolability) pain assessment tool*

Categories	Scoring		
	0	**1**	**2**
Face	No particular expression or smile	Occasional grimace or frown, withdrawn, disinterested	Frequent to constant quivering chin, clenched jaw
Legs	Normal position or relaxed	Uneasy, restless, tense	Kicking or legs drawn up
Activity	Lying quietly, normal position, moves easily	Squirming, shifting back and forth, tense	Arched, rigid or jerking
Cry	No cry (awake or asleep)	Moans or whimpers; occasional complaint	Crying steadily, screams or sobs, frequent complaints
Consolability	Content, relaxed	Reassured by occasional touching, hugging, being talked to or distracted	Difficult to console or comfort

 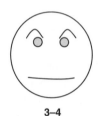  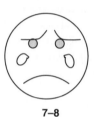 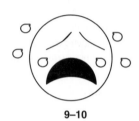

| 0–2 | 3–4 | 5–6 | 7–8 | 9–10 |

Figure 5.1 *The faces scale*

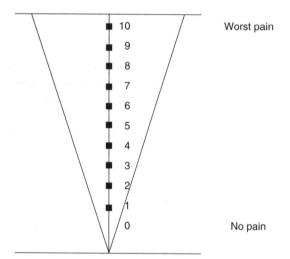

Figure 5.2 *Vertical scale*

From about 8 years: A vertical scale (Fig. 5.2) can be used for older children up to teenage. Vertical scales are better than horizontal scales for children.

Methods of pain management

SUGAR-COATED DUMMIES

- Significantly decrease crying after heel prick and venepuncture in infants aged 1–6 days.

- The effect increases with an increased dose.
- The effect is probably due to the presence of solution in mouth because of the rapid response.
- They cause activation of endogenous opioids and the response can be blocked by naloxone.
- A pacifier is better than sucrose or glucose but sucrose followed by a pacifier is best. The pacifier provides sensory dominance and is accepted by most neonates.

Sucrose is safe and effective for reducing procedural pain from single painful events (heel lance, venepuncture). The optimal dose of sucrose in preterm and/or term infants has not been identified but lies within the range of 0.012–0.12 g. It appears to be a useful adjunct but should not be used as the sole analgesic or anaesthetic.

PARACETAMOL

Paracetamol has a 36–37 per cent morphine-sparing effect and should be used wherever possible for pain management to reduce opioid-related side effects.

Metabolism

There is a gradual change in pharmacology of paracetamol with age. The young conjugate paracetamol into the sulphite metabolite and there is a gradual change into the glucuronide metabolite that reaches adult levels by 12 years. The glucuronide metabolite is responsible for liver damage and this change in metabolism correlates well with the increase in toxicity seen in children over the age of 12 years. Toxicity after a single dose does not occur until a level of 120 µg/mL is reached four hours after ingestion. The toxic dose is 250 mg/kg per day but hepatic compromise may be seen at 100 mg/kg per day.

Neonates have lower levels of cytochrome P-450 enzyme which may confer some protection against liver damage, but the reduced clearance rate means the maximum dose in neonates should be 60 mg/kg per day.

Dose (Box 5.2)

The therapeutic blood concentration for analgesia is not well established but it is widely accepted as 10–20 µg/mL. Little analgesia is produced below this level.

The dose of paracetamol in adults is generally accepted as 1 g although this dose may not produce therapeutic levels in many. Difficulty arises when prescribing for children over 25 kg for rectal paracetamol and 50 kg for oral paracetamol assuming the paediatric dose is 40 mg/kg and 20 mg/kg, respectively. Children over 25 kg receiving 1 g paracetamol rectally do not have blood levels within the therapeutic range; this dose may be insufficient for the majority of children over 25 kg but further work needs to be done to confirm this.

Paracetamol 1 g rectally may be insufficient in the majority of children over 25 kg but further work needs to be done to confirm this.

BOX 5.2 Paracetamol – recommended doses

- Oral: 30 mg/kg preoperatively, then 20 mg/kg four hourly.
- Rectal: 30–40 mg/kg eight hourly to a maximum of 100 mg/kg per day and review at 48 hours. Rectal absorption is erratic and delayed and the half-life is prolonged. Absorption may be between 25 and 85 per cent and the peak effect occurs at 2.5–3.5 hours.
- Neonatal: The maximum dose should be 60 mg/kg per day.

NSAIDs

Aspirin should be avoided in children under 16 years because it may, rarely, lead to Reye's syndrome. NSAIDs should not be used in infants under 6 months because of concerns about renal and cerebral perfusion.

Studies have shown that oral diclofenac two hours preoperatively significantly reduces rescue analgesia requirement postoperatively after tonsillectomy compared with rectal

Table 5.2 *Comparison of morphine metabolism at birth and in adulthood*

	Birth	Adult
Volume of distribution	80 L/70 kg	136 L/70 kg
Total body clearance	14.5 L/h per kg	71 L/h per 70 kg

BOX 5.3 Morphine – recommended doses

Loading dose
- <1 month – 25 µg/kg
- 1–3 months – 50 µg/kg
- >3 months – 100–150 µg/kg given in 50 µg/kg aliquots

Infusion rate
- 0–1 month – 5 µg/kg per hour
- 1–3 months – 10 µg/kg per hour
- >3 months – 20–40 µg/kg

---

diclofenac at induction. Children should receive NSAIDs preoperatively where possible and regularly postoperatively.

OPIOIDS

Codeine in children

Codeine may be particularly unsuitable for use in the younger child because of reduced metabolism, difficulty in pain reporting and assessment and unpredictable effects. Young children may be more liable to experience side effects and get less analgesia. The enzyme CYP2D6 is switched on at birth. Levels are low in neonates and infants. By five years of age the activity of CYP2D6 is 25 per cent. Codeine should not be used in neonates or infants.

Morphine

Morphine is the opioid of choice for use in children with severe pain because there is a large amount of experience of its use. It can be given orally, rectally or intravenously.

At six months the clearance of morphine-6-glucuronide (M-6-G) and morphine-3-glucuronide (M-3-G) is 80 per cent of that in an adult. By 5–6 months babies have normal response to opioids. See Table 5.2 for changes in morphine metabolism with age.

Dose (Box 5.3)

A mean steady-state serum concentration of 10 ng/mL can be achieved in children after non-cardiac surgery with morphine with the following doses:

- Birth to term neonate – 5 µg/kg per hour (3.3 kg)
- 1 month – 8.5 µg/kg per hour (4 kg)

- 3 months –13.5 µg/kg per hour (6 kg)
- 1 year – 18 µg/kg per hour (10 kg)
- 1–3 years – 16 µg/kg per hour (12–18 kg)

Morphine levels are also affected by bilirubin levels and the higher the bilirubin the higher the serum morphine level.

These doses are only guidelines for the first few doses of morphine. The dose required by an individual is the dose required to alleviate pain, provided there are no significant side effects, and this dose may vary widely. Morphine should always be titrated to produce the required response.

'Opioid jerks'

Restlessness and twitching may be seen in infants receiving continuous morphine. It may be due to accumulation of M-3-G (stimulatory) and it responds to reduced infusion rate.

USE OF PATIENT CONTROLLED ANALGESIA IN CHILDREN

Patient selection

Children must be **able to understand** the patient controlled analgesia (PCA) (see Chapter 4) instructions and able to push the PCA button. This requires explanation and comprehension preoperatively. Patient controlled analgesia has been used in children as young as 4 years. Indications include surgical procedures when a child is expected to remain hospitalized longer than 24 hours and will require intravenous opioid analgesia.

Dosage guidelines

- Morphine 1 mg/kg in 50 mL normal saline = concentration 20 µg/kg per mL up to a maximum of 1 mg/mL.
- A child over 50 kg may use 50 mg morphine in 50 mL with 1 mg bolus (as in adults).

Initial setup

- Bolus dose – 1 mL (i.e. 20 µg/kg)
- Lockout interval – five minutes

There is no evidence that PCA increases nausea and vomiting or that it is related to the dose of opioid received.

Transfer from infusion/PCA mode to per rectum (PR)/ per oral (PO) analgesics. Consider the following criteria:

- pain level mild to moderate
- no immediate interventions planned
- low use of intravenous opioids or epidural infusion
- child able to take oral medication.

Preoperative instruction to the patient/parent should include:

- rationale for PCA
- use of the machine
- explanation of the safety features
- explanation of the monitoring, e.g. pain scores and sedation scores
- likely duration of treatment.

NURSE CONTROLLED ANALGESIA

Occasionally a child does not require a background infusion of morphine but needs frequent boluses of opioid for movement, physiotherapy or dressing changes. If the child cannot use the PCA button, for example because of injury to both hands, nurse controlled analgesia can be prescribed. The nurse, rather than the patient, is responsible for pressing the button. This technique can be safe provided protocols for use are followed.

FENTANYL

If a child is not tolerating morphine it is worth switching to fentanyl but the patient should be monitored in a high-dependency area because of the risk of respiratory depression. Fentanyl is often used in the ITU, and it is has advantages for use in children with pulmonary hypertension. It can be given intravenously, transmucosally and transdermally, and epidurally. It may be the drug of choice in children with renal failure but it may show tachyphylaxis.

Guidelines for use of fentanyl infusions

- Children who have an allergy or unusual response to morphine.
- Children in whom morphine does not appear to produce analgesia despite increasing the dose.
- Children undergoing surgery when an epidural infusion cannot be used and morphine is contraindicated as above.
- In children with renal failure or impairment, where morphine is likely to cause increasing respiratory depression because of accumulation of its active metabolites.
- No other opioid by any other route should be prescribed while the child is on fentanyl infusion.
- Sedative drugs such as diazepam should be used with caution.
- The child should be monitored and remain in a high-dependency area for a minimum of four hours after discontinuation of fentanyl infusion.

Dosage

- Loading dose – 1–10 µg/kg
- Infusion rate – 0.5–2 µg/kg per hour (see Table 5.3 for drug concentrations)

Table 5.3 *Fentanyl dosing chart*

Weight of patient (kg)	Amount of neat fentanyl required + amount of saline to be added	Concentration of fentanyl (μg/mL) in 50 mL syringe
10–14 kg	500 μg (10 mL + 40 mL saline)	10 μg/mL
15–19 kg	750 μg (15 mL + 35 mL saline)	15 μg/mL
20–24 kg	1000 μg (20 mL + 30 mL saline)	20 μg/mL
25–34 kg	1500 μg (30 mL + 20 mL saline)	30 μg/mL
35–39 kg	1750 μg (35 mL + 15 mL saline)	35 μg/mL
40–44 kg	2000 μg (40 mL + 10 mL saline)	40 μg/mL
45–49 kg	2250 μg (45 mL + 5 mL saline)	45 μg/mL
50 kg or more	2500 μg (50 mL neat fentanyl)	50 μg/mL

Drug concentration

The infusion should be made up as given in Table 5.3.

- Remember that the concentration of neat fentanyl = 50 μg/mL.
- Dilute the fentanyl with 0.9 per cent saline.

Side effects include sedation, respiratory depression and itching. **Also prescribe regularly** (unless contraindicated):

- Paracetamol 20 mg/kg six hourly orally
- Ibuprofen 5 mg/kg (or other NSAID)

INTRANASAL DIAMORPHINE

The relative potency of intranasal diamorphine compared with an intramuscular dose is 50 per cent. It has been used in emergency departments in children and provides as rapid an effect as an intramuscular dose but with better parental acceptability.

Diamorphine is diluted and placed in a metered spray bottle with one to two puffs up the nose. It is not yet licensed for use in children. The onset is immediate and lasts 15–20 minutes so analgesia and sedation set in fairly quickly.

Side effects of diamorphine include nasal irritation and vomiting. It should be used while the tetracaine (Ametop®) is working, so then a cannula can be sited and further intravenous analgesia given. Often the child will not require more analgesia.

Because of its rapid onset and sedation diamorphine may be useful for dressing changes or removal of sutures, etc.

Dose

1 Use the weight of the child to the nearest 5 kg.
2 Add saline in the amount shown in Table 5.4 to 10 mg diamorphine.

Table 5.4 *Diamorphine dilution chart*

Weight of child to nearest 5 kg	Volume saline (mL)
15	1.3
20	1.0
25	0.8
30	0.7
35	0.6
40	0.5
50	0.4
60	0.3

3 Draw up 0.2 mL and give via a 1 mL syringe or metered spray.
4 The dose is approximately 0.1 mg/kg in 0.2 mL saline.

NALOXONE

If severe respiratory depression has occurred from an overdose of an opioid drug the effects can be reversed with intravenous naloxone in the following manner:

1 Dilute ampoule of naloxone (400 μg/mL) with saline to 10 mL (80 μg/mL).
2 Give 2–4 μg/kg every two to three minutes until respiratory depression is reversed.
3 Dose may need to be repeated or an infusion started because the effects of naloxone last only about 20 minutes, but the opioid may last one to two hours.

Overdose of naloxone may cause vomiting, hypotension or severe pain due to reversal of the analgesic effect of the opioid drug.

CAUDAL EPIDURALS IN CHILDREN

Caudal anaesthesia can provide both intraoperative and postoperative analgesia for procedures up to the umbilicus, especially orchidopexy, circumcision, inguinal herniotomy, lower limb and pelvic orthopaedic procedures and lower abdominal surgery in neonates. The block extends over a wider area than for adults possibly because of the lower density of epidural fat. It is relatively easy to perform as anatomical abnormalities rarely appear before the second decade.

Dose

The dose depends on the size of the child and the level to be blocked (Table 5.5). There is a linear relationship between the dose in millilitres, the dermatome to be blocked and age:

- Up to 7 years – 0.056 mL/kg per dermatome
- Children <6 months – 1 mL/kg; 0.125 per cent will block lower thoracic dermatomes
- At 6 months – 0.25 per cent will block inguinal dermatomes if the child is <20 kg
- At 20 kg the results are inconsistent
- Sacral dermatomes will be blocked by 0.3–0.5 mL/kg at all ages

Age may provide better accuracy but with many neonates with variable weights requiring surgery, it is easier to use mL/kg. Aim to avoid motor block as children do not like paraesthesia or being unable to move. Use less than 20 mL of local anaesthetic.

Side effects

Urinary retention is rare when using 0.25 per cent bupivacaine and hypotension is rare in children under 8 years. Itching can be severe when using an opioid and is often best to use just local anaesthetic. Opioids are used in adults to reduce sympathetic effects of the local anaesthetic but these are rare in children and therefore they do not need opioids.

EPIDURALS

Epidurals (see also Box 5.4) can provide excellent analgesia in children for major procedures but are rarely essential. In neonates and infants the fat in the epidural space is spongy and loculated with spaces between the lobules allowing the passage of a catheter from the sacral region to any level. This becomes more difficult with increasing age because of the development of the lumbar lordosis and the increased density of epidural fat. The lobules become more densely packed and connected by fibrous strands. If the procedure is difficult then it should be abandoned.

Epidurals are good for major surgery, children with respiratory disease and ex-premature babies. The differences between paediatric and adult epidurals are:

- Children have reduced sympathetic tone and therefore less hypotension.
- Blood volume in the splanchnic circulation and lower limbs is less in children.
- Children show more cardiovascular stability with epidural analgesia.
- Children over 8 years have a variable reduction in heart rate and blood pressure but it may be severe with hypovolaemia.

Dose

There are many infusion regimens and none is superior to the others. The main concern is to keep the total dose low to minimize systemic toxicity. The combination of local anaesthetic and opioid minimizes the dose of each drug. The following are examples of combinations and doses that can be used:

- Bupivacaine 0.25 per cent = 4 mg/kg per day total
- Bupivacaine 0.125 per cent + fentanyl 1 μg/mL. Maximum 0.5 mL/kg per hour and aim for 0.2 mL/kg per hour
- Bupivacaine 0.125 per cent + diamorphine 50–160 μg/mL 0.1–0.5 mL/kg per hour
- 0.125 per cent bupivacaine + fentanyl 2 μg/mL run at 0.2–0.3 mL/kg per hour
- 0.125 per cent bupivacaine + 2.5 μg/mL clonidine run at 0.2–0.3 mL/kg per hour. Reduces nausea from fentanyl and better for muscle spasms, e.g. for cerebral palsy or scoliosis

---

Table 5.5 *Various caudal epidural blocks for children*

Block	Volume (mL/kg)	Time
Armitage recommends using 0.5% bupivacaine		
Lumbosacral	0.5 mL/kg (circumcision)	6–8 hours
Thoracolumbar	1.0 mL/kg (hernia)	6–8 hours
Mid-thoracic	1.25 mL/kg (orchidopexy)	>3 hours

BOX 5.4 **Depth of the epidural space in the lumbar region**

- Neonates – 4–15 mm
- 4 years old – 10–30 mm
- <20 kg – 10–30 mm
- Guide – 1 mm/kg between the ages of 6 months and 10 years.
- Over 10 years there is a poor correlation.

Side effects

- Fits with prolonged bupivacaine use.
- Urinary retention (increases with age).
- Air embolus may occur with use of loss of resistance to air so saline is better.
- Hypotension is rarely a problem in children <8 years but may occur in older children.
- Generally no low molecular weight heparin or heparin is given to children so the risk of epidural haematoma is less of a problem than in adults.
- The overall incidence of complications is 0.45 per cent.
- Serious complications occur in 1:5000 especially with multiple traumatic attempts.
- Age less than 3 months is associated with more complications.

MANAGEMENT OF ITCHING

When opioids are used epidurally some children will become very itchy. Management is not always effective and the best treatment is to remove the opioid from the infusion. However, the following can be tried to alleviate the itching but they have variable effects:

- Chlorphenamine orally or intravenously:
  - <2 years 1 mg/kg PO twice daily
  - 2–5 years 1–2 mg PO three times daily
  - 6–12 years 2–4 mg PO three times daily
  - >12 years 4 mg four times daily
- Ondansetron 0.1 mg/kg orally or intravenously
- Naloxone 0.5 μg/kg intravenously

SPINAL ANAESTHESIA

The injection is usually given at the level of L4/5 or L3/4. In children under 5 years there is little change in heart rate or blood pressure with spinal anaesthesia. At 6 years and above changes in heart rate and blood pressure are variable.

Technically spinal anaesthesia is difficult in small children and it does not prevent the distress associated with traction on the spermatic cord or the peritoneum. The duration is short and is only suitable for procedures lasting less than an hour.

Spinal anaesthesia used to be recommended for ex-premature babies or premature babies for hernia repair for example, but modern anaesthetic techniques are now so good that general anaesthesia is no longer contraindicated. Spinal anaesthesia requires skill, practice and sufficient awareness of the complications that is difficult to develop with the small number of procedures carried out in this age group.

LOCAL ANAESTHETIC BLOCKS FOR CHILDREN

Penile block

This is one of the methods for providing analgesia for penile surgery, particularly circumcision.

Nerve supply of the penis

Nerve supply is from the second, third and fourth sacral nerve roots. The fibres run in the dorsal nerve of the penis (terminal branch of the pudendal nerve, Fig. 5.3). The nerves run with the artery along the inferior ramus of the pubis through the suspensory ligament of the penis and under the pubic arch where they lie in the floor of the suprapubic space before entering Buck's fascia which is the fibrous tissue that invests the corpus cavernosum. The autonomic nerve supply arises from the inferior hypogastric plexus in the pelvis.

Technique

1. Place a finger under the pubic symphysis in the midline.
2. Raise a skin wheal and insert a 23 G 5 cm needle in the midline vertical to the skin.
3. Pass the needle under the pubis and into the suprapubic space.
4. Inject first to one side of the midline and then the other.
5. 0.2–0.3 mL/kg of 0.5 per cent bupivacaine (**plain**) gives 6–12 hours analgesia.

Complications

- Oedema – makes surgery difficult.
- Arterial compression with forced injection into Buck's fascia may lead to gangrene.

Inguinal nerve block

An inguinal nerve block should be used whenever a child undergoes a hernia repair. The technique is similar to that in

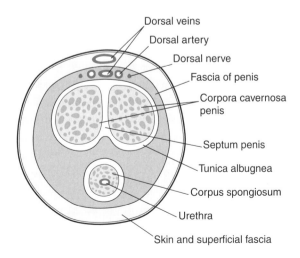

Figure 5.3 *Cross-section of the penis*

an adult and the dose is 0.5 mL/year of age of 0.25 per cent bupivacaine. The block will last approximately four hours. There is a small but significant risk of weakness of the legs due to femoral nerve blockade.

COGNITIVE BEHAVIOURAL THERAPY

Good preparation of the child before surgery is important so they understand what is happening to them. The child and the family should be encouraged to come to the ward before an elective procedure is planned. It is also important to discuss the procedure and the methods of pain relief to reassure the family that pain control is an important part of the overall management. It is especially good for procedure-related pain. This preparation can be carried out on the ward by a play therapist.

When a child has suffered a traumatic incident and is admitted as an emergency, pain control is extremely important. If pain is poorly managed the child grows to fear movement and procedures, the anticipation of the pain can make the situation very difficult. Simple pain relieving measures may not be sufficient and the child becomes extremely anxious and distressed. Cognitive behavioural therapy at this stage can:

- improve pain control by teaching specific pain reducing strategies
- modify any behaviour (child or staff) that intensifies pain
- reduce the child's emotional distress by decreasing the aversive significance or meaning of pain to the child or family.

Methods

- Reinforcement/incentive.
- Behavioural rehearsal.
- Active coaching by parent or staff.
- Distraction and attention: child's attention fully involved with an activity or topic, music, lights, toys, conversation, computers, movies.
- Guided imagery: the child is guided to recall or vividly describe a previous positive experience, story or sensation. The more vividly they experience it the less pain they feel.
- Behavioural therapy: exercise and relaxation – relaxing and loosening a fist, rhythmically raising and lowering a leg, deep breathing, etc. all minimize pain.

Improving acute pain management in children

- Remember the different psychological needs of children, their differing physiological development and reserve,

the differing pharmacokinetics and pharmacodynamics and the specific complications in children.

- Preparation and support during painful events is essential. Parental presence may be of more benefit than any other single measure, providing reassurance and distraction.
- Environment and personnel should be non-threatening and child friendly.
- Avoid prolonged starvation and dehydration.
- Encourage parental involvement, e.g. cooling and rubbing, massage.
- See Boxes 5.5–5.7.

BOX 5.5 Doses of commonly prescribed analgesics

Opioids

- Morphine – 0.15–0.20 mg/kg (titrate in 50 μg/kg aliquots to avoid nausea and vomiting) intravenously two to four hourly; 10–40 μg/kg per hour by intravenous infusion
- Morphine suppositories – 1 mg/2.5 mg/5 mg/10 mg available; 1 mg/kg per 24 hours; <1 year = 1 mg maximum
- Oral morphine 0.2 mg/kg four hourly (not for neonates)
- Codeine phosphate 1 mg/kg PO four to six hourly (NOT to be given intravenously)
- Cocodamol one effervescent tablet = 500 mg paracetamol: 8 mg codeine
- For children >7 years – half to one tablet PO four to six hourly

Non-opioids

- Paracetamol 30 mg/kg preoperatively PO **then** 20 mg/kg PO four hourly; OR 30–40 mg/kg PR eight hourly (maximum recommended dose 100 mg/kg per day)
- Review treatment at 48 hours

NSAIDs

- Diclofenac suppository prep – 12.5 mg/25 mg/50 mg/ 100 mg tablets; 25 mg/50 mg dispersible tablets; dose is 12 mg/kg with maximum recommended dose 3 mg/kg per day by any route; **caution** with **asthma, renal impairment** and with **low platelets**
- Ketorolac intravenous preparation – dose 0.2–0.5 mg/kg single intraoperative dose
- Ibuprofen tablets – 200 mg or elixir 20 mg/mL; dose 5 mg/kg six hourly; 20 mg/kg per day maximum dose

BOX 5.6 Intravenous morphine infusions

Give an adequate loading dose of morphine (see below) before starting the continuous intravenous infusion. The infusion rate can be adjusted with reference to the patient's pain score. The intravenous infusion should be given via a separate cannula or a one-way valve (Cardiff valve). Remember it is the intravenous fluid and **not** the morphine that goes through the valve.

Dosage

- 1 mg/kg made up to 50 mL with normal saline
- 1 mL/h = 20 μg/kg per hour
- Initial setting – 5–10 μg/kg per hour
- Maximum – 15–20 μg/kg per hour
- Loading dose –
   <1 month = 25 μg/kg;
   1–3 months = 50 μg/kg;
   >3 months = 100–150 μg/kg given in 50 μg/kg
       aliquots
- Intravenous infusion – maximum doses are
   0–1 month = 5 μg/kg per hour;
   1–3 months = 10 μg/kg/hour;
   >3 months = 40 μg/kg/hour

BOX 5.7 Commonly prescribed adjuvant drugs

- **Respiratory depression** – intravenous naloxone 4 μg/kg repeated as necessary is the routine prescription for all patients receiving intravenous opioids
- **Nausea/vomiting** – PO/intravenous ondansetron 0.1–0.2 mg/kg eight hourly
- **Pruritus, urinary retention** – intravenous naloxone 0.5 μg/kg repeat every 10 minutes; maximum × 4 = routine prescription for all patients receiving intravenous opioids. Chlorphenamine – 0.1 mg/kg intravenously eight hourly for resistant pruritus via sedative effect

Children with learning disabilities

THE PAIN EXPERIENCE

Information about pain in children with cognitive impairment is lacking. It is possible that the pain experience may be different in children with learning disabilities and studies have demonstrated elevated pain thresholds in 25 per cent of patients with cerebral palsy. Alterations in motor, sensory and autonomic systems may have a profound effect on the experience of pain. Conditions such as cerebral palsy may affect the ability to comprehend and communicate pain but whether this reflects a true insensitivity to pain is not certain.

PAIN ASSESSMENT

Most parents feel that healthcare providers have difficulty in assessing and treating pain in these children. Parents and carers are often the best people to assess the child's distress and can help with differentiation between hunger, anxiety, discomfort and other causes of distress.

Assessment is difficult because of problems of communication. Behavioural indicators such as facial grimacing, groaning or altered sleep patterns may be present in the non-pain state. Children with mild to moderate cognitive impairment have been described as directly communicating their pain in a similar way to those without impairment.

Little work has been done on producing good tools to measure pain in the adult or child with learning disability, and indicators of pain in cognitively impaired children can be significantly different from unimpaired children and between themselves. The following have been found to be related to pain and all seven changes improve as pain decreases postoperatively:

- Tense face
- Grimace
- Corner of the mouth turned down
- Eyes almost closed
- Eyes squeezed
- Frightened/fearful look
- Looks or turns red

MANAGEMENT

Identify problem

- Is there a possibility of pain?
- Maintain high index of suspicion.
- Adequate assessment and reassessment.
- Consider trial of analgesia.
- Physiologic changes/behaviour/grimacing.
- Cognitive evaluation – how well the patient expresses pain.

Consider possible causes of pain

- Intravenous infusion
- Sore throat
- Headache
- Full bladder
- Anxiety/fear
- Fatigue
- Absence of parent or guardian

It is important to differentiate pain from hunger, anxiety, discomfort from positioning and other causes.

PRINCIPLES OF TREATMENT

- Use communication aids where possible.
- The use of a questionnaire for parents and carers detailing how the child communicates and how they react to pain and hunger and other situations may help one work out what is wrong.
- Respect the opinions of parents and carers. They may be aggressive but this is often as a result of previous experience, stress, frustration, anger or guilt.
- Manage pain the same as for all other patients.
- Analgesia should be based on the regular assessment of pain.
- Use analgesic ladder ± benzodiazepines.
- Use antispasmodics as necessary.
- Do not prescribe drugs on an 'as required' basis as the children do not ask.
- Titrate the dose to the effect. Give small amounts at frequent intervals.
- Use regional and local anaesthesia where indicated.
- Monitor side effects.

PAIN MANAGEMENT IN ELDERLY PATIENTS

Pain management remains a peripheral focus in the management of elderly patients (see also Box 5.8).

Reasons

- Lower expectations of the impact of analgesia in the elderly patient.
- Fears of overmedication by patient and healthcare staff.
- Increased side effects from medication.
- Resource issues – pain assessment is labour intensive.
- Lack of research – research excludes patients over 65 years.
- Many elderly patients appear apathetic or depressed.
- There may be irritability because of intellectual disability, visual defects and hearing problems.
- Many elderly patients have a fear of being a nuisance and try not to complain. They often do not mention pain.
- Communication barriers.
- Poor pain assessment tools for the demented patient.

Management

Adhere to key principles of pain pharmacology and use analgesic drugs as for all other groups of patients. Treatment strategies should be individualized.

BOX 5.8 Physiological differences in the elderly patient

- Pain perception and response to acute pain stimulus are not diminished in cognitively impaired or elderly patients. No evidence that those over 70 years feel less pain. Similarly in Alzheimer's but slower cortical processing of nociceptive input
- No evidence that pain causes less change in ventilation or behaviour disturbance than in the young
- Effects of analgesics and narcotics are greater in the elderly. More side effects from NSAIDs
- Volume distribution is smaller especially when the drug is strongly protein bound (i.e. may need smaller doses)
- Most morphine in the body is found in the muscle. If there is less muscle there is more free morphine available (i.e. may need smaller doses)
- Biotransformation and excretion less effective because of decreased blood flow to liver and kidneys
- Poor renal function so slower clearance of drugs. NSAIDs may contribute to renal failure
- Increased central nervous system depression with opioids further increased by cerebral hypoxia from arterial thickening
- Epidural anaesthesia more widespread for a given volume or mass of drug
- Reduced ventilatory responses to hypoxia and hypercarbia

Drug treatment

MORPHINE

Opioids are good for pain management in the elderly but they usually require a reduced dose. The initial dose should be calculated as: 100 − age in years = 24 hour morphine dose. The metabolite M-6-G accumulates in renal failure and the elderly patient may have poor renal function. Opioid use requires care in the elderly over a period of time.

PETHIDINE

Do not use pethidine in elderly patients: the metabolite nor-pethidine accumulates because of its long half-life and causes fits, especially with reduced renal function.

NSAIDs

The risk of side effects from NSAIDs is very much increased in elderly people. The risk of death in the over 65 year age group with long-term treatment with conventional NSAIDs is 1:1200. Recent research has shown that the COX-2 NSAIDs are associated with significant problems, especially when patients have cardiac problems or hypertension. NSAIDs of any kind are best avoided in the elderly except for very short-term treatment.

Other treatments

Because of the side effects caused by many analgesic drugs in elderly patients it is best to use regional/local blocks and consider non-pharmacologic methods wherever possible. Consider regional techniques (e.g. spinals for fractured hips); caudals (e.g. for vaginal hysterectomy, haemorrhoids, etc.); femoral cannula for fractured neck of femur; micro-waveable hot water bottle for pain; transcutaneous electrical nerve stimulation (TENS); aromatherapy; ultrasound; music; acupuncture; topical preparations; massage; reflexology; relaxation; and distraction.

Confusion in elderly patients

Confusion in the elderly is not usually due to opioids. Many other causes are more likely to be responsible including hypoxia, sleep deprivation, other drugs, sepsis and an unfamiliar environment.

Pain in elderly patients with dementia

DO PATIENTS WITH DEMENTIA EXPERIENCE PAIN?

- Communicative dementia patients' reports of pain tend to be as valid as those of cognitively intact individuals.
- A moderate decrease in pain occurs in cognitively impaired elderly with neuroanatomy changes.
- Assessment scales developed so far require improvement in accuracy and facility.

PAIN MANAGEMENT

Pain management should be the same as in the elderly cognitively intact patient. As assessment of pain is difficult, it is often worth a trial of analgesia to see if the patient improves.

Pain is poorly managed in patients with dementia and pain assessment is the cornerstone of pain management. Cognitively impaired patients are less likely to report problems with pain. It is possible to assess pain by a combination of interview and interpretation of reactions during activity but this can be very time consuming; physical examination is a valuable complement to this process.

Fear and confusion can interact with pain to cause resistance and aggression. Moderate cognitive impairment might exacerbate the impact of pain on the depressed affect. Cognitively impaired patients may experience greater affective distress as a function of their pain than do more intact patients. Aggression scores are higher in cognitively impaired patients with pain.

PAIN MANAGEMENT IN PATIENTS ON LONG-TERM OPIOID USE

Patients with cancer will often be prescribed opioid analgesics and may take up to 6 g morphine a day. Patients with non-malignant pain may also be prescribed long-term opioids to manage their chronic pain and may be taking large doses.

Postoperative opioid prescribing in opioid-tolerant patients

Partial agonists should be avoided because they may precipitate withdrawal. For patients on long-term opioids (Fig. 5.4), it may be necessary to convert oral morphine/fentanyl, etc. to parenteral morphine in the perioperative period. These patients usually have much higher post-operative requirements than non-opioid-treated patients. An exception to this would be if the operation removed their 'original' pain. If this is the case, cessation of opioid therapy will need to be monitored to avoid acute withdrawal effects but, in practice, if the patient has been taking MST (slow release morphine) in a dose just sufficient to relieve their pain it is rarely a problem.

Because of the doses (and volumes) of morphine involved it is sometimes impractical to use PCA or intramuscular injections in this group of patients. Therefore, if the patient is nil by mouth an intravenous infusion of morphine in the immediate postoperative period provides the appropriate amount of morphine. If the patient is absorbing orally, MST can be continued with PCA for additional analgesia. A fentanyl patch can be continued throughout the perioperative period, with PCA for postoperative pain. These patients may require a larger bolus than normal but this should be assessed on an individual basis.

Guidelines for the management of acute pain in drug abusers

The aims of pain management in drug abusers are to provide good pain relief and prevent symptoms of signs of withdrawal during the postoperative period.

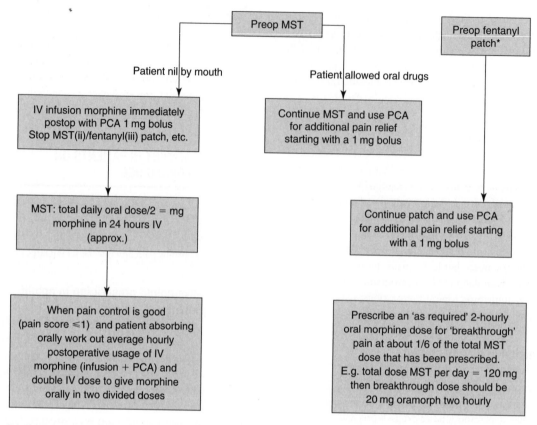

Figure 5.4 *Pain management for patients on long-term opioid treatment.* *Fentanyl 25 μg patch = 100 mg oral morphine/24 h = 50 mg IV/24 h. MST, slow release morphine; IV, intravenous; PCA, patient controlled analgesia*

THE PROBLEMS

- There is often associated disease including hepatic damage, and difficult venous access.
- There is often increased agitation postoperatively.
- Postoperative hypotension may be a sign of bleeding but also of drug withdrawal.
- The postoperative period is not the time to discuss treatment programmes for withdrawal.
- Patients may also be addicted to other drugs, e.g. alcohol, barbiturates, benzodiazepines.
- Signs and symptoms of withdrawal from these drugs must be monitored – agitation, delirium tremens, etc.
- The patient can be very demanding of analgesia and may injure him- or herself or the staff.
- In an emergency situation, overdose or withdrawal may be present on arrival in hospital.

THE MANAGEMENT PLAN (FIG. 5.5)

- Drug and alcohol rehabilitation services may need to be involved.

- Treat signs of withdrawal with methadone.
- Use regional anaesthesia where possible.
- Agree with the patient and adhere to a treatment plan, dose of the drug and timing.
- PCA is good because of possible large opioid requirements – ensure it is tamperproof and use the minimum reservoir possible. It avoids staff–patient confrontations about pain relief.

Why use methadone?

Withdrawal from opiates is not life threatening. However, the symptoms of withdrawal can be extremely uncomfortable. Methadone can help control these withdrawal symptoms. The methadone that is prescribed may not feel the same as regular drug use, as it is designed to act over a longer period of time. However, it does act in the same way as other opiates and so will stop the withdrawal symptoms.

How is it prescribed?

Sometimes it is necessary to ask the patient to sign a methadone contract (see Box 5.9). This outlines what the

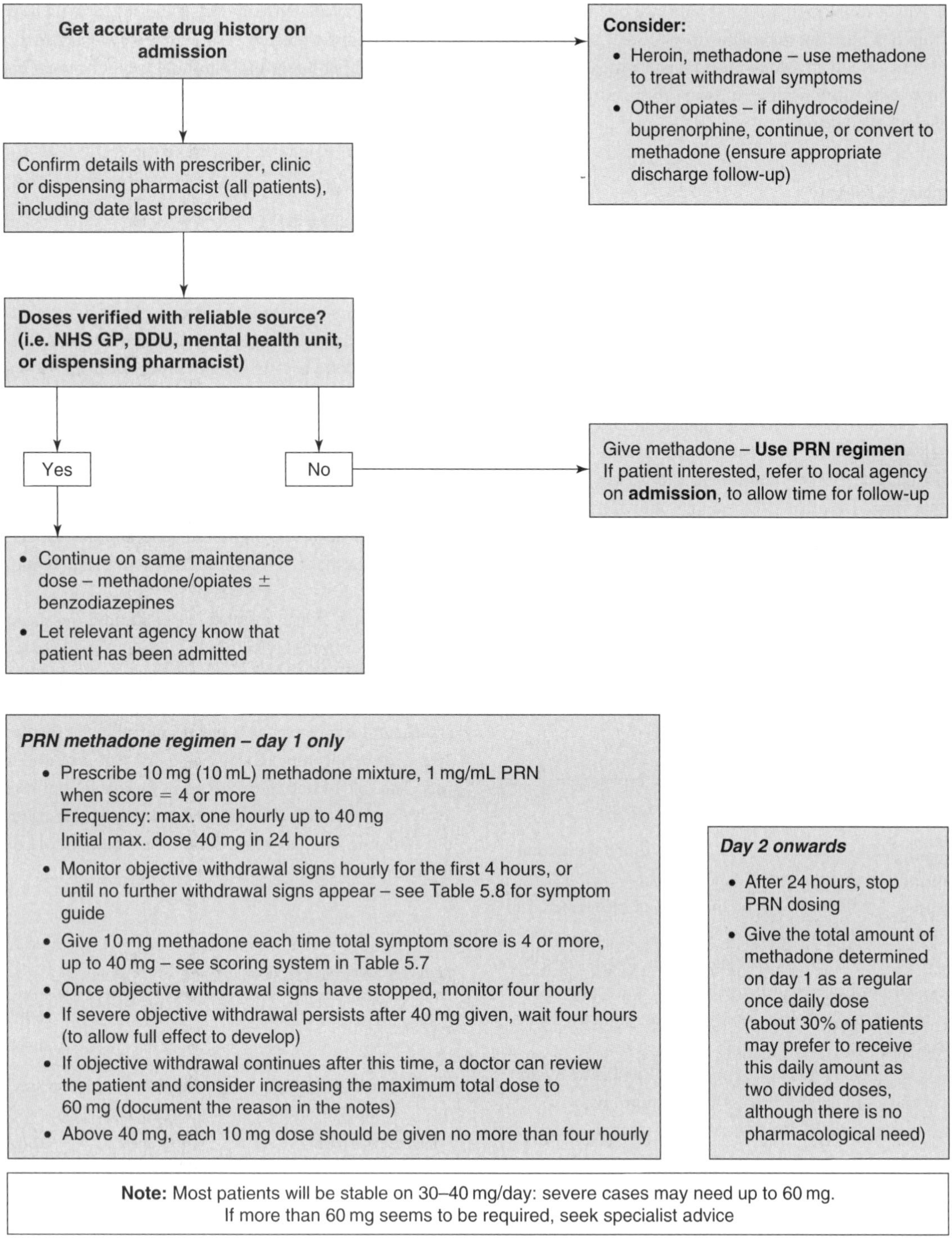

Figure 5.5 *Management of opioid drug users/methadone programme patients. DDU, drug dependency unit*

patient's and the hospital staff's responsibilities are while prescribing methadone. If the patient is already in a methadone maintenance programme, and the current dose can be confirmed with the prescribing agency, the same amount of methadone should be continued. If the methadone cannot be confirmed, an assessment of withdrawal symptoms should be made on day 1 of the admission and an appropriate amount of methadone prescribed. There is a set maximum limit, above which more methadone should not be given. In the UK, this has been set according to national guidelines at 60 mg daily. The methadone must be consumed in front of the nurse who administers the drug. This is a requirement for all controlled drugs.

Prescribing methadone

Heroin or other opioid (Table 5.6)

Ask how much drug the patient is using. It is important to find out how much they use and not how much they buy. They will often share the drug among friends, but only give information of how much they buy. Most bags of street heroin are packed as 0.2 g = 15 mg methadone. This will cost about £10, so if you know how much they spend, you can calculate how much they use. Sometimes the size of the bag will vary, and the patient will usually know how much they get for their money. You must ask how much is in the bag. Heroin 1 g is roughly equivalent to 60 mg methadone.

The methadone should be given in the morning. About a third of patients will not have 24 hours benefit from a single dose. If they are distressed by the morning, the methadone dose can be split into two doses.

When the patient is admitted an adequate dose of methadone should be prescribed to prevent opiate withdrawal symptoms (calculated as above). If the patient is nil by mouth and requires pain relief PCA should be set up as normal, starting with a 1 mg bolus and 5-minute lockout time. This may need to be altered later. If oral analgesia can be used, consider paracetamol, and an NSAID regularly with cocodamol 30/500 or Oramorph 10 mg two hourly as required.

Buprenorphine (Subutex®)

Buprenorphine is a synthetic opioid drug. It is a partial μ opioid agonist that is being increasingly used in the treatment of opioid dependence because it is associated with milder withdrawal symptoms on dose reduction. It is safer than methadone because of its ceiling effect on the respiratory depressant effects. Buprenorphine withdrawal is easier and safer but should be overseen by a specialist drugs team so all patients presenting on this treatment will be known to a drug team that can be contacted to plan further treatment. The typical addiction dose used is 4–16 mg daily. As with methadone, however, buprenorphine should not be used for the treatment of pain, only to manage withdrawal symptoms.

A relatively large number of μ opioid receptors are occupied by buprenorphine, which limits the access to these receptors by other opioid agonists such as morphine. The high affinity of buprenorphine for the receptors means that it is difficult for other opioids such as morphine to displace it – 16 mg buprenorphine blocks 79–95 per cent μ opioid receptors. The role of buprenorphine in this area is continuing to evolve but it may cause difficulty when a patient requires opioid analgesia. Specialist help should be requested when dealing with these patients wherever possible.

BOX 5.9 Methadone administration contract

I .... understand that as an inpatient on Ward .... at .... Hospital, I will be given methadone as prescribed in accordance with my clinical need.

I have been shown the scoring system that is used to assess my clinical need for methadone, and understand that methadone will only be given to me in accordance with this system.

If I experience withdrawal symptoms, I will inform my nurse and allow them to assess these symptoms.

I also understand that I will not receive methadone if I:

- threaten to discharge myself from hospital
- behave in an aggressive or threatening manner to other patients or staff.

If I break the terms of this prescription contract, I may be asked to leave ward.

Signed .... (Patient)
Signed .... (Nurse)
Date ....

Table 5.6 *Methadone conversion table*

Drug	Dose	Methadone equivalent
Street heroin (diamorphine)	Purity varies, 1 gm is roughly 50–80 mg methadone	
Pharmaceutical heroin	10 mg tablet	20 mg
	30 mg ampoule	60 mg
Morphine	10 mg ampoule (oral)	10 mg
Dihydrocodeine	30 mg tablet	3 mg
Pethidine	50 mg tablet	5 mg
	50 mg ampoule	5 mg
Codeine phosphate	30 mg tablet	2 mg
	60 mg tablet	3 mg
Dextromoramide	5 mg tablet	5–10 mg

Problems may occur when a patient has taken their buprenorphine dose for the day and then requires opioid analgesia for pain relief. Most people can use analgesics on top of the buprenorphine and still get some effect but there may be some clinically significant effects of the opioid receptor blockade by buprenorphine. There is very little experience in the management of these patients but it appears that short-acting opioids and PCA can be used safely to treat severe pain. The best way to manage both pain and withdrawal is therefore similar to those patients taking methadone – use the buprenorphine to manage the symptoms of withdrawal and morphine to treat pain.

Equivalent doses

Equivalence tables are very complex and can only be used as a rough guide to doses required:

- Buprenorphine dose used to treat pain 0.2–0.4 mg three times daily
- 1 g of heroin is equivalent to approximately 8–12 mg buprenorphine
- Methadone 30–40 mg is equivalent to 4–8 mg buprenophine
- Methadone 60 mg is equivalent to 8–12 mg buprenophine

Benzodiazepines

Benzodiazepines are the least addictive drugs. High doses for a long time are necessary to cause physiological dependence, e.g. 500 mg/day (compared to physical withdrawal within weeks of using opioids).

- Use for 2–3 years – 25 per cent will have physical withdrawal
- Use for 8–9 years – 75–80 per cent will have physical withdrawal

Most patients do not need these high doses and will not withdraw although they may become agitated. Fits and delirium tremens can occur but this is very rare. It is often necessary to negotiate but it should never be necessary to supply more than 30–60 mg a day.

Crack cocaine

Crack cocaine is a very short-acting drug. There should be no physical withdrawal. Depression and psychosis may occur but these are rare. There may be a rebound reduction in mood and they may become sleepy. Supportive psychological care is usually all that is necessary but symptomatic treatment may rarely be required. Appetite usually improves when the drug has been stopped. If there is any question that the patient is using street drugs while in hospital, the pathology laboratory can carry out a urine immunological screen for confirmation.

GENERAL MANAGEMENT

- Check for signs of infection:
  - Viral hepatitis
  - Hepatitis B and C
  - HIV
  - Bacterial endocarditis
  - Tuberculosis
  - Septicaemia, pneumonia, deep vein thrombosis, pulmonary embolism, abscess, dental disease
- Enquire about alcohol dependence
- Avoid all partial agonist drugs such as nalbuphine and buprenorphine for pain management and avoid initiating benzodiazepines if possible.

MANAGEMENT OF POSTOPERATIVE PAIN

Pain tolerance remains low for years after drug addiction and the patient is more likely to become addicted on challenge with narcotic drugs so use regional analgesia if possible (Box 5.10). If opioid drugs must be used they should be withdrawn as soon as possible. **Avoid** using methadone to treat pain.

The use of patient controlled analgesia

Patients often need a larger than average PCA bolus dose and they may benefit from a background infusion. When the patient is a drug abuser the opioid intake is usually variable because street drugs are never pure. The patient often has a

---

BOX 5.10 Management of pain in drug abusers

Mild to moderate pain

Methadone as per guidelines

- + NSAIDs
- + paracetamol
- + regional/local technique where possible – will not prevent withdrawal. Prescribe methadone as per guidelines also

Severe pain

Methadone as per guidelines

- PCA – allow unrestricted use for 24 hours within set parameters. May need to increase the bolus dose. May need background infusion to prevent withdrawal if methadone cannot be taken orally
- Epidural – will not prevent withdrawal. Prescribe methadone as per guidelines also

fear of withdrawal and being without access to an opioid can make them very agitated even though they are not experiencing withdrawal. Allowing them to decide when they use the PCA and avoiding confrontation with medical staff can improve management of pain in these patients.

Oral analgesia should be started as soon as possible. Restart methadone orally at the normal dose if the patient is already on a methadone programme and prescribe additional oral analgesia as necessary.

If a patient is a reformed drug abuser

- He or she may tolerate a considerable amount of pain without opioid treatment in order to prevent relapse into dependency.
- Be sensitive to the fact that relapse to opioid abuse may result from opioid medication.
- Discuss the pain control options with the patient.

Withdrawal can occur in patients who have had large doses of opioids for as little as two weeks. The severity of withdrawal IS NOT necessarily related to the quantity of drug consumed. Untreated heroin withdrawal reaches its peak at 36–72 hours after the last dose and subsides substantially after five days. Methadone withdrawal peaks at 4–6 days subsiding at 10–12 days.

Discharge from hospital

- If a patient is receiving prescriptive treatment from a general practice/specialist services it is essential they have early notification of the discharge date.
- If the patient is on an opioid substitute it is essential to liaise with the general practice/specialist services to agree a discharge plan.
- Patients should not be discharged on combination analgesics because of the risk of potential paracetamol overdose.
- Where opioid intake has been reduced, warn the patient against returning to preadmission street drug dose. Tolerance to respiratory depression will have decreased.

What happens when the patient leaves leave hospital?

While the patient is in hospital he or she should be given the opportunity to contact a local drug treatment agency to arrange their own continuing care. Methadone should not be prescribed for the patient to take home. They will need to contact the local drug treatment agency for an appointment if they would like to begin a community detox or maintenance programme. If the patient intends to restart heroin or non-prescribed methadone they must be warned of the risk of overdose. Tolerance for a certain drug builds

Table 5.7 *Withdrawal symptoms 1: vital signs and corresponding scores*

Symptoms	Score
Pupils dilated $\geq 5\,mm$	2
Pinned pupils $\leq 2\,mm$	−2
Restlessness	1
Drowsy	−1
Sweating	2
Skin goosebumps	1 = barely palpable
	2 = readily palpable
Pallor	1
Yawning	1
Runny eyes (1 = eyes watery; 2 = eyes streaming)	2
Runny nose (1 = sniffing; 2 = profuse)	2
Pulse rate 20 beats or faster than baseline	1
Pulse rate 30 beats or faster than baseline	2
Pulse rate 20 beats or slower than baseline	−2
BP 20 points or more above baseline	1
BP 30 points or more above baseline	2
BP 20 points or more below baseline	−2
Tremors	1

BP, blood pressure.

up over time; tolerance may have decreased while in hospital. Half the usual dose may be as much as the body can cope with.

Many general practitioners (GPs) are unhappy about patients being discharged on methadone and will refuse to prescribe it. Do not give any drug abuser more than one day's supply of methadone at discharge – it is a very dangerous drug when taken in large quantities. If the patient is discharged at a weekend, or when their GP is unavailable and they need a longer supply, each methadone dose must be prescribed on a separate script so they can only get one dose at a time. The pharmacist will give this dose.

Vital signs to observe for withdrawal (Table 5.7)

A score of 4 or more indicates significant withdrawal and methadone should be given.

Other withdrawal symptoms

See Table 5.8.

Primary withdrawal symptoms

Temperature, blood pressure, pulse and pupil size are not affected by alcohol or benzodiazepine withdrawal; if pupils are constricted then previous opioid is still affecting the patient.

Table 5.8 *Withdrawal symptoms 2*

Opioid		Benzodiazepine	
Moderate	**Severe**	**Moderate**	**Severe**
Muscle aches and pains	Vomiting	Anxiety	Feelings of unreality
Pupil dilatation	Piloerection (hair standing on end)	Sweating	Abnormal sensation of movement/body
Nausea	Tachycardia	Insomnia	Hypersensitivity to stimuli
Yawning	Elevated blood pressure	Headache	Psychosis
			Epileptic seizures
		Tremor	
		Nausea	

Most challenging symptoms to treat

These are the symptoms that can persist several weeks into a methadone programme – do not increase the methadone but treat the symptoms themselves:

- Insomnia – avoid benzodiazepines; if absolutely necessary try oral promethazine 25–50 mg at night but review before discharge.
- Aches/pains – use NSAIDs/paracetamol if appropriate.
- Diarrhoea – try loperamide 2 mg as required, up to 16 mg/24 h.

For patients admitted on dihydrocodeine/codeine or other opioids (other than for pain relief) follow the same process as for methadone, confirming the dose with a National Health Service (NHS) prescriber or dispensing pharmacist. If still current, continue the confirmed dose. If unconfirmed or non-current, start with a reasonable baseline dose (e.g. 60 mg eight hourly) and titrate to objective withdrawal symptoms.

ANALGESIA FOR NEUROSURGERY

Orthostatic or low-pressure headache

A low-pressure headache is usually a global headache, made worse by sitting up and associated with nausea and/or vomiting and sometimes dizziness or diplopia, sixth nerve palsy and tinnitus.

OTHER FEATURES

- The time to onset of the headache on standing is immediate to 265 minutes.

- The time to resolution on lying ranges from 0 to 15 minutes.
- The more sudden the onset of the headache the greater the severity of the pain.
- Those who have migraine and headaches are more susceptible to postural headaches.
- These headaches are more common in younger women.
- The onset can be from 15 minutes to 12 days after initiating event.
- The average duration of pain is four to eight days.
- Pain is not affected by the amount of fluid removed, or the number of times the fluid is removed.

MECHANISMS OF PAIN

Cerebral and meningeal vessels are pain sensitive; brain parenchyma, choroid plexus and the dura are less sensitive. The aetiology of low-pressure pain remains speculative. Low pressure may lead to traction on pain sensitive structures. Magnetic resonance imaging (MRI) reveals abnormalities such as descent of the cerebellar tonsils, and MRI scans with gadolinium reveal changes in 90 per cent of patients. Radio-isotope scans may reveal the site of the leak.

CAUSES

Low-pressure headache is usually seen in patients following the loss of a large volume of cerebrospinal fluid (CSF) as in:

- Lumbar puncture (there may be recurrence of the headache up to six months after an epidural blood patch)
- Surgery
  - Trans-sphenoidal hypophysectomy
  - Foramen magnum decompression
  - Microvascular decompression of cranial nerve V
  - Head/back injury

The pain may be exacerbated by:

- Intercourse
- Sneezing
- Coughing
- Exercise
- Nose blowing

TREATMENT

The most effective treatment appears to be:

- Intravenous fluids (to supplement oral intake, aiming for 3 L total daily input).
- Regular laxatives.
- Bed rest.

Table 5.9 *Differential diagnosis of pain of neurosurgical procedures*

Major pain	Intermediate pain	Minor pain
Complex cervical surgery	Craniotomy, cranioplasty	Intracranial pressure bolt insertion
Cervical laminectomy	Posterior fossa decompression	Burr hole biopsy
Complex thoracic surgery	Transphenoidal hypophysectomy	Trigeminal thermocoagulation
Thoracic laminectomy and fusion	Ventroperitoneal shunt (local should be used in abdominal wound)	Drainage of chronic subdural haematoma
Complex lumbar surgery	Anterior cervical decompression	Carpal tunnel decompression
Lumbar laminectomy	Lumbar microdiscectomy	Ulnar nerve transposition
Foramen magnum decompression	Spinal cord stimulator	Muscle biopsy
	Deep brain stimulator	

BOX 5.11 Analgesic regimens for neurosurgical pain

Major and intermediate pain (pain score 2–3)

- Regular analgesia
- Paracetamol 1 g four times daily orally and NSAIDs orally (if not contraindicated)
- Morphine intravenous PCA or codeine phosphate 60 mg or tramadol 50–100 mg four times daily if unable to use PCA

Minor pain (pain score 1–2)

- Regular analgesia
- Paracetamol 1 g four times daily
- NSAIDs
- Codeine phosphate 60 mg or tramadol 50–100 mg four times daily (given with paracetamol)

- Regular antiemetics (cyclizine can be very useful).
- Patients who fail to respond to conservative treatment may need an epidural blood patch.
- Caffeine in the form of Coca-Cola® (not the decaffeinated variety!), strong tea or coffee. For an unknown reason, low-pressure headache often improves with caffeine but it may lead to insomnia. Give:
  - caffeine 300 mg orally or
  - caffeine 500 mg IV.
- Theophylline 300 mg orally may help.

Classification of pain of neurosurgical procedures

See Table 5.9 and Box 5.11. Tight head bandages can also be a source of headache.

Intracranial surgery and morphine

Used carefully, morphine is safe to use after intracranial surgery. Patients with abnormal pupils usually have neurological reasons and the use of morphine does not interfere with this finding. Patient controlled analgesia is to be recommended but if necessary intramuscular morphine can be prescribed for this group of patients with care: >60 kg–10 mg; 45–60 kg–7.5 mg and <45 kg–5.0 mg. These doses should be 'tailored' to the patient's neurological status.

Important pain-relieving adjuvants include:

- neck roll to support back of neck, and arm support to reduce weight of arms in patients following complex cervical spine surgery.
- warm pack, cold pack, airline eye covers (for severe headache and photophobia), physiotherapy, moral support, etc.
- a small dose of benzodiazepines prescribed regularly can be very effective in reducing muscle spasm, e.g. 2 mg diazepam (remember synergism with opioids).
- wound infiltration – postoperative infiltration of the wound with bupivacaine 0.25 per cent with 1:200 000 adrenaline can significantly reduce initial postoperative pain especially; infiltration of the abdominal wound in theatre is particularly effective following insertion of ventriculo peritoneal shunts.
- scalp blocks with 0.5 per cent bupivacaine also reduce postoperative pain.

Scalp blocks

LOCAL INFILTRATION

Bupivacaine 0.25 per cent with 1:200 000 adrenaline infiltrated into the pin sites before fixation, around the incision site subcutaneously preoperatively and at the end of the procedure has been shown to lower heart rate and to reduce pain

Table 5.10 *Scalp blocks for pain of neurosurgical procedures*

Nerve	Technique
Greater, lesser and third auricular nerves	5 mL using 22 G needle infiltrate along the superior nuchal line, approximately half-way between the occipital protuberance and the mastoid process
Supraorbital and supratrochlear nerves (terminal branches of the ophthalmic branch of the trigeminal nerve)	2 mL to each nerve as it emerges from the orbit above the eyebrow with a 22 G needle perpendicular to the skin
Auriculotemporal nerves (terminal branch of the mandibular branch of the trigeminal nerve)	5 mL 2.5 cm anterior to ear at the level of the tragus with needle perpendicular to the skin; 2.5 mL to the deep fascia; and 1.5 mL superficially as the needle is withdrawn
Postauricular branches of the greater auricular nerves	2 mL between the skin and bone 1.5 cm posterior to the ear at the level of the tragus
Zygomaticotemporal (terminal branch of the maxillary branch of the trigeminal nerve)	

scores for at least one hour postoperatively. Scalp blocks performed with ropivacaine or bupivacaine have been shown to have the following beneficial effects:

- reduction in postoperative pain compared with placebo
- no rise in blood pressure during head pinning
- blood coagulability is increased by 20–30 per cent on incision of skin but this effect is attenuated by scalp block.

PROCEDURE

See Table 5.10 and Fig. 5.6. Use 20 mL of 0.5 per cent bupivacaine with or without 1:200 000 adrenaline.

Analgesia regimen for patients with subarachnoid haemorrhage

Most patients with subarachnoid haemorrhage (SAH) are in the 'major' pain category:

- Regular oral paracetamol 1 g six hourly.
- Regular oral codeine phosphate 60 mg or tramadol 100 mg six hourly.
- NSAIDs – only according to the following guidelines:
  - pre-angiography – **no NSAIDs**
  - 'angiogram-negative' SAH – NSAIDs may be introduced 12 hours post-angiogram
  - 'angiogram-positive' SAH – (i.e. patient has aneurysm or arteriovenous malformation) no NSAIDs preoperatively/embolization
  - postoperative clipping/coiling of aneurysm – NSAIDs may be introduced 12 hours postoperatively if the aneurysm has been successfully clipped.

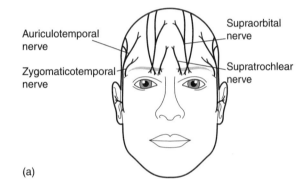

(a)

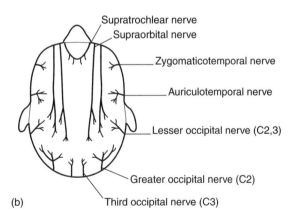

(b)

Figure 5.6 *Scalp innervation: (a) facial view and (b) coronal view*

Also consider:

- regular lactulose 20 mL twice daily
- airline eye covers/ear plugs
- morphine PCA if the patient can manage it, but confusion and vasospasm may limit its use. Start with 1 mg bolus and increase as necessary.

PAIN MANAGEMENT FOR DAY-CASE SURGERY

Pain following discharge from day surgery influences the time taken to return to normal activity and may lead to further unplanned hospitalization. Successful day surgery is dependent on the management of postoperative pain.

Use a protocol for prescribing

Patient education is important, both oral and written as patients are often reluctant to take drugs. Written information for patients, parents and carers improves compliance with analgesic drugs. The information should provide the following information:

- description of drug
- when it should be taken
- how long it should be taken
- side effects of each drug
- who to contact in event of problems.

Patients' expectations of analgesia are low and they expect to have pain. A protocol allows nurses to check drugs and contraindications in patients and avoids duplication. It also allows optimization of analgesia regimens and makes prescribing easy. Other features include:

- all patients are provided with analgesia (not selective)
- preload patient with oral analgesia prior to discharge
- advise patients to take analgesia before local anaesthetic wears off
- use a multimodal approach to analgesia
- when treatment is standardized audit is more straight-forward
- standardized treatment reduces the number of drugs kept in the day surgery unit
- use a similar method for adults and children.

Pain management

- Good pain assessment.
- Preoperative analgesia should be given where possible and when indicated including:
  - regional blocks
  - local infiltration
  - NSAIDs wherever possible
  - paracetamol
  - opioids.
- Use local anaesthetic where possible and use long-acting agents like bupivacaine but beware the long action of some

blocks causing reduced mobility. Spinals are fine as long as there is time for good recovery.
- Use short-acting opioids during surgery as long-acting drugs like morphine increase the risk of nausea and vomiting and hence admission. Low-dose morphine (0.1 mg/kg) may be helpful.

DISCHARGE ANALGESIA

Give NSAIDs, preferably long-acting because there is better compliance. Give paracetamol with or without codeine. Tramadol may be considered but be aware that this may cause nausea and dizziness. Oral opioids may be necessary for some patients.

PAEDIATRIC DAY SURGERY

Use a protocol similar to the adult one but with paediatric doses. Pain assessment is more difficult and parents find pain assessment difficult. Regional and local techniques are very useful. Toys, televisions and videos can distract a child from their discomfort and help with pain management.

STANDARDS

Arrange telephone follow-up after discharge and record:

- pain scores
- number of patients discharged with analgesics
- incidence of severe pain in first 48 hours
- incidence of no pain or mild pain
- number of patients satisfied with pain management.

MANAGEMENT OF PATIENTS WITH FRACTURED RIBS

High-risk patients

These patients have a high morbidity and mortality if not treated actively, and 50 per cent of these fractures will not be detected in chest radiographs. Therefore a high index of suspicion and careful clinical assessment are essential. (NB 35 per cent will develop pulmonary complication and 10–15 per cent will die.) These patients include:

- smokers and patients with respiratory disease
- obese or poorly nourished patients
- patients over 60 years
- patients with multiple trauma, especially head injuries, abdominal injuries, fractures of the pelvis and multiple limb fractures
- flail segment, pulmonary contusion or other chest injuries.

If inadequately treated these patients will develop pulmonary complications about 24–48 hours post injury.

MANAGEMENT

Inform

- Acute pain service
- On-call ITU registrar out of hours, or for patients in the high-risk category or those with multiple trauma
- Ward physiotherapist and when appropriate the on-call physiotherapist.

Monitor

In addition to routine observations, all these patients should have the following recordings:

- regular pain and sedation scores
- pulse oximetry
- respiratory rate.

Analgesia

Analgesia should be instituted as soon as possible after admission and must be adequate to allow the patient to take deep breaths and cough. This will help prevent pulmonary complications.

Suggested analgesic regimen: AIM for a pain score of 1 to enable deep breathing and coughing.

Simple fractures

Patients with simple fractures who have none of the risk factors given above will probably manage with the following regimen of oral analgesics:

- diclofenac 50 mg eight hourly
- paracetamol 1 g six hourly
- codeine phosphate 60 mg six hourly given with the paracetamol or oral tramadol 50–100 mg, four to six hourly. Tramadol should be avoided in patients with epilepsy or those taking monoamine oxidase inhibitors.

Patients who have indigestion with NSAIDs may benefit from lansoprazole 30 mg orally daily.

Moderately severe fractures

Patients who have other risk factors, pain scores greater than 2 and those whose ability to cough is seriously impaired by pain should have:

- morphine intravenously via a PCA

  or

- thoracic epidural with bupivacaine ± opiate

  with

- diclofenac 150 mg daily as tablets or suppositories, provided there are no other contraindications.

Patients requiring epidurals should have these inserted in theatre recovery areas or anaesthetic rooms where there are the facilities and staff to look after them until they are stable enough to return to the ward.

Severe injuries

These patients should be seen by the anaesthetic team on admission and go to either theatre or ITU at first, but may return to the ward some days later with an epidural or PCA as above.

OXYGEN

Oxygen should be given, via nasal cannulae or a face mask at 2–4 L per minute to maintain SaO_2 above 95 per cent. If oxygen flows greater than 4 L per minute are needed it suggests pulmonary complications and the ITU registrar should be informed. Oxygen flow rates greater than 5 L per minute require humidification.

PHYSIOTHERAPY

Early assessment is essential and physiotherapy can only be given if pain control is adequate. To maximize lung function, patients should be encouraged to sit up in bed, sit out and mobilize with supervision.

DIETARY ADVICE

These patients have increased nutritional requirements. Adequate nutrition should be given to preserve lean tissue and diaphragm mass. A referral should be made to the dietician if a patient is unable to meet their nutritional requirements.

THROMBOEMBOLIC PROPHYLAXIS

Provided there are no contraindications patients should be started on subcutaneous low-dose heparin daily.

SICKLE CELL DISEASE

Sickle cell disease is an inherited blood disorder. Abnormal haemoglobin causes the red blood cells to change into a sickle shape in several circumstances including:

- dehydration
- infection

- stress
- fatigue
- menstruation – worse in the first week after menstruation
- puberty in boys – there is often a clustering of events around this time that correlates with the increase in haemoglobin levels. Some centres undertake venesection at this time
- pregnancy
- cold (including air conditioning)
- swimming
- overexertion.

Pain is the most frequent problem seen in patients with sickle cell disease and the painful events are known as **sickle cell crises**. Red blood cells clump together to block normal blood flow through blood vessels, leading to occlusion of blood vessels, hypoxia, ischaemia and infarction. The area becomes inflamed and painful, organ damage can occur and the blood cells die, producing anaemia.

Symptoms may begin in infancy and may affect any region in the body. They vary in severity and may last from hours to weeks. The onset can be rapid or gradual as can the resolution. The most painful episodes are due to musculoskeletal pain in the low back and extremities. Visceral pain may occur from the spleen, liver and lungs and the pain can migrate. Some patients may have 40 or more crises per year whereas others have none or one. Only 20 per cent of patients with sickle cell disease present with these pains. The number of painful crises is an indication of the severity of the disease.

Most patients have painful episodes affecting bones or joints. It may affect single or multiple sites and may be symmetrical, for example in both arms and legs. It may involve the central skeleton, especially the spine, after adolescence. It may present as painful swelling of the backs of the hands or feet (hand-foot syndrome (dactylitis)).

Unfortunately the pain may mask life-threatening events that also present with pain. Chest pain may lead to acute chest syndrome and respiratory failure. The patient with chest pain should be transferred to hospital immediately.

Management

Families should be included in the development of pain management plans because the pain will cause lifelong problems.

DRUG TREATMENT

- Apply the World Health Organization (WHO) analgesic ladder (see Chapter 4)
- NSAIDs (see below)
- Paracetamol
- Opioids

- Tricyclics
- Epidurals – may help acute chest syndrome and may be life saving by providing adequate analgesia without hypoventilation but long-term treatment in this way may cause epidural adhesions at the treatment site
- Try to avoid pethidine
- TENS
- Heat
- Positioning
- Splints – for painful extremities
- Fluids – >3 L/day for adults and 80–100 mL/kg per day for children
- Oxygen
- Antibiotics – broad spectrum
- Cold exacerbates vaso-occlusion and worsens pain so do not use
- Psychology

Risks of NSAIDs with sickle cell disease

Blood loss from occult gastritis may destabilize the precarious haemodynamic compensation in chronic anaemia. Long-term analgesia can cause nephropathy especially as the patient is already at risk of renal failure from their disease.

Opioids

Doses required are often higher than expected because of their frequent use and the very severe nature of the pain. It is often described as being more severe than postoperative pain. The dose should be titrated rapidly to be effective. Oral opioids may be enough but vomiting may preclude their use. The incidence of addiction among patients with sickle cell disease is often overestimated. Having the disease neither increases nor decreases a patient's vulnerability to addiction – the incidence parallels the general population.

PSYCHOLOGY

Although genetic and physiological factors determine the disease severity, psychosocial factors and coping skills interact with the pathophysiology to determine the severity of the pain and its impact on the individual and the family. Some patients function well despite frequent and intense painful episodes and others do not.

Children and adolescents may miss out on schooling because of their illness which leads to school avoidance, failure or drop-out. Patients whose functioning is impaired often display psychosocial dysfunction by adolescence and often show the following:

- increased number of hospitalizations
- increased school absences

- school failure
- increased use of analgesics
- family discord
- mood changes.

Consistency with treatment reduces anxiety surrounding the crisis. It is important to reinforce self-efficacy and control during each crisis.

SPECIFIC THERAPY FOR CRISIS

Hydroxyurea reduces the number of poorly formed red blood cells in the circulation. Purified poloxamer 188 (PP188) reduces the duration of painful crises. The patient is 50 per cent more likely to be pain free in one week. It appears to allow blood cells to slip around each other and it reduces the thickness of the blood and blood components allowing the rigid crescent shaped cells to move through more easily. Greater benefit is seen in children and in those already taking hydroxyurea. This suggests there may be a fundamental difference in the nature of the painful crises in children and adults.

PAIN MANAGEMENT IN CRITICAL CARE

Problems

Pain and agitation are common in critically ill patients. It is estimated that 49–64 per cent of patients in ITU suffer with severe pain at some time during their stay, and 14.9 per cent of these patients are unhappy with their management.

The stress response causes tremendous neurohumoral elevations of plasma catecholamine, cortisol, glucose, antidiuretic hormone and acute phase protein levels. These elevations can result in tachycardia, hypertension, vasoconstriction, increased oxygen consumption, salt and water retention, and blunting of the immune response. The primary goals of sedation and analgesia are to relieve pain and anxiety, attenuate the stress response, and improve compliance with care.

Assessment

Assessment is difficult because patients are sedated, intubated, frightened, confused and often at the extremes of age. Reliable, objective measures of pain are unavailable and underlying disease or medications may alter blood pressure and heart rates, which are commonly used indicators in non-communicative patients. The visual analogue scale is a useful tool for assessing pain in patients who are awake and communicative, which is often not the case in ITUs.

Pain may be due to:

- primary disease
- procedures and treatment
- disrupted sleep
- anxiety
- prolonged immobility
- painful joints, contractures, ulcers
- neuropathic pain – spinal cord injury.

In patients with multiple organ system derangements, treatment of pain may compromise other system functions (causing, for example, respiratory depression or hypotension), and agents must be chosen with this in mind. Analgesia must be considered along with required sedation. The following also need to be taken into account:

- environment
- positioning
- boredom
- vital signs
- blood pressure
- pulse rate (difficult when the patient requires inotropic support).

Behavioural clues to pain include posture, vocalization and grimacing.

General management

Make the patient as comfortable as possible by using sedative drugs where necessary, controlling noise in the environment as much as possible and keeping the environmental temperature comfortable.

Pain management

Manage pain as for all other acute pain situations:

- WHO ladder
- regular paracetamol
- NSAIDs where possible (Box 5.12)

OPIOID ANALGESIA

Opioid analgesics are the drugs of choice for pain relief in the critically ill by intermittent bolus or continuous infusion. The intravenous route is preferred because absorption may vary with other routes.

BOX 5.12 NSAIDs in ITU

Advantages

- Antipyretic
- Anti-inflammatory activity
- Inhibit platelet aggregation
- Do not cause sedation
- No respiratory depression
- No hypotension

Disadvantages

- Platelet dysfunction
- Renal dysfunction
- Gastrointestinal ulceration or irritation

Intravenous infusion ± PCA

- Morphine 1–5 mg/h. Care with morphine in renal dysfunction because it is not removed by haemodialysis.
- Fentanyl 1–4 μg/kg per hour. Despite the drug's short half-life, redistribution into peripheral tissues occurs and can cause prolonged effects due to saturation of its distribution sites. Fentanyl accumulates with infusion. This effect is independent of renal function. Rapid tolerance to fentanyl can occur and chest wall rigidity can cause a problem with ventilation.
- Alfentanil 25–50 μg/kg per hour. Alfentanil is 90 per cent metabolized in the liver and has no active metabolite. It has a rapid and predictable recovery after infusion. It is useful in renal failure but is more expensive than morphine. The action is prolonged by liver failure but not affected by renal dysfunction.
- Remifentanil 0.1–0.25 μg/kg per hour (good but expensive).
- Pethidine is not removed by haemodialysis.

Extra analgesia must be prescribed for procedures such as turning, physiotherapy and placement of lines.

CLONIDINE

Clonidine is used as a sedative and an analgesic in ITU and the neonatal and paediatric ICU. It stimulates opioid receptors and it can also be used to control opioid withdrawal. It can be given orally or intravenously. An overdose of clonidine can be reversed by naloxone.

LOCAL AND REGIONAL TECHNIQUES

Regional anaesthetic blocks can reduce or eliminate the need for narcotic analgesics, control postoperative pain, attenuate the neurohumoral response to stress, and provide analgesia and anaesthesia for invasive procedures.

Epidurals are superior to opioids in the critical care environment in terms of analgesia and recovery. They have been shown to reduce ITU and hospital stay in patients undergoing oesophagectomy. Extubation occurs earlier and there is reduced risk of mortality.

ROLE OF EPIDURAL ANALGESIA

There is no level 1 or 2 evidence (see Chapter 4 for definition of levels of evidence) to support the perceived clinical benefit of epidurals in ITU. Studies are small and they have produced conflicting results. They may be beneficial in certain well defined groups, for example they have been shown to reduce ITU and hospital stay in patients undergoing oesophagectomy. Extubation occurs earlier and there is a reduced risk of mortality. No evidence exists to allow this to be extrapolated to other groups.

Improved pulmonary function tests and decreased postoperative pulmonary complications have been found in postoperative patients with continuous epidural analgesia compared to systemic opioid therapy. Although these benefits do not translate into improved outcome there is some evidence of the potential benefit of epidural analgesia. It would seem unlikely that the benefits of epidural analgesia are going to be submitted to a large randomized controlled trial in ITU patients and therefore good evidence confirming or refuting proposed benefits or harm will not be gathered.

Advantages of epidurals in ITU

- Epidurals allow the patient to be awake, mobile, cooperative and pain free.
- Useful in renal failure as the risk of opioid accumulation is avoided.
- Most patients on ICU have invasive cardiovascular monitoring that allows early recognition and prompt treatment of epidural-related cardiovascular instability.
- Ease of access to experienced medical back-up means that inadequate analgesia or side effects of the epidural can be rapidly and correctly treated.

Disadvantages

- Epidural analgesia may adversely affect splanchnic perfusion in critically ill patients.
- Epidural analgesia does not result in earlier or more successful enteral feeding compared to systemic opioid analgesia.
- The major disadvantages of epidural analgesia are the rare but catastrophic complications that can occur including infection and haematoma. The signs are difficult to detect in a sedated patient. The intrathecal or epidural route should probably be avoided in critically ill patients who are immunocompromised or who have coagulopathy.

Absolute and relative contraindications to epidural analgesia in critically ill patients are poorly defined with marked regional variation in practice. The incidence of serious complications is at best an estimate as neither the number of patients receiving epidural analgesia nor the number of complications that occur is accurately recorded.

Neuropathic pain

This is not well studied in the ITU environment but is most likely fairly common because of the high incidence of trauma and surgery, and the likelihood of associated nerve damage and compression. If the patient appears uncomfortable it is always worth trying tricyclic or anticonvulsant drugs.

Chronic pain

Of those patients reporting severe pain in ITU, 40 per cent have pain at six months. There is a 38 per cent incidence of chronic pain in patients with acute respiratory distress syndrome (ARDS). Pain in hospital is most strongly associated with pain after discharge so good pain management may help to reduce the incidence of chronic pain.

ANALGESIA FOR CARDIOTHORACIC SURGERY

The main argument against using epidural analgesia for coronary artery bypass grafting (CABG) surgery is the possible increased risk of epidural haematoma because these patients receive high-dose heparin immediately before bypass. This perceived increased risk cannot be quantified but the incidence of epidural haematoma following catheter insertion without heparinization is in the region of 1 in 10 000, i.e. 0.01 per cent. Given the overall incidence of 4 per cent stroke and 2 per cent mortality for CABG and the 10-year survival, the risk may be offset by the benefits. A recent large prospective study confirmed that perioperative morbidity is significantly lower with epidural analgesia. In a number of small studies epidural analgesia:

- improved haemodynamic stability
- reduced myocardial oxygen consumption
- reduced intra- and postoperative myocardial ischaemia
- abolished the catecholamine response
- diminished the cortisol response
- improved analgesia
- improved pulmonary function
- allowed patients to be extubated earlier.

Analgesia may promote earlier ambulation and discharge if continued into the postoperative period and there are fewer complications overall.

Analgesia

Thoracic epidural anaesthesia has been shown to be superior to other forms of analgesia for most types of surgery including cardiothoracic surgery. Patients often prefer the analgesia an epidural provides compared with PCA morphine.

PULMONARY EFFECTS

- There is up to 50 per cent reduction in the incidence of proved lower respiratory tract infection with epidural analgesia.
- Patients are extubated significantly earlier with epidural analgesia.
- Greater mean maximum inspiratory lung volume with epidural analgesia.
- Pulmonary function is preserved, probably a result of several factors, which include superior analgesia (allowing the patient to cooperate more fully with physiotherapy), the avoidance of opioids and their mood altering effects.

CARDIAC COMPLICATIONS

- Lower incidence of *new* supraventricular arrhythmias requiring treatment probably as a consequence of this sympathetic blockade.
- Postoperative infarction occurs in between 10 and 25 per cent of patients following CABG. In animal models epidural analgesia has been shown to reduce myocardial infarct size.
- There may be fewer cerebrovascular accidents in the epidural group.

RENAL FAILURE

- Significant reduction in the incidence of acute renal failure in patients receiving epidural analgesia.

All patients should receive additional oral ibuprofen every eight hours and paracetamol every six hours.

PAIN MANAGEMENT IN THE EMERGENCY ROOM

A variety of problems present to the emergency room including the acute abdomen, renal colic, burns, trauma and chest pain. Patients can be adults or children. The principles of pain management remain the same. Important points to consider are:

- The patient may require surgery.
- Trauma may delay gastric absorption and intravenous pain relief may be better than oral.
- It is often stated that the use of analgesia may interfere with clinical signs and should be avoided until a diagnosis is established. There is no evidence to support this and it is usually easier to examine a patient who is comfortable.
- Similarly a diagnosis of compartment syndrome is said to be hindered by an absence of pain and good analgesia should be withheld so a diagnosis can be established. Other signs are always present including raised pressure and adequate pain relief should not be withheld.
- The patients may be unknown and unconscious and caution needs to be exercised in case of:
  - hypovolaemia.
  - trauma or dehydration may compromise renal function.
  - renal failure.
  - asthma. The evidence against NSAIDs in asthmatics is tenuous. They should be avoided only in those on regular bronchodilators and moderate to severe asthma. In all cases, the risk and benefit accruing should be weighed.
  - coagulopathy. As NSAIDs inhibit prostaglandin synthesis, they can exert additional or synergistic effects on concurrently administered anticoagulants.
  - peptic ulcers. NSAIDs and steroids should be used with caution, especially when used simultaneously.

Pain management

- Always use the WHO analgesic ladder.
- Consider the most appropriate method of administration for the analgesia given.

PARACETAMOL

If able to take orally, all patients should receive paracetamol. Alternatively, the rectal or intravenous route should be considered.

NSAIDs

NSAIDs should be prescribed provided there are no contradictions. They can be administered orally, intravenously or rectally as appropriate but the intramuscular route should be avoided where possible.

OPIOIDS

Intramuscular versus intravenous: contrary to common perception, intravenous opiates are far safer than the intramuscular route. This is because titration is better achieved and the effect is more predictable. Intramuscular administration should be avoided.

Contraindications: there are no major contraindications to opioids apart from previous hypersensitivity reactions to the drug.

LOCAL ANAESTHETICS

Unfortunately this modality is underused. Nerve blocks and local infiltration are suitable for treating limb pain. Anaesthesia only lasts from four to 24 hours (depending on site and procedure), so one must consider alternative modes of analgesia for when the local anaesthetic wears off if the patient is to be discharged home.

GUIDELINES FOR MANAGEMENT OF BURN PAIN

The pain experienced by patients when they have been burned can be severe, longlasting and multifaceted. A range of strategies are necessary for managing these patients at different times. They require a combination of treatment for nociceptive and neuropathic pain. The pain will persist at least until the wounds are healed, and often into the rehabilitation stage.

Effective analgesia should be provided as soon as the patient is haemodynamically stable. Approximately a third of patients admitted with burns may not immediately require analgesia. Requirement for analgesia must be assessed on admission and at frequent intervals thereafter.

Emergency phase (first 72 hours)

- Pain control used at this time depends on the condition of the patient.
- Reassurance and information are important.
- Consider the presence of other mood altering drugs.
- Analgesia at this stage may improve cooperation between doctor and patient, allowing completion of evaluation of the patient.

Healing phase (after 72 hours)

The healing phase continues until the wounds are closed. Until this occurs the pain will continue and fluctuate in intensity. Analgesia needs to be continued as above as necessary. When the patient is tolerating food or enteral feed, consider changing to oral opioids for background pain but continue with the PCA if there is significant incident pain (movement, physiotherapy, etc.). Also consider:

- day-to-day background discomfort
- pain due to surgical discomfort (including donor site pain)
- pain associated with dressings and other procedures
- may continue for weeks or months (1–1.5 days/per cent burn)
- carefully planned strategies are required based on regular assessment and tailored therapy as no two patients are alike in their response.

PSYCHOLOGY

The perception of the pain experience can be affected significantly by the psychological response to the trauma. It may be necessary to introduce psychological help for those who are experiencing difficulties coping with the trauma. A play therapist should be involved with all the children.

OTHER DRUGS

Benzodiazepines

Lorazepam can be useful for anxiety – 2–4 mg orally. Midazolam nasal spray 0.2–0.4 mg/kg has a 10–15-minute onset.

Tricyclics

Burns are often complicated by the development of neuropathic pain. It may occur in the acute phase, or it may occur later and persist often for many years. It may be due to abnormally regenerated nerve endings, deficiencies in the re-innervation of the scars or possibly more central mechanisms. Consider amitriptyline 10–50 mg at night for adults.

Anticonvulsants

Topical phenytoin speeds wound healing and decreases pain. Sodium valproate, carbemazepine and gabapentin can all be used for neuropathic pain.

Intravenous lidocaine

The euphoric actions of lidocaine may help to ameliorate anxiety and it can help reduce neuropathic pain. The dose is 1 mg/kg bolus and 40 μg/kg per minute infusion (2 g lidocaine in 500 mL saline up to three days).

See Table 5.11 for a summary of pain management in the emergency room for children and adults.

ITCHING

Itching occurs in up to 85 per cent of patients. It can persist for years. It occurs in burns of all depths and in donor sites but most commonly in partial thickness wounds. It can be especially severe at night, during bed rest and especially in the lower limbs. It is worse if the wound takes more than three weeks to close.

Treatment

- Antihistamines may give some relief but mainly because of the sedative effects
- Cool compresses
- Emollients
- Pressure garments
- TENS
- Doxepin cream
- Gabapentin

PAEDIATRIC BURN PAIN

Children aged between birth and four years old represent approximately 20 per cent of all hospitalized burn patients. Several studies show that procedural burn pain in children is largely underestimated and under-treated. However, these shortcomings can be overcome by adhering to protocols similar to those used for adults. Accidental overdosage mostly occurs because of the difficulties of pain evaluation (overestimation) in children rather than the actual pharmacodynamic specificity of a drug. In addition, special attention should be paid to the child's environmental conditions. For instance, a parent's presence and participation in the procedure can have a highly beneficial effect.

Analgesic requirements vary considerably among patients. When skin coverage is complete children reduce their morphine use spontaneously and wean off morphine without any problems. The morphine dose does not bear any relation to extent of burns and the dose should be titrated to achieve the desired effect.

PROCEDURAL PAIN

Pain can be caused by many procedures during hospital treatment including halo adjustment and physiotherapy, but dressing changes particularly for burn wounds can be a major cause of prolonged pain over a long period of time. Patients undergoing repeated painful procedures may come

Table 5.11 *Management of pain in the emergency room in children and adults*

	Children	Adults
Emergency phase (first 72 hours)	**Bolus IV** morphine to control pain **IV morphine infusion** with or without PCA Regular **paracetamol** Burns <10% commence **NSAID** immediately on admission (5% in babies under 6 months) Burns >10% do not give **NSAIDs** for 48 hours after (5% in babies <6 months) Inform play therapist as soon after admission as possible	**Bolus IV** morphine to control pain **IV morphine infusion** with or without PCA Regular **paracetamol** Do not give NSAIDs for 48 hours after admission
Healing phase (after 72 hours)	**For all children with <10% burns:** Regular **paracetamol** until comfortable Commence **ibuprofen** after 48 hours if necessary **Children with burns of >10%** Regular **paracetamol IV morphine** infusion **or PCA** morphine + IV morphine infusion. Begin with 10 µg/kg per hour infusion and increase by 50% if demand on PCA exceeds three times successful bolus rate. Regular **NSAID** unless there is sepsis, or compromised renal function	Regular **paracetamol** **IV morphine** infusion **or PCA** morphine + IV morphine infusion Increase PCA bolus dose by 50% if demand on PCA exceeds three times successful bolus rate Regular **NSAID** after 48 hours unless there is sepsis, or compromised renal function
Regional techniques	Consider the use of regional analgesia in burns where possible but be aware of the risks of infection	Consider the use of regional analgesia in burns where possible, but be aware of the risks of infection

IV, intravenous; NSAID, non-steroidal anti-inflammatory drug; PCA, Patient controlled analgesia.

to anticipate pain before anything is done and this exacerbates the pain experience. Under-treated pain during these procedures can result in non-compliance with hospital treatment which may disrupt care, increase the risk of post-traumatic stress disorders and the patient may lose confidence in the care team.

The issue of pain at dressing changes is often overlooked but it is necessary to ensure optimal control of pain from the outset of care and application of the first dressing, through to the end of treatment. Managing pain adequately during the first procedure the patient experiences usually helps reduce anxiety associated with future procedures.

Stages of wound dressings

The most painful stage of a dressing change is the removal of the innermost layer of gauze, which usually adheres to some degree to the wound. This is followed by debridement and

topical applications; 86 per cent have severe pain during these procedures even with routine opioid cover.

Time course of pain

It is important to note that post-dressing background pain intensity is always greater than the pain experienced before a dressing change. The time it takes to change the dressing will depend on the extent of tissue damage, but dressings applied to the face and hands will take longer than those applied to other parts of the body. The choice of pain management depends on many factors including:

- the nature of the procedure
- whether the patient has an indwelling cannula
- where the procedure is to take place
- patient age
- condition of the patient.

BOX 5.13 Requirements for optimal analgesia at burn dressing changes

- Ensure an adequately staffed and safe environment in which to care for sedated patients
- Control severe acute pain due to nociception (inflammatory response) during the painful stages of the dressing (i.e. dressing removal, wound cleansing) by titrating analgesia to patient's individual requirements
- Avoid oversedation during and following the dressing change, but ensure adequate post-procedural analgesia through frequent pain assessment and monitoring of vital signs such as respiratory rate and sedation level
- Avoid prolonged fasting whenever possible as adequate nutrition and hydration are essential for the healing process

---

SKIN GRAFTING

The excision of non-viable tissue and the application of skin grafts decrease the duration of a patient's pain. Not only will these procedures reduce the number of painful dressings changes required, but the wound itself will also feel less painful, despite having undergone a surgical procedure. The donor sites are likely to be painful for a minimum of 48–72 hours.

ASSESSMENT OF PAIN INTENSITY

It is important to establish the severity of pain and the effectiveness of analgesia. The pain experienced by burn patients varies greatly from patient to patient. For this reason treatment protocols stipulate low starting doses of analgesia, and allow for adjustments to be made based on the individual pain assessment (Box 5.13).

DRUG MANAGEMENT

Analgesia

Paracetamol and NSAIDs should provide background analgesia.

Opioids

- If a cannula is present opioid can be given intravenously as a bolus or via PCA or nurse controlled analgesia.
- **Morphine** is often used as a background infusion with a PCA and this may be sufficient for pain relief. If the dressing does not take long morphine may be too

longlasting, causing sedation at the end of the dressing. Fentanyl or alfentanil provide a quicker acting alternative and both may have a shorter duration of action. Short-acting medications such as fentanyl, alfentanil and remifentanil may be more appropriate for pain relief in patients with burns.

- **Alfentanil** is a fast-acting medication, reaching peak effect in one minute. There is rapid pain relief and a relatively short duration of action (mean half-life 90 minutes). A starting dose of 10 μg/kg is appropriate, and can be repeated every minute according to the level of pain. Combining repeated boluses with a continuous infusion of 2 μg/kg per minute is effective in improving pain relief.
- **Remifentanil** is even shorter acting but because of its short action it has the disadvantage of not being capable of providing lasting post-procedural pain relief.

The use of intravenous opioids for severe procedural pain does, however, have its drawbacks in that some patients may require such high doses of analgesia that there is an increased risk of apnoea and loss of consciousness.

Oral route

If there is no intravenous cannula available then the opioid can be given orally about 30 minutes before the procedure. The delayed onset of action (10 minutes) of morphine and the longlasting effects (several hours) do not allow for the analgesic therapy to be adjusted easily to meet individual needs. Oral morphine takes 30–90 minutes to reach peak effect and can be administered at least 60 minutes before the dressing change: it is widely used in adults and children. The recommended starting dosage is 0.3 mg/kg in children although clinical experience suggests that 0.5–1 mg/kg may be more appropriate. The main drawbacks of oral morphine are:

- its reduced and uncertain bioavailability (15–50 per cent)
- it is not possible to give extra doses in response to severe pain during the procedure (delay for peak plasma concentration: 30–90 minutes)
- the usually long post-procedural sedation.

Sedation

Midazolam and various anxiolytics act synergistically with opioids to potentially increase the risk of respiratory depression and reduced mental awareness. They should, therefore, be used to treat anxiety only, which is usually anticipatory and can be reduced considerably with efficient analgesia and thoughtful pre-procedure preparation of the patient.

The addition of a benzodiazepine may potentiate the respiratory depression and sedation so use low doses of both.

Midazolam

Midazolam is the drug of choice for dressing changes. Its effects include reduction of skeletal muscle spasms, reduction of anxiety and amnesia. It has a rapid onset and a short half-life (1–12 hours).

Midazolam can be given intravenously, orally or intranasally. When using midazolam orally it should be given 30–45 minutes prior to procedure. The intranasal dose will lead to sedation in five minutes and it will last about 60 minutes. An intravenous dose should be given three minutes before the procedure. The first dose should be one-third of the normal dose if opioids are also used and the dose then titrated to effect. Once sedation has been achieved give additional doses of 25 per cent of dose required to produce sedation.

Paediatric midazolam dose:

- Intravenous – 0.03–0.1 mg/kg
- Oral – 0.5–0.75 mg/kg

Flumazenil

- Children – 0.01 mg/kg loading dose and 0.005 mg/kg per minute until awake to a maximum of 1 mg
- Adults – 0.1–0.2 mg over one to three minutes and 0.2 mg at 60 second intervals to a maximum of 1 mg.

Other drugs for sedation

Ketamine

The option of involving a skilled anaesthetist in order to use anaesthetic agents such as ketamine or propofol should be considered for achieving 'conscious sedation' versus general anaesthesia. Subanaesthetic doses of ketamine have been used extensively for many years, especially in children in whom its unpleasant dysphoric side effects are less pronounced. Oral ketamine has also been used, although its effects can be unpredictable. The recommended dosage is 10–20 mg/kg.

Propofol

Low-dose propofol has also been suggested for short procedures but its safety at the bedside remains questionable.

Entonox®

Nitrous oxide and oxygen (Entonox) is one of the most popular and safest anaesthetic agents used in patients with burns. It has a rapid onset of analgesia and can be used for the duration of the procedure. However, it has a limited analgesic potency and although it is widely prescribed there is no up-to-date published research on its use in burns. Its use should be restricted to an hour per day.

Fentanyl lollypops

These are a more interesting alternative: they have a rapid onset of action (within a few minutes) and a longer-lasting effect than intravenous fentanyl due to their double mechanism of absorption (transmucosal and gastric).

If sedation is insufficient the patient should undergo procedure under general anaesthetic.

NON-PHARMACOLOGICAL THERAPIES

Recent research on the effects of distraction therapies in reducing burn procedural pain shows that anticipation of pain increases pain intensity and discomfort, which can be decreased by diverting the patient's attention. Distraction through use of interactive computerized virtual reality for example, can have a significant analgesic effect.

The same is true for hypnosis, which is used extensively by a number of burn teams. These supportive techniques may be time consuming, but they can help to reduce the feelings of fear and anxiety, especially during long procedures. However, they must always be used in conjunction with pharmacological treatments, and should never replace them.

Distraction techniques

Some suggestions

- Hypnosis
  - Decreases anxiety and pain
  - Requires trained hypnotists
  - Not all people hypnotizable
  - Some people do not like it
- Relaxation
- Massage
- Meditation
- Video games

Ambulatory patients

About 95 per cent of burn patients are treated on an outpatient basis, but only 75 per cent of these patients receive medication at dressing changes. There is scant literature on the subject and, unfortunately, there are no published guidelines for best practice. Protocols involving short-acting intravenous opioids used at the bedside are suitable for use in the outpatient setting provided there are facilities for post-procedural surveillance.

PAIN MANAGEMENT IN MYOCARDIAL INFARCTION

The pain, distress and anxiety that accompany myocardial ischaemia will increase sympathetic tone and release catecholamines. This induces a tachycardia, dysrhythmias and hypertension which in turn increases myocardial work, worsens ischaemia and hastens cell death. Opioid analgesia reduces pain and thereby improves cardiovascular function. Morphine also produces vasodilatation probably via histamine release, which will further reduce myocardial work. The mood elevating effect allays anxiety. It should be given intravenously, not intramuscularly, because of the preceding thrombolytic therapy. The drug of choice is diamorphine and patient controlled analgesia may provide more immediate relief than nurse administration.

Problems

Nausea and vomiting may antagonize the benefits of pain relief so antiemetics should be given. Dysphoria produced by opioid therapy may lead to restlessness and agitation and counteract the beneficial effects of therapy.

RENAL COLIC

The pain of renal colic is caused by stretching of the ureteral muscle as the ureter contracts around the stone during peristalsis. The resulting ischaemia causes pain, which is referred through T11, T12 and L1. Hyperalgesia may occur in the cutaneous distribution of these nerves. The stone obstructs the flow of urine leading to increased wall tension and pressure. The result of this is the release of prostaglandins and the subsequent vasodilatation causes a diuresis. This in turn further increases the pressure. Prostaglandins are also directly produced as a result of smooth muscle spasm.

Treatment

- High fluid input to maintain high fluid output.
- Paracetamol.
- NSAIDs – prostaglandins appear to be involved in the smooth muscle contraction seen in renal and biliary colic, conditions in which these agents are particularly effective. NSAIDs are the preferred treatment for colicky pains because they are associated with fewer side effects than opioids. Patients receiving NSAIDs achieve greater reductions in pain scores and are less likely to require further analgesia in the short term than those receiving opioids, particularly pethidine.
- Antispasmodics.
- Opioids.
- Contrary to popular belief the use of morphine does not increase ureteric spasm and is a good analgesic agent to

manage the pain of renal colic. Pethidine certainly confers no advantages.

USE OF INTRAVENOUS MORPHINE IN THE RECOVERY WARD

It is the responsibility of the anaesthetist to ensure that their patient is free of pain or has an acceptable pain score during their stay in the recovery ward. Nursing staff in the recovery ward can give intravenous morphine to patients with severe pain, but only as prescribed by the anaesthetist.

Morphine should be given according to an algorithm similar to the one shown in Fig. 5.7. The dose(s) and time(s) at which morphine is given by the nursing staff must be recorded next to this prescription. **It is unacceptable for patients to be sent back to their ward in pain and the recovery ward staff should not discharge patients if their pain score is more than 1.**

Monitoring

- Respiratory rate
- Heart rate
- Blood pressure
- SaO$_2$
- Pain scores
- Sedation scores
- Nausea and vomiting scores

If pain is not settling consider:

- an NSAID if not given
- paracetamol if not given should be administered intravenously
- benzodiazepine if the patient is very anxious but take care if using opioids.

If a drug is given by the oral or rectal route it will not act for about 30 minutes. If morphine is given during this time the additive effects may produce unexpected respiratory depression so it is important to keep the patient in recovery for at least 45 minutes after the last dose of any drug.

SUMMARY

When considering pain management in any situation it is important to follow the same basic mechanism (Fig. 5.8) and monitor the outcome.

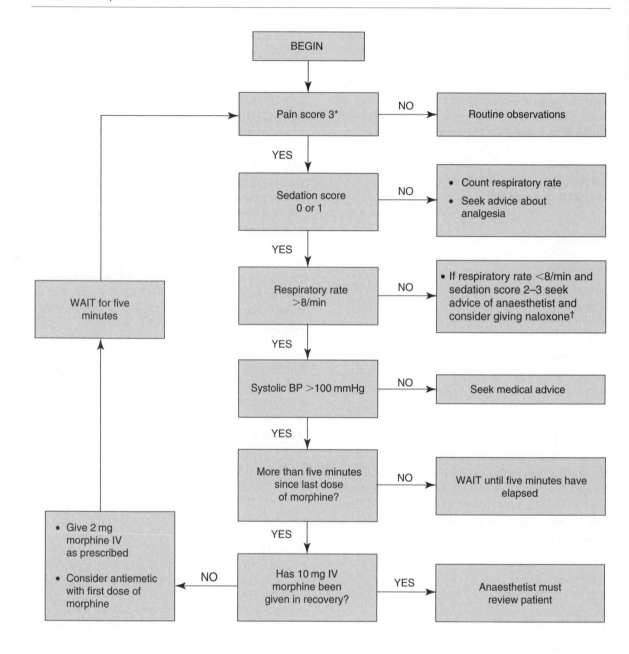

*Pain and sedation scoring system

Pain score (R = rest; M = movement)   Sedation score

3	Severe pain	3	Unrousable
2	Moderate pain	2	Asleep/rousable
1	Mild pain	1	Drowsy
0	No pain	0	Awake
†	Naloxone IV 100–400 µg slowly IM 400 µg		

Figure 5.7 *Algorithm for the use of intravenous morphine in the recovery ward. IV, intravenous; IM, intramuscular*

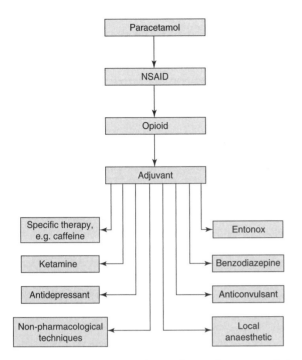

Figure 5.8 *Summary flowchart of the basic steps in management of pain. NSAID, non-steroidal anti-inflammatory drug*

CASE SCENARIO

A 24-year-old woman is admitted with an infected abscess in her groin secondary to intravenous heroin abuse. The abscess requires surgical debridement. Discuss postoperative management of her drug requirements and pain relief.

Management

The patient is at risk from drug withdrawal. It is important to ascertain:

- how much she uses
- when she last had a dose
- what other drugs she uses
- what are her plans as regards drug abuse on discharge.

Management of withdrawal

Prescribe methadone for prevention of withdrawal symptoms. She admits to spending £500 per week. Currently the cost of

heroin is about £10 per bag so this is 50 bags per week or seven per day. Most bags are 0.2 g (variable purity) so she is using approximately 1.4 g heroin per day. A bag is equivalent to 15 mg methadone – 1 g of heroin is 50–80 mg methadone. It is rarely necessary to give more than 60 mg methadone per day and it should be given in a single dose in the morning.

Management of pain

- Paracetamol orally or intravenously will reduce opioid requirements.
- Use an NSAID whenever possible.

The abscess and surgery will be painful. Consider regional techniques where possible, for example an epidural. However, there is already an established infection that may prevent regional techniques being used. Also such patients often wish to be off the ward and prefer to mobilize. Methadone must still be given to prevent withdrawal symptoms.

If opioids are required the use of patient controlled analgesia may prevent any arguments between the patient and nurse about how much analgesia is required. The initial dose should be 1 mg bolus with a 5-minute lockout but the bolus dose may need to be increased. Monitoring is important as patients who abuse opioid drugs often have a low pain threshold and use the PCA excessively.

Further management

If the patient requires help with their addiction they can be given the telephone number of the local drug team and encouraged to contact them on discharge. The patient should not be discharged on methadone unless they were admitted on methadone or they have started on a rehabilitation programme and a named person is in charge of the patient on discharge. The patient should be warned to use a reduced dose of heroin because their tolerance may have reduced while in hospital and they run the risk of taking an overdose by mistake.

FURTHER READING

Department of Health. *Drug Misuse and Dependence – Guidelines on Clinical Management.* London: The Stationery Office, 1999.

6 Acute Back Pain and Sciatica

INTRODUCTION

Back pain is a common experience of mankind, and has probably been a universal experience ever since human beings assumed the upright posture. As such, it could be argued that back pain should not be termed a disease; and yet it is one of the commonest causes of distress, disability and loss of livelihood in the developed countries of today. Since industrialization the problem has been more prominent, and over the past 50 years has rapidly escalated.

The UK Department of Health OPCS Omnibus Survey in 1993 identified 37 per cent of adults aged 16 and over who had experienced back pain lasting more than a day in the previous 12 months. Only 7 per cent of these back pain sufferers claimed this as their first episode of back pain; the rest had experienced previous or ongoing back pain. Fourteen per cent of respondents were suffering from back pain on the day of interview. For almost a fifth the pain had lasted all year, suggesting that 7 per cent of adults have back problems throughout the year. This survey revealed that 16 per cent of all adults had visited their general practitioner (GP) about their back pain. In the four weeks prior to interview, 3 per cent of all adults had spent days lying down because of back pain and 11 per cent had restricted their activities in other ways. About 4 per cent of adults had taken time off work or been unemployed because of back pain during the 4-week period. Thirty-five per cent of people suffering from back pain felt that their pain was related to work; either to the nature of the work or to some accident or work-related injury. Sports injuries, pregnancy and arthritis were cited as other commonly attributable causes.

It is estimated that, in the UK, because of back pain about 52.6 million working days are lost each year and that back pain results in about 2.4 million medical consultations and treatments. The cost to quality of life and the economy is enormous.

The cause for most back pain is obscure and the treatment is poorly understood. The inability of 'scientific medicine' to manage back pain effectively has encouraged the flourishing of multiple forms of therapy and therapists in the alternative or complementary medical fields: many of these may reflect conventional medicine's incomplete understanding of back pain, but several clearly exploit the demand for solutions where there is a void, and invoke implausible and untested or unproved ideas which defy logical examination.

Modern medicine has a need to describe the pathology of diseases so that appropriate treatment can be prescribed. The failure to effectively identify a disease process underlying much back pain increases the difficulty of providing effective treatment and has led to either unnecessary and sometimes harmful surgical intervention or a dismissal of the reality of patients' symptoms, attributing them entirely to behavioural and personality problems, when the medical model of disease fails to provide an answer.

In the 1930s it was discovered that back pain and sciatica may be associated with herniation of intervertebral discs. The notion of the 'slipped disc' entered the public consciousness. After several millions of surgical interventions on prolapsed discs, we can see that many patients have undoubtedly been relieved of their symptoms, yet many have found that their symptoms persisted after technically successful surgery and some even became worse. Modern imaging techniques show that many patients whose symptoms are suggestive of a prolapsed disc do not have any misplaced disc tissue, whereas some patients who are shown to have disc displacement have no symptoms. The popular manipulative treatments for disc problems are similarly difficult to explain by demonstrated pathology. Although the correlation between cause and effect remains elusive, surgical intervention has become much more selective in recent years and conservative non-surgical management of back pain and sciatica is often the first choice.

Alternative causes for back pain may be degenerative or arthritic changes in the spinal joints. Most of the older population will have some radiological evidence of degenerative change, but not all suffer from back pain. Some back pain may arise in the muscles and soft tissues, and many people with back pain present with tender and stiff muscles. This may be a primary myofascial pain problem, or may be secondary to underlying skeletal pain. The results of treatment aimed at this type of pain are unpredictable and difficult to relate to specific diagnostic signs.

Non-medical therapists of many disciplines suggest other causes of back pain, possibly involving abnormal spinal balance, posture and movement, which require various manipulative and physical therapies. Although such approaches often result in beneficial therapeutic effects, the theories supporting them seem to rely more on the results of such treatment, rather than verifiable scientific explanations. The wide range of theories, potential therapies and the general poor results of most interventions for back pain should perhaps steer us away from medical interventions, to regard the majority of back pain as a maladaptation and concentrate on the restoration of normal function, and on the cognitive and behavioural aspects of management to minimize disability and distress.

ACUTE BACK PAIN

Back pain, usually of sudden onset, which may or may not be related to an episode of trauma, and which lasts from two to 12 weeks, is generally termed 'acute pain'. However, this may represent an acute episode against a background of chronic pain or be a recurrent problem. The majority of acute back pain, and/or sciatica, resolves spontaneously, although many sufferers go on to develop recurrent episodes or chronic pain at a later date. Until recent years the recommended treatment for acute back pain/sciatica was a prolonged period of complete bed rest, often lasting for many weeks. It is currently believed that prolonged immobilization for acute back pain is generally unnecessary and indeed may be detrimental to the long-term prognosis. Early restoration of function is important and the usual practice now is to allow a maximum of 48 hours rest if necessary to enable some of the painful muscle spasm to settle before starting a programme of mobilization and graded activity. This approach has been shown to reduce long-term morbidity and improve the chances of a return to work.

Acute back pain may be accompanied by sciatica or other symptoms suggestive of possible nerve root compression. Symptoms and signs of serious pathology should be excluded before starting a mobilization programme. Analgesics should be used to relieve some of the acute pain and enable the patient to mobilize. This may include the use of paracetamol and a non-steroidal anti-inflammatory drug (NSAID) (if tolerated) on a regular basis, and not 'PRN' (when required). If pain is severe, opiate analgesics should be considered. This often takes the form of weak opiates such as codeine-based analgesics or tramadol, but it is quite reasonable to consider oral morphine (on a timed administration) for several days when pain is severe.

Patients with acute back pain and muscle spasm are often prescribed diazepam to relieve muscle spasm and to enable an anxious and stressed patient to rest. However, many patients are given diazepam for too long a period and may develop some dependence. Muscle relaxants such as baclofen or methocarbamol may be preferable to avoid the sedative and anxiolytic effects of benzodiazepines.

It is important to exclude serious pathology that may require urgent medical or surgical attention when assessing acute back pain. A list of symptoms, the so-called 'red flags', is often used to exclude such conditions before a more conservative line of management is undertaken. This should exclude acute inflammatory disease, neoplastic spinal disease and conditions presenting a major threat to the structure and function of the spinal cord and nerve roots.

Red flags when assessing back pain

POSSIBLE SERIOUS PATHOLOGY

- Non-mechanical pain
- Thoracic pain
- Previous cancer, human immunodeficiency virus (HIV), steroids
- Unwell, weight loss
- Widespread neurology
- Structural deformity
- Onset <20 or >55 years

CONDITIONS SUGGESTING CAUDA EQUINA SYNDROME AND REQUIRING URGENT SURGICAL REFERRAL

- Sphincter disturbance
- Saddle anaesthesia
- Progressive motor weakness/gait disturbance

Yellow flags when assessing back pain

In addition, there are a number of psychological elements to consider which may have an important bearing on the longer-term management of back pain. These are often described as 'yellow flags':

- a belief that back pain is harmful or potentially severely disabling
- fear avoidance behaviour and reduced activity
- tendency to low mood and withdrawal from social interaction
- expectation of passive treatment.

Management of acute back pain

The majority of acute back pain and/or sciatica is initially managed in the primary care setting. General practitioners assess the patient and exclude the likelihood of serious pathology which requires urgent medical or surgical attention. Treatment consists of a short period of rest if necessary, rarely more than two days, with administration of analgesics. Mobilization is started early with encouragement to return to normal activities as soon as possible. If progress is slow, early help from a physiotherapist or chiropractor can be beneficial. Unless there is concern that there may be more serious pathology present, plain radiographs or magnetic resonance imaging (MRI) scans are not generally useful or necessary at this stage.

Referral of the patient to a specialist centre should be considered when symptoms persist for more than six weeks without making any progress, or when there are persistent symptoms and signs of nerve root compression. If pain is unmanageable or the signs of nerve root compression are severe and prevent mobilization then further help and assessment should be sought earlier. Signs suggesting possible cauda equina syndrome (see Red flags above) indicate an urgent surgical opinion.

EPIDURAL INJECTIONS FOR ACUTE SCIATICA

Persistent nerve root pain which is not resolving with conservative management or is causing prolonged immobility will require further investigation, preferably with MRI. Evidence of disc prolapse with nerve root compression may require surgical decompression. Surgical discectomy may relieve symptoms but is not always successful and long-term results may be no better than of those treated more conservatively.

An alternative is to offer such patients a series of epidural steroid injections. Disc prolapse will usually result in inflammatory changes in the nerve root from compression or chemical irritation from extruded disc material. It is possible that the inflammatory response is responsible for much of the pain and accompanying muscle spasm associated with acute disc prolapse. Injection of steroid (usually + local anaesthetic) to the epidural space reduces inflammation and oedema of affected nerve roots, relieving acute pain and thereby allowing earlier mobilization.

Patients with acute sciatica may be given up to three steroid epidural injections at intervals of one to two weeks. The injections may be given by the lumbar or caudal route, depending on which is most easily accessible (the technique is described in Chapter 8). The results are comparable with either route. Epidural steroid injections make little difference to long-term prognosis after acute prolapsed disc, but the procedure usually allows earlier resolution of pain and promotes improved mobility during the acute stage. Patients in whom pain and altered sensory and motor function persist after epidural injections should be reassessed for surgery.

CARE PLAN FOR ACUTE BACK PAIN

See Box 6.1.

BOX 6.1 Care plan for acute back pain

Simple back pain, e.g. lumbosacral buttocks and thighs

- Mechanical pain (movement)
- Patient well
- Onset usually 20–55 years

Or

Nerve root pain

- Unilateral leg pain
- Pain, numbness, paraesthesia to foot/toes
- Straight leg raising causes leg pain

✔ radiograph not usually required
GP advice:

- Avoid bed rest >2 days
- Regular analgesics
- Early return to work, normal activity and progressive exercise
- Back education
- Pain not resolving after four weeks – consider physiotherapy, manipulation
- Pain still severe at six weeks – refer to back pain service/surgical opinion; consider epidural injections for sciatica
- **Possible serious pathology** (red flag) – surgical referral within four weeks
- **Possible cauda equina syndrome** – emergency surgical referral
- **Possible inflammatory disorder** – refer to rheumatology, e.g:
  - Gradual onset
  - Marked morning stiffness
  - Widespread reduction of range of movement
  - Peripheral joints affected
  - Iritis, skin rash, colitis, urethritis
  - Family history

DEVELOPMENT OF CHRONIC PAIN

It is important at this stage to try to prevent an acute back pain developing into a chronic condition. The current belief is that early return to normal activity and the minimal medicalization of the problem will help to reduce this progression. Patients who are subject to repeated episodes of acute back pain and who consequently struggle to cope with their employment and generally managing to lead a normal lifestyle may benefit from attending courses, usually organized by physiotherapists with a particular interest in back pain rehabilitation. Such programmes aim to help sufferers to understand repeated back pain, how to look after their backs, and how to cope with the episodes of pain which they continue to experience.

CASE SCENARIO

Barbara is a 43-year-old woman who works as a receptionist in a medical practice. She has previously been fit and well although she has had occasional self-limiting episodes of backache over the past three years. While lifting some files at work she experiences a sudden sharp lumbar pain. The pain persists and later that day she is sent home from work to rest.

Over the subsequent 24 hours Barbara's pain becomes more intense and involves the right leg with some feeling of numbness and tingling radiating down to her big toe. Attempts to get out of bed result in increased pain and spasm of the lumbar muscles. She is a little hesitant passing urine but does not experience any incontinence. Her GP prescribes cocodamol analgesia and advises that after 48 hours' rest she should get up and start to mobilize.

After 48 hours Barbara is becoming distressed with pain, muscle spasm and inability to stand without severe pain, although the numbness in her leg has decreased a little. Her lack of mobility and the signs of nerve root involvement lead her GP to refer her to hospital for further assessment.

Examination demonstrates signs of fifth lumbar nerve compression. There are no signs of perineal numbness, progressive muscle weakness or urinary incontinence, but she is referred for an urgent MRI scan to confirm the diagnosis. The MRI confirms the presence of a small right-sided disc prolapse but no nerve root compression. A decision is made not to embark on immediate surgery and Barbara is seen by the pain clinician who suggests a course of steroid epidural injections.

An epidural injection is administered via the caudal route (sacral hiatus) consisting of 20 mL of 1 per cent lidocaine combined with 40 mg of triamcinolone. The following day Barbara is in less pain and starts to mobilize. A second epidural injection is given one week later as symptoms continue to improve and she starts a gentle exercise regimen.

Barbara is discharged from hospital with arrangements to return as an outpatient in two weeks' time for a third epidural injection. Pain continues to subside with less numbness in the leg and no further muscle spasm. She is referred to the physiotherapy department for further back strengthening and mobilizing exercises before she is able to return to work four weeks later.

Section Three

7 Treating Chronic Pain: Use of Drugs

PERSISTENT PAIN

The description 'chronic pain' describes the temporal aspects of pain and its value as a label is limited. It is generally taken to refer to symptoms of pain which persist over a longer period than any pain related to immediate trauma or active nociception would be expected. The definition is arbitrary, but is often considered to be a condition which has persisted for longer than three months. However, many conditions of nociception may continue for longer periods, and pain which is not apparently directly associated with ongoing nociceptive processes may have been present for lesser periods. Moreover, 'chronic pain' is a term often used to describe specific conditions which may be longlasting, but the description also has implications about the aetiology of the pain. The descriptions of 'acute pain' and 'chronic pain' are therefore imprecise and it is controversial whether there is a rationale for separate consideration of these two conditions.

How does pain become chronic? To answer this we must consider what types of pain may present in the long term. A disease process may continue to provoke nociceptive activity. This may associated with a long-term tissue damaging process, such as a painful non-healing wound, burn or ulcer. Inflammatory arthritis or an invasive tumour will similarly produce ongoing nociceptive stimulation. Should this be given the contradictory description of 'acute pain of long duration'?

The more difficult concept arises when this pain of nociception continues to cause distressing symptoms after the healing process has been apparently completed, the inflammatory process has resolved or the invasive destructive process has been removed. Continuing pain may be provoked by active stimulation of the structure involved or when some mechanical abnormality results in normal use of the part provoking pain.

Following prolonged nociceptive stimulation there are apparent changes that develop in the way sensory information is received and processed by the nervous system. The development of 'wind-up' in the dorsal horn of the spinal cord is a mechanism postulated to increase the response to continuing nociception (see Chapter 1), but there are many longer term effects which may cause pain to persist. There may be a process of peripheral sensitization and changes in the dorsal horn which increase the receptive field of afferent input as well as altering the response of wide dynamic range (WDR) neurones so that the response to non-noxious stimuli is perceived as painful. There are also changes in cortical representation as pain becomes long term.

Persistent pain is often the result of damage to or malfunction of a part of the peripheral or central nervous system, and pain is then described as neuropathic, although 'neurogenic' may be a more appropriate description. This type of pain may be quite obviously related to direct damage to neural tissue as in trauma or surgery, or following vascular catastrophes. There may be more subtle neurological injury/disease such as herpetic infection, metabolic neuropathies or degenerative neuropathy (multiple sclerosis?). Moreover, some degree of neurological dysfunction appears to play a role in many longer-term pain conditions resulting in some of the characteristics of neuropathic pain although the direct connection with neurological damage or disease may not be clear.

An important aspect of any long-term pain is its effect on a person's behaviour, cognition and functional levels. Chronic pain usually results in suffering and frequently in disability. These factors will normally affect behaviour. The degree of behavioural response to chronic pain may have a considerable effect on the perception and maintenance of pain and should be considered as an important area of interaction in planning the most appropriate means to relieve suffering and disability.

However much we postulate on the causes of long-term pain, there are always patients who present with persistently painful symptoms in whom we cannot explain the possible causes for pain. Sometimes these pains fit into recognized pain syndromes which have been consistently described, and yet it remains impossible to describe the condition in terms of recognized physiology. It has been commonplace in medical practice to dismiss such unexplained pain syndromes as being a result of a disordered psyche or even sheer malevolence or malingering on behalf of the patient. Such a response is unhelpful in our attempts to relieve distress in our patients, whatever its cause, and also illustrates the shortcomings in our ability to understand the complexities of the mechanisms of pain perception. It is accepted that all other physiological systems are vulnerable to malfunction; why should pain perception, which is known to be a remarkably complicated and as yet incompletely understood system, be any different?

Managing chronic pain demands a series of problem-solving exercises, and the assessment process should provide some answers to these questions:

- What is the nature of the pain of which this patient complains?
- What physiological system is affected by the symptoms of pain?
- Is there an identifiable disturbance of function or structural integrity which may be generating the pain?
- How is the function and wellbeing of this person affected by the perception of pain, and what effect does it have on their life and the lives of those around them?

The answers to these questions should indicate the most likely path of managing pain and the effects of pain. Treating the symptom of pain will frequently require several different approaches to have an effect on the multiple factors involved in the experience of pain. Understanding of the neurophysiology and pharmacology of pain has made significant advances in recent years, but it remains incomplete and appears increasingly complex. Nevertheless, the use of drugs in the treatment of pain has for generations held a prime position in the provision of analgesia. Recent advances in knowledge of neurotransmitters has not only helped us to explain why analgesic drugs do not always provide a complete answer to the need for pain relief, but also helped to direct further work to develop more effective analgesics.

Physical methods for treating pain have also been used since the earliest days of mankind's development, and early records of ancient techniques often have an echo in the present day. The concept of stimulating part of the sensory system to modify activity in another part has often found a role in the management of pain. The attempt to improve and modify physical function has seen many changes to the present day, but has for long played a useful part in the management of chronic pain.

The behavioural effects of pain and the attempt to modify the cognitive experience of pain has come to play an increasingly important role in the management of chronic pain, but perhaps some of the more ancient practices suggest that there has long been an appreciation of the psychological component of pain management.

USE OF DRUGS IN CHRONIC PAIN

Lay parlance refers to 'pain killers'. This term carries connotations of 'DRUGS'. Drugs are things which may mask symptoms enabling an underlying disease to cause unbridled harm

and possibly allow people to tolerate pain so that they may unknowingly cause further harm to themselves. They may be associated with terminal hopeless disease states or terrible side effects. Finally, of course, drugs are associated with abuse and addiction. These popular beliefs are either misconceptions based on the erroneous ideas about the nature of chronic pain or, in the case of the last two points, ideas may be influenced by inappropriate use or misuse of drugs without adequate supervision and monitoring of response.

Many patients will express the feeling that they do not want to take 'pain killers' indefinitely, and although there is a well-made point that continued medication is seen as some type of burden, there is also frequently a feeling that this is not a right and ethical approach to life. There are, of course, many people who crave as much medication as they can get, for a chance to support the insoluble problems in their lives, and this is often a situation which leads to inappropriate drug use. However, the use of drugs to produce analgesia remains one of the most important and widely used methods of providing pain relief for both short- and long-term pain: after all, the term 'analgesic' means 'no pain'.

Negative aspects of drug therapy

The use of analgesic drugs is associated with some negative aspects. Drugs may be expensive and demand continued use of resources. They may cause unpleasant or intolerable side effects, and the long-term effects on health may be detrimental. There is also the problem of ensuring adequate patient compliance with drug regimens.

Positive aspects of drug therapy

The positive side seems perhaps more impressive. Most drugs produce a predictable and controlled response, which, most importantly, is nearly always reversible. Drugs used for pain relief can be gradually developed and modified in accordance with advances in understanding of the neurophysiology of pain and can therefore be more accurately targeted. This has to be contrasted with more invasive and destructive methods of producing pain relief. Surgical redesign of the musculoskeletal system or ablation of components of the nervous system cannot be reversed and can rarely be completely free of unwanted effects. Destructive methods of pain relief are sometimes more widespread and drastic in states where there is restricted access to potent analgesic drugs.

The original, naturally occurring agents used for analgesia, opiates, cannabis and alcohol, have a direct effect on the central appreciation of pain. Modern research has demonstrated that for the first two of these, there are naturally occurring receptors in the nervous system and elsewhere which can modify the transmission of painful sensations. Later discoveries of natural products, such as salicylate, were found to modify the production of pain generation following trauma and inflammation. Other vegetable products have long been used to block neural transmission and provide local anaesthesia. Later developments to design synthetic molecules for drugs based on these natural products led to more refined drugs with an improved side effect profile that have become the mainstay of analgesic medication. Many other groups of drugs have been added to these, which act on different aspects of pain perception systems. Many were originally designed for use in other areas of medicine and subsequently found to have analgesic use. More recently drugs have been designed with the specific aim of modifying pain physiology.

Selection of drugs for analgesia

It is helpful, when trying to determine the most effective medication to treat pain, if the pain can be categorized. Pain may be nociceptive, neurogenic, unknown/idiopathic or a combination of any of these. The requirements of an analgesic drug regimen are:

- It should be appropriate for the type of pain.
- It should be easy to administer.
- It should have acceptable levels of unwanted effects with no long-term harmful effect.

The division of drugs in this way is rarely perfectly defined. Anti-inflammatory drugs have central analgesic activity as well as the more obvious peripheral effects. Opiates can affect the nature of pain perception as well as having a direct effect on receptors involved in neurotransmission and modification. There used to be a strong belief that opiate drugs were not helpful in the management of neuropathic pain, but later work has shown that this is not completely true. Neuropathic pain is relatively resistant to opiate analgesia but there is frequently some response even though this may only become apparent at dose levels which are above the level at which intolerable side effects are manifest.

NON-STEROIDAL ANTI-INFLAMMATORY DRUGS

The pain of arthritis presents a number of problems. Although there is perhaps implicit in the term 'arthritis' that there is an inflammatory process involved, this is quite obviously far from a universal situation. Many arthritides have a continuing inflammatory process and treatment may be directed at reducing inflammation and presumably inflammatory-mediated pain production, as well as specific treatments aimed at modifying the disease process. However, much joint pain is seen after apparent cessation of active inflammatory activity, as in osteoarthritis and degenerative joint disease, where there is no classic inflammatory response with the expected chemical mediators of inflammatory pain. Other pain-generating mechanisms are clearly operating which may involve complex neural responses to chronic injury. Anti-inflammatory analgesics are unlikely to alter the disease process but are widely prescribed for managing joint pain, whether or not there is an active inflammatory process. There is often a moderately good response to anti-inflammatory analgesics, and it may be that the centrally acting analgesic properties of this group of drugs are more important than their anti-inflammatory effects.

The important side effect profile of NSAID drugs limits their use, particularly in the relatively vulnerable older patients who are afflicted with joint pain. The more recent introduction of selective cyclo-oxygenase (COX)-2 inhibitor drugs has increased the tolerance of NSAIDs but adverse effects, particularly on the gastrointestinal tract and renal function, may still be major restrictions on their use. Recently determined cardiac effects may limit future use of the COX-2 drugs.

Simple analgesics like paracetamol, with or without weak opioid drugs, will usually be the mainstay of analgesia in most arthritic pain. In severe pain which is poorly relieved by these measures, stronger opioids, such as tramadol, buprenorphine, or morphine and oxycodone, may be used where there is a demonstrable response, and the drug is tolerated without excessive side effects such as sedation, dizziness and nausea. The use of more potent opiate analgesics always has to be carefully considered in regard to the benefits opposed to the short- and possible long-term adverse effects, and the social and legal restrictions surrounding opiate drugs.

OPIOID ANALGESICS

Opioid analgesics are typically prescribed for their use in relieving nociceptive pain, although as previously mentioned, this is not an exclusive indication. Traditionally the use of opioids carries a medical and social stigma. The associations with drug abuse and the social and legal consequences of opioid use have tended to restrict their use, even for medical purposes. In many parts of the world the legal use of opioid analgesics is severely restricted or even prohibited as a result of misguided legislative attempts to control the illicit drug trade. The wider acceptance of opioid use for managing pain in cancer has slowly developed over the past few decades, but there is still widespread scepticism and mistrust of the use of strong opioid analgesics for managing pain in non-life-threatening conditions. The fact that chronic pain often responds only poorly to opioid analgesia reinforces the negative views of this therapeutic approach. The development of tolerance and dependence on opioid drugs is often seen as a major obstacle. However, there is often some beneficial analgesic response to opioids in musculoskeletal pain as well as other predominantly nociceptive conditions, and when this is apparent without unacceptable side effects, the use of strong opioids may be reasonably considered where other analgesics have proved inadequate to improve the quality of life of the patient in pain. Tolerance to true analgesia is unlikely to be a problem. Although some physical dependency may develop (necessitating gradual withdrawal if it is decided to change therapy), psychological addiction is rarely a problem in the patient who is taking opioids for a genuine analgesic effect. Careful assessment of the patient and their response to opioid analgesia with continued monitoring is essential for patients given strong opioid analgesics.

WEAK OPIOID ANALGESICS

The so-called 'weak' opioid analgesics are, in contrast, widely prescribed. Their use rarely provokes the sort of concerns associated with morphine and similar related drugs, and yet their efficacy is often more dubious and side effect profile troublesome. Codeine and dihydrocodeine are common either as single use analgesics or in combination with paracetamol. Codeine appears to have a low ceiling analgesic effect, but a higher relative adverse effect. So, increasing the dose of codeine may not increase analgesic effect, but will almost certainly increase unwanted effects, such as sedation, dizziness, nausea and perhaps the most complained of effect in patients with chronic pain, constipation.

Codeine will undoubtedly remain a frequently used analgesic because it is effective for many patients. It may enable a reduction in the use of anti-inflammatory drugs, and it is free of prescribing restrictions and the social and medical stigmata of strong opioids. Its limitation, however, should be borne in mind. Patients with chronic pain who are to be maintained on a codeine-based drug are frequently prescribed a combined preparation, such as cocodamol 8/500 or 30/500, two tablets four times daily. It is important that patients recognize the limitations of this medication and are not allowed to increase the dose in a desperate, but fruitless, quest for greater analgesia.

TRAMADOL

Tramadol represents a possible step further up the analgesic ladder. It may not be a more effective analgesic than codeine and dihydrocodeine, but it is often better tolerated, there may be a little more flexibility in dose, and there is some evidence that it may have analgesic properties over a slightly wider range of pain. As well as having effects on the μ opiate receptors, this synthetic opioid is thought to enhance the descending inhibitory activities in the central nervous system. This may give it some useful properties in the management of neurogenic pain. Long-term maintenance of patients with musculoskeletal or mixed types of pain with slow-release tramadol is often well tolerated, especially with a lesser tendency to cause severe constipation than with other opioids.

The traditional practice for the use of opioid analgesics has been to work up the 'analgesic ladder' (see Chapter 3), starting with weak analgesics and progressing to stronger opioid analgesics if this is inadequate. In practice, this progression may be shortened or modified depending on the response both in terms of analgesia and side effects. A codeine-based analgesic may be replaced by tramadol, where this presents a more acceptable side effect profile, although this may in some circumstances represent an increase in potency. Progression to 'strong opioids' such as morphine, oxycodone or fentanyl may represent increased analgesic efficacy, but may be considered when a low dose of potent opioid could have the same analgesic effect but with lower side effects than a large dose of weak opioid analgesic.

PRESCRIBING OPIOID ANALGESICS FOR NON-MALIGNANT PAIN

Before prescribing strong opioid analgesics for patients with chronic non-life-threatening pain the patient and the object of the prescription should undergo a careful assessment. It is recommended that the following points should be considered:

- The prime object of prescribing opioid analgesics in persistent pain is to provide pain relief.
- Opioids should not be used primarily as anxiolytics or sedatives. However, improvements in physical and social function, as well as sleep, may occur as a secondary benefit from improved pain relief.
- Opioid analgesics may form only part of an overall strategy aimed at physical and social rehabilitation of the patient with persistent pain.
- The selection of patients for opioid therapy should usually only be made after alternative medication strategies have been fully explored, particularly the use of anticonvulsants and antidepressant drugs when the pain is considered to be neurogenic.
- The assessment of patients should include the patient's beliefs, fears and expectations about their pain and about what they expect the opioids can and cannot do.

A history of drug abuse or psychiatric disorder indicates a particular need for careful assessment of the patient and their behaviour in response to opioid treatment, but it is not an absolute contraindication to the use of opioid analgesics. Ensure adequate supervision of the patient over the long term when opioid analgesics are prescribed, and it is important that the drugs are usually prescribed from a single source.

Practical points in prescribing opioid analgesics

- Opioids should generally be given as modified-release preparations, either orally or transdermally. Short-acting opioids tend to predispose to drug-seeking behaviour and are less suitable for long-term use, but may be useful during the process of titrating the dose of opioid initially, or occasionally for managing breakthrough pain in clearly defined situations.
- Injectable opioids are rarely appropriate for use in long-term non-cancer pain. Demands by patients for this form of medication are more likely to be associated with drug abuse than genuine analgesic effects.
- Patients should be advised of the controlled legal status of these drugs. They should be stored safely and the quantity of medication should be accounted for. Accounts of the tablets 'falling down the toilet', or 'the dog eating the prescription', etc. should be treated with a degree of scepticism.
- Drug doses should be increased at fixed intervals until pain relief is achieved or side effects are unacceptable. Controlled-release drugs and transdermal drugs require several days before stabilization on each dose.
- Patients should be regularly monitored during the titration process for pain relief, changes in mood, sleep, physical and social function, as well as assessment of unwanted side effects such as nausea, constipation, somnolence and dysphoria.
- If pain relief is not achieved and there is no overall improvement in function with opioid therapy, then it should be accepted that it has failed. Some patients may benefit from switching to an alternative opioid, but if this is not the case, the medication should be discontinued and alternative means of pain management explored.
- Patients taking long-term opioid medication need regular reassessment. They will need special consideration when they undergo surgery or suffer trauma (see Chapter 5). Concerns about opioid use should arise with the presentation of:
  - early requests for repeat prescriptions
  - claims of lost prescriptions
  - intoxication
  - frequent failure to keep appointments
  - use of other scheduled drugs.
- Unfortunately, analgesics, even potent opioids, may have limited benefits in managing pain on movement. The pain of weight-bearing on an arthritic hip is only partially modified with heavy analgesic use.

ISCHAEMIC PAIN

Ischaemic pain, as experienced in peripheral vascular disease, is to a large degree, nociceptive. In chronic states there may be an element of neuropathy contributing to pain, but the nociceptive pain of ischaemia may respond to opioid analgesics. This is especially useful for night-time ischaemic rest pain, where the sedative effect of opioids may be a valuable additional property. Patients with these problems often tend to be elderly and frail, so that there may be a relative intolerance of opioid drugs that cause excessive sedation. Careful titration of dose against effect is important, and possibly the trial of different analgesics in combination with other analgesic drugs may be required to achieve maximum benefit with minimal tolerated side effects.

NEUROPATHIC PAIN

Neuropathic pain or what has been described as 'neurogenic pain' presents different problems in management. The nature of neurogenic pain is complex (Chapter 1). We can describe the symptoms and signs: there are changes in normal sensory function, with loss of, or exaggerated response, to normal stimulation. These features may present simultaneously. Numbness, hyperalgesia, allodynia may all be present with a complaint of shooting, lancinating, burning or dysaesthetic pain. The causes may be central or peripheral but the pain is generated within the nervous system as a result of damage, malfunction or a disordered processing of sensory information. There may be a peripheral neuropathy with degeneration of peripheral tracts, or a structural and functional change in the dorsal horn or central tracts, or disorder of central structures in the nervous system, as may follow a cerebrovascular accident or direct trauma or degeneration of the central nervous system. The common feature of neurogenic pain is the relative insensitivity to simple, anti-inflammatory and opioid analgesics. Medication for treating neurogenic pain includes a wider range of pharmacological activities, using many drugs which were usually developed for activities other than analgesia.

There is little firm evidence to support the use of peripherally acting drugs in the management of neuropathic pain. However, while the pain of, for example, post-herpetic neuralgia is thought to be centrally generated, some pain relief may be provided with the use of topically applied anti-inflammatory analgesics or local anaesthetics. Is this a result of reducing any existing nociceptive input which normally results in an exaggerated and painful sensation because of the defect in normal neural function?

Drugs used to manage neuropathic pain

Neurogenic pain is often managed with drugs originally developed as anticonvulsants, drugs developed as antidepressants or a combination of the two. The analgesic properties of these drugs are largely unrelated to their anticonvulsant effects or treatment of depression, but the effect of these drugs on neurotransmitters may influence seemingly unrelated symptoms (Chapter 3). The general principle is to stabilize neuronal function, reduce central sensitization and possibly enhance intrinsic inhibitory systems.

ANTIDEPRESSANT DRUGS

The antidepressants with the most proved effects in neuropathic pain belong to the group known as 'tricyclic antidepressants'. It is likely that this effect is the result of changes in several transmitter systems. Antidepressants which are 'cleaner' in activity, such as serotonin reuptake inhibitors, are generally less effective as analgesics than the 'dirtier' drugs which are known to have effects on several transmitters. Unfortunately this means that these drugs generally have a poorer side effect profile, and it may be more difficult for the patient to tolerate an effective dose. On occasions, side effects may be a valuable adjunct to treatment, and the night sedative properties, or the anxiolytic and even antidepressant effects may provide a valuable addition to analgesia in the management of patients with chronic pain.

The most widely used drug in this group is **amitriptyline**, but there is a high rate of intolerance to its sedative effects, sometimes perhaps surprisingly more so in younger patients. **Nortriptyline** provides a less sedating alternative, or dosulepin (dothiepin) may be effective when some night sedation and anxiolysis would be useful but with less hangover effect than amitriptyline. **Desipramine** and **imipramine** further extend the range of properties. The analgesic effect of these drugs is usually evident at doses lower than those which would normally be used to treat depressive illness, although some patients do require higher doses. It is usually beneficial to start at a low dose and increase gradually according to response and tolerance.

Patients treated with amitriptyline should be started on a dose of 10–25 mg at night. If this dose is tolerated without excessive daytime sedation, a gradual increase can be made in weekly increments of 10 or 25 mg (depending on age and general fitness). It is unusual to require a dose of more than 75 mg daily. The whole dose can be given as a single dose one or two hours before bed, in order to minimize daytime sedation.

Patients should be warned about the enhanced effect of alcohol when taking amitriptyline, although this is not an absolute contraindication to moderate consumption if that is the patient's usual habit. The effects on ability to drive or operate dangerous machinery should be discussed and given careful consideration. Similar practice should be followed with the other tricyclic antidepressant drugs. Patients should be warned about the most frequent side effect: a dry mouth. These drugs are relatively contraindicated for patients with severe ischaemic heart disease or prostatic symptoms.

ANTICONVULSANT DRUGS

Anticonvulsants have a long association with treating pain. Initially older drugs such as phenytoin were widely used. The use of carbamazepine for treating trigeminal neuralgia was discovered by association and has since been extended to other neuropathic pain states. The more recent introduction of drugs like gabapentin for use in neuropathic pain suggests that this group of drugs may not represent a homogeneous mode of activity, and effects on neurotransmission unrelated to anticonvulsant activity are likely to be responsible.

The strong connection between carbamazepine and the effective management of trigeminal neuralgia led to a common practice of reserving the use of anticonvulsant drugs for the management of lancinating or shooting pain. Although this is a valid observation, it has become apparent that anticonvulsant drugs can be useful in the management of different neuropathic pain symptoms. Trials in the use of gabapentin demonstrated the range of efficacy of this drug in a variety of neuropathic pain syndromes.

Carbamazepine

This has long been established as a first-line treatment for trigeminal neuralgia and is widely used for other types of neuropathic pain. The drug needs to be taken regularly to be effective but dose requirements and tolerance vary widely among individuals. It is usual to start on a dose of 100 mg three times a day, or even once a day in the elderly. The dose is then increased in stages until an effective dose is achieved or side effects are intolerable. The dose may need to reach 400 mg three times daily, but side effects such as sedation, ataxia and gastrointestinal upsets are common at higher dose levels.

Thrombocytopenia and bone marrow depression are rarer side effects of carbamazepine and occasional blood counts are advisable during long-term use. The drug should be withdrawn gradually if discontinuation is necessary, to reduce the risk of epileptic attacks, as with other anticonvulsants.

Sodium valproate

This is a useful alternative to carbamazepine. It may be less toxic and better tolerated. The dose is started at 100 mg three times a day, and gradually increased according to response and side effects. A dose of 600 mg three times a day may be required. Side effects are most frequently gastrointestinal, but dizziness and sedation may occur. Alopecia occasionally occurs, and liver function may be disturbed (detected by change in hepatic enzymes).

Clonazepam

This is a benzodiazepine. It may be helpful in managing lancinating pain. It can be given as a night time dose of 0.5–2 mg. The sedation produced by clonazepam is often unacceptable and long-term use may cause problems of habituation.

Clobazam and **flecainide** are further examples of membrane-stabilizing drugs occasionally used in this way. More recently introduced anticonvulsant drugs have been used in the management of neuropathic pain. **Lamotrigine** may be effective in this type of pain and may be used alone or in addition to other anticonvulsants such as carbamazepine for the management of trigeminal neuralgia.

Gabapentin

This has an established role in the treatment of chronic neuropathic pain. This effect is likely to be unrelated to its anticonvulsant properties. It is relatively well tolerated, but sedation, dizziness and ataxia limit its use in some patients. More serious side effects such as muscle and joint pain or blood dyscrasias are uncommon.

Gabapentin is better tolerated if it is introduced gradually. A frequently used regimen is to start with 100–300 mg once daily for four days, then twice daily for four days, and then increasing to 300 mg three times daily. If well tolerated, the dose can then be increased in further increments to 600 mg three times daily or even further to 900 mg three times daily in some situations.

Gabapentin or the other anticonvulsant drugs may be combined with tricyclic antidepressant drugs in the management of neuropathic pain.

NMDA RECEPTOR BLOCKERS

Transmitter and receptor systems concerned with the modulation and perception of pain within the central nervous system may be an important area to target new pharmacological approaches to the management of pain. The role of NMDA (*N*-methyl-D-aspartate) receptor activation in the propagation of chronic pain, particularly neurogenic pain, makes it an attractive target. Several older drugs have been found to have NMDA-blocking properties which may have use as analgesics. Ketamine, used as a dissociative anaesthetic, has long been known to provide analgesia. Some of this activity may be related to its effect on NMDA receptors.

Ketamine

Ketamine is a difficult drug to use for ambulant patients, as apart from its general anaesthetic potential, it produces dysphoria and hallucinations, even at subanaesthetic doses. Ketamine can be given by intravenous infusion (a benzodiazepine such as midazolam may be given in addition to reduce the incidence of hallucinations) and may continue to reduce neuropathic pain for days or sometimes weeks after a single dose. The alternative is to administer the drug sublingually; when oral ketamine is swallowed its bioavailability is only about 15 per cent. Patients can learn to administer small regular doses of ketamine sublingually (the taste is a problem). There is a difficult margin to achieve between effective analgesia and unacceptable side effects, and with many patients this is an unachievable compromise.

Other drugs with NMDA-blocking activity and potential as analgesics include **amantadine** and **dextromethorphan**. The former is usually given by intermittent intravenous infusion and the latter by oral administration. Both have been helpful in some patients for reducing the intensity of neuropathic pain, but are perhaps disappointing in the predictability of beneficial effects. **Methadone** also has NMDA-blocking properties. It is difficult to know how important this is in clinical use, but it may help to explain why methadone can sometimes demonstrate a more potent analgesic effect than other μ agonist opioids in comparable doses.

CAPSAICIN

Capsaicin applied as a topical preparation can be used to reduce the pain of post-herpetic neuralgia. It can also provide relief from the pain arising in scar tissue where there seems to be a neuropathic component, and has been used to relieve the pain of peripheral arthropathy, when pain is considered to be essentially nociceptive. Capsaicin produces a burning sensation when applied. This is usually mild when applied to intact skin, but severe when it comes into contact with damaged skin or mucous membranes. However, the effect of capsaicin is believed to be different from the 'counter-irritant' effect of other rubefacients. Absorption of capsaicin is believed to affect C fibres and deplete them of the neurotransmitter 'substance P', which is implicated in peripheral neuropathic pain (see Chapter 1).

LOCAL ANAESTHETICS

The application of local anaesthetics to the skin (as a gel or patch) as well as peripheral nerve blocks with local anaesthetic can provide relief from peripheral neuropathic pain. This may again be by reduction in unpleasant sensory stimuli affecting the perception of pain. This seems to be an 'active' process.

Simply severing the nerve supply to a dermatome that is affected by neurogenic pain may produce an area of numbness, but will rarely get rid of the pain, and may result in a more intense or unpleasant painful experience in the long term. The preservation of some functioning afferent nerve supply seems to be important when trying to modulate the sensory experience, whether that is by stimulating or actively blocking that residual sensory function.

FURTHER READING

Recommendations for the Appropriate Use of Opioids for Persistent Non-cancer Pain. A consensus statement prepared on behalf of the Pain Society, the Royal College of Anaesthetists, the Royal College of General Practitioners, and the Royal College of Psychiatrists. London: The Pain Society, 2004.

8 Treating Chronic Pain: Nerve Blocks

INTRODUCTION

There is a long history of attempts to relieve pain by denervating the painful area of the body. Cutting or burning nerves, or injecting toxic chemicals into nerve tissue, may result in a change in the painful sensation but can also result in motor paralysis, the development of new painful sensations (e.g. anaesthesia dolorosa), and unpleasant numbness and dysaesthesia. Perhaps worse, is the frequent return of the original pain, but often in conjunction with these other unpleasant consequences. Perfect pain relief after destruction of a nerve tract could only be theoretically achieved if the pain perception systems behaved like a 'hard-wired' electrical circuit, rather than a plastic adaptable system where the sensory experience is the summation of effect from many different activities of the nervous system with modulation and adaptation at many levels.

The ability to block nerves is a tempting way of providing analgesia, often in the short term, and is perhaps the reason why it was anaesthetists who became some of the main practitioners of pain medicine. A nerve block will often stop or temporarily suspend a painful afferent stimulation, and it is common experience that chronic pain is often moderated for a longer period than would be expected simply from the duration of the local anaesthetic effect. Perhaps relief of chronic pain can be achieved by moderating central activity when peripheral afferent nerves are blocked or there is a change in stimulation of afferent activity.

INDICATIONS FOR NERVE BLOCKS

Nerve blocks may be used in a diagnostic or therapeutic role:

- Relief of pain following a successful nerve block may provide information about the source of pain.
- Blocking nociceptive input with local anaesthetic can produce prolonged pain relief.

Sometimes a more specific effect is required, such as when steroid is injected to relieve nerve root compression. Destructive procedures are mostly only applied to small peripheral nerves for a clearly defined local effect, as for example the radio-frequency lesioning of nerves to spinal facet joints (see Chapter 9) or the local neurolysis of abdominal cutaneous nerves which have become entrapped. Larger procedures include neurolysis of the major sympathetic trunks or of the trigeminal ganglia for relief of trigeminal neuralgia. Occasionally in palliative care it is acceptable to perform destruction of a major nerve trunk or tract when other methods of pain relief have proved inadequate, and the potential benefits are considered to outweigh the hazards. It must be remembered that in these situations that pain may return, so that it is usually only considered justifiable to perform a procedure such as cordotomy in patients with limited life expectancy.

EPIDURAL INJECTIONS

Indications and mechanism of action

It is widespread practice for anaesthetists to provide epidural injections for back pain and sciatica as well as other spinal complaints. This derives from the supposition that pain arises as a result of nerve root compression or irritation by protruding disc material. Nerve roots can become swollen and inflamed by both mechanical compression and chemical irritation. It seems logical to suggest that the injection of steroids into the epidural space will result in reduced swelling and inflammation and thereby relieve pain. Unfortunately, nerve root pathology cannot be demonstrated in most people with back pain or in the majority with sciatica or nerve root symptoms. Steroids have many effects, and one possible role is that of causing shrinkage/atrophy of connective tissue. It is possible that epidural steroids produce a reduction in fatty and connective tissues within the spinal canal, leaving a little more room for neural structures.

Risks

The use and benefits of epidural steroids are not universally accepted. There is always the risk that substances injected in close proximity to the central nervous system could cause neurological damage. Most preparations of depot steroids contain other potentially neurotoxic chemicals, preservatives and emulsifiers, and there have been suggestions that these may be associated with the development of arachnoiditis. Although this remains an important consideration, in practice it seems most of the well-documented cases of arachnoiditis have followed intrathecal injection of steroid preparations and it is difficult to find convincing evidence of a properly placed epidural injection producing this disastrous consequence.

Outcome

Studies have generally shown that epidural steroids produce a short-term benefit in relieving pain in cases of proved disc prolapse with nerve root signs. The long-term benefits are more difficult to demonstrate convincingly, and it may be that in such cases, the epidural injection results in earlier pain relief and mobilization of the patient than occurs with entirely conservative management. This early pain relief can be dramatic and is increasingly offered as an early alternative intervention to surgery. The long-term results of both interventions may not be very different. The use of epidural steroids where there is no clear radiculopathy, and for more chronic pain syndromes, is, as expected, less useful. Nevertheless, there remain a small number of patients who do respond in a limited way, enough to justify the procedure in situations where there seems to be little else which is of benefit.

Symptoms of spinal claudication resulting from spinal stenosis is one example of a condition which may improve for a period following epidural steroid injection, giving the patient a valuable respite where surgery is not possible, or is to be delayed. Less clearly defined benefits may be seen in patients suffering from spinal collapse or spondylolisthesis.

Although relief following epidural steroid injection may be relatively short term, some practitioners will offer selected patients epidural injections at repeated intervals of perhaps six months or a year for maintenance in chronic conditions. This is not a universally acceptable procedure, but it is more widespread practice than many will admit.

Technique

The technique for 'therapeutic' epidurals is essentially the same as that used for anaesthesia. The route chosen will depend to some extent on the experience of the operator but there are some other considerations. An epidural injection for pain associated with lumbar or sacral nerve roots is probably as effective whether given by the lumbar or the caudal approach. A lumbar epidural is often a more familiar technique to many anaesthetists and will allow a relatively small volume of anaesthetic and steroid to reach the affected nerve roots.

However, many patients presenting for this treatment will already have undergone spinal surgery with consequent scarring, and probable distortion or obliteration of the epidural space, making the precise identification of the epidural space more uncertain. This may result in a slightly higher incidence of inadvertent dural puncture. Not only does this result in the usual problems of post dural puncture headache, but it increases the risks of intrathecal injection of local anaesthetic and also depot steroid, which may be neurotoxic.

A caudal injection, using the sacral hiatus to reach the epidural space, almost always avoids the possibility of dural puncture, but there is a higher rate of failure to enter the epidural space. Some patients may have an excessive covering of subcutaneous tissues over the sacral hiatus and there is wide anatomical variation in the position, shape, and even patency of the sacral canal. The injection of fluid into the sacral epidural space seems to be associated with pain or discomfort more frequently than the lumbar epidural space.

Epidural injections should only be performed by a skilled operator who is competent in resuscitation. Informed consent should be obtained. The presence of infection or a history of abnormal bleeding or warfarin therapy should be regarded as contraindications. Intravenous access should be available. The procedure should be performed as a sterile procedure with nursing assistance and appropriate facilities for resuscitation. The patient should be monitored by trained nursing staff following an epidural injection, until normal function has returned and all observations are stable.

LUMBAR EPIDURAL

A lumbar epidural can be performed with the patient sitting in the forward flexed position or lateral flexed. After skin preparation and draping, infiltrate local anaesthetic into the skin and subcutaneous tissues overlying the site of injection, which can be midline or paramedian. Advance a Tuohy needle into the chosen site, using saline or air (saline is safer) to test for loss of resistance on entry to the epidural space. When the space is positively identified, inject 8–10 mL of 1 or 1.5 per cent lidocaine mixed with 40 mg of depot steroid preparation. The steroid frequently used is triamcinolone. The injection may produce some discomfort but if it is very painful then the position should be checked. If severe pain continues on injection, then it is probably wise to discontinue. The injection may be made with steroid suspended in saline, instead of local anaesthetic. This reduces the incidence of hypotension and does not result in any numbness or weakness of the legs after the injection, so making the 'recovery' period much shorter. Opinion is divided about whether the local anaesthetic plays any useful role in the therapeutic effect of the epidural injection. It does make the injection less uncomfortable for the

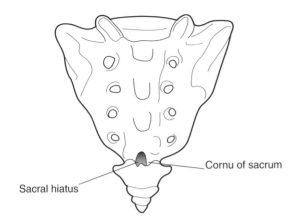

Figure 8.1 *Anatomy of the sacrum showing the common position of the sacral hiatus*

patient, and it provides a useful indicator of the possible spread of the injected material.

CAUDAL EPIDURAL

An epidural injection via the sacral hiatus (Fig. 8.1), a caudal block, is usually straightforward and is much less likely to produce any cardiovascular effects than a lumbar injection. It is often easier and likely to result in a successfully placed injection if this procedure is performed with the patient lying prone. The patient can be asked to evert their heels in order to open the natal cleft and improve access. The skin is sterilized, taking care not to allow skin preparation solution to run down the natal cleft to the perineum. The sacral hiatus can be identified by palpation in the majority, although there is wide variation in the size and orientation of this structure. Particularly in male patients, the hiatus can occasionally be surprisingly low down and shallow angled. The skin over the hiatus can be anaesthetized using a fine gauge (27 G) needle. The author then uses a 5 mL syringe containing 1 per cent lidocaine with a 21 G (1.5 or 2 inch) needle to infiltrate down to the hiatus (Fig. 8.2), using this needle to explore at the same time. Entry to the sacral epidural space should be accompanied by easy injection of local anaesthetic with a check aspiration that is negative for blood or cerebrospinal fluid (CSF). The syringe can then be changed with the needle *in situ*, and 15–20 mL of 1 per cent lidocaine or saline mixed with 40 mg triamcinolone injected.

The injection should be given slowly with occasional repeated gentle aspirations. Rapid injection may be painful and results in unpleasant sensations of pressure in the spine and sometimes in the head. There is often some discomfort on injection, especially in patients who have constricted nerve roots from disc prolapse or scar tissue and adhesions. If the patient complains of severe pain or paraesthesiae, tinnitus,

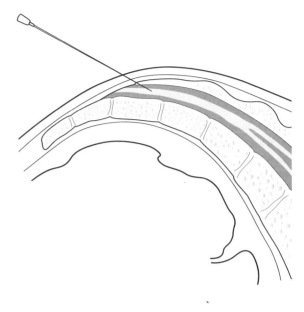

Figure 8.2 *Caudal block. The position of the needle within the caudal canal*

or faintness, the injection should be stopped. Following the injection, the patient should be turned supine and stay flat for 30 minutes, with blood pressure monitored at 5-minute intervals.

THORACIC EPIDURAL

Thoracic epidurals are less frequently performed for therapeutic indications. The technique used is the same as for a thoracic epidural performed for anaesthesia, using the midline or paramedian approach. When the epidural space has been identified, 6–10 mL of local anaesthetic or saline with steroid are injected.

CERVICAL EPIDURAL

Cervical epidural injections present particular difficulties and hazards. The spinal cord is particularly vulnerable at this level and the landmarks used in this block are more difficult to identify. There is also the possibility that a high spinal block could result in cardiovascular consequences. The accuracy and safety of the injection are increased by carrying out the procedure under radiological screening. Good intravenous access must be established.

The patient is positioned in the lateral position with the neck gently flexed. The skin is infiltrated in the midline at the chosen interspinous level, usually between C5 and C6 or C6 and C7. A lateral view on the image intensifier will confirm that the infiltrating needle is at the correct level, aiming between the spinous processes. An 18 G Tuohy needle can then be advanced through the anaesthetized superficial tissues towards the interspinous space. Saline injection is used to test for loss of resistance and the position of the needle relative to the spine can be checked with radiographic screening intermittently. The spinal ligaments in the cervical region offer less resistance in contrast with the lower spine and therefore the endpoint for identification of the epidural space is less clear. It is easy to get a false-positive result when testing for loss of resistance. A radiological check of the position of the needle relative to the lamina will help to confirm a false result. It is also helpful to inject a small amount of radio-contrast medium (<0.5 mL of Omnipaque 240) which will clearly show whether the injection is spreading into connective tissue or epidural space. This provides great reassurance for the operator to continue advancing the Tuohy needle until true loss of resistance is discovered. Placement in the epidural space can be confirmed by injecting a further small volume of radio-contrast medium and observing the spread within the epidural space as well as excluding an intrathecal injection. If there is any suspicion that the dura has been breached, then the injection should not proceed. If placement is satisfactory, then an injection of 2–3 mL 1 per cent lidocaine mixed with 20 mg of triamcinolone can be given. The patient is carefully monitored after the procedure until it is certain that there are no cardiovascular or neurological changes.

An alternative technique would be to introduce an epidural catheter into the upper thoracic spine, and then using radiographic imaging, pass the catheter in a cephalad direction until its tip lies in the lower cervical epidural space. The injection can then be made through the catheter to reach the epidural space.

LUMBAR SYMPATHETIC BLOCK

The lumbar sympathetic chain lies on the anterolateral aspect of the vertebral bodies in a fascial compartment. It is separated from the somatic nerve roots by the psoas sheath and is posterior to the retroperitoneal fascia.

Indications

The main indication for blocking the lumbar sympathetic chain is pain in the lower limbs mediated by the sympathetic system. In particular, this is most usual for severe ischaemic pain in the lower limbs. This block is most appropriate for rest pain. There may be some improvement in perfusion following sympathetic blockade, but whether this is responsible for the relief of pain remains open to doubt. The pain of claudication is not usually an indication for sympathetic block, and this symptom may even deteriorate after sympathectomy,

because of a 'steal effect' diverting blood supply from muscle to skin. Lumbar sympathetic block may be indicated for managing pain of the complex regional pain syndrome (CRPS), pelvic pain of malignant origin, and possibly some types of spinal pain where there is considered to be a major neurogenic component. Lumbar sympathetic block may be used as part of the management of CRPS and for the management of Raynaud's disease.

Lumbar sympathetic block can be performed with local anaesthetic, which although resulting in a short-term block, can produce pain relief for an extended period. If a permanent neurolytic block is required, often called a 'chemical sympathectomy', then phenol is injected onto the sympathetic chain. Radio-frequency thermocoagulation is sometimes used to produce a prolonged block.

LUMBAR SYMPATHETIC BLOCK AND CHEMICAL SYMPATHECTOMY – TECHNIQUE

Secure venous access prior to performing this procedure. The injection can then be given with local anaesthetic infiltration and occasionally light sedation if the patient is particularly anxious or uncomfortable.

The patient should be positioned on a radiolucent table with a C-arm image intensifier to provide accurate localization of the injection. The procedure is easier if the patient lies prone with a small pillow under the lower abdomen, and this allows easy access when a bilateral procedure is carried out. If the patient is unable to lie prone, the lateral position is satisfactory, with the affected side uppermost. If the block is to be bilateral, the patient must be turned for the second side.

The image intensifier is positioned to give an anteroposterior view of the vertebral levels to be injected. Usually the second, third or fourth lumbar vertebral levels are selected. The skin is cleaned and draped. A local anaesthetic wheal is raised about 5–8 cm lateral to the midline of the level that is chosen. The exact distance will vary according to the build of the patient. Insert a 15 cm 20 or 22 G needle through the wheal at an angle of about 15° laterally from the perpendicular, infiltrating with local anaesthetic as it is advanced, aiming for the lateral border of the vertebral body, and keeping the bevel of the needle (marked by a notch on the hub) facing medially. Bone may be encountered at a depth of 5 cm or so, usually indicating that the transverse process has been contacted. Check the view on the image intensifier and redirect the needle towards the vertebral body. When contact is made and the position is confirmed radiologically, withdraw the needle slightly and redirect it to pass immediately off the anterolateral border of the vertebral body and advance until the tip of the needle appears just medial to the lateral border

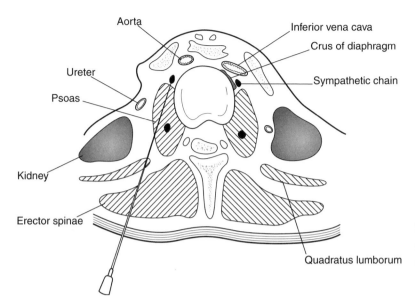

Figure 8.3 *Transverse view showing anatomical positioning of needle for lumbar sympathetic block*

Labels: Aorta, Inferior vena cava, Crus of diaphragm, Ureter, Sympathetic chain, Psoas, Kidney, Erector spinae, Quadratus lumborum

of the vertebral body. The position is then checked with radiological screening in the lateral plane. The needle should lie immediately posterior to the anterior margin of the vertebral body when viewed in this plane (Fig. 8.3).

The position of the needle should now be checked with the injection of a radio-contrast medium such as Omnipaque. Inject 1–2 mL of contrast and observe the spread of the medium. If the injection is correctly positioned, the medium will be seen to spread as a broad 'smudge' parallel to the line of the spine in the anterolateral projection. In the lateral view, the contrast forms a narrow band in line with the spine and along the anterior margin of the vertebral bodies (Fig. 8.4). If the contrast is seen to spread laterally, the tip of the needle probably lies within the psoas sheath and injection of a neurolytic solution in this position will result in damage to motor and sensory nerves. The needle must be repositioned more ventromedially and the position again checked radiologically to ensure that it is not within the psoas compartment.

If a trial or local anaesthetic block is required, inject 6–10 mL of 0.25 per cent bupivacaine through the correctly sited needle. For a neurolytic block, inject 3–6 mL of 6 per cent aqueous phenol. When phenol is used, flush the needle with 1–2 mL of saline prior to withdrawing the needle to avoid leaving a track of neurolytic solution. Larger volumes of injectate are unnecessary if the needle is in the correct fascial compartment. Some recommend using a needle at two or three separate levels and restricting the volume of phenol to 2 mL to reduce unwanted spread. The procedure is repeated on the opposite side for bilateral blocks.

After a neurolytic block, the patient should remain prone for 20 minutes to minimize the risk of phenol spreading onto

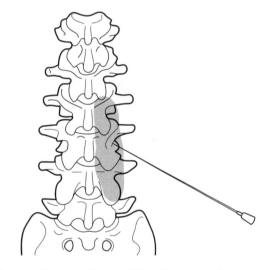

Figure 8.4 *Diagrammatic representation of the radiographic appearance of the injected contrast medium during a sympathetic block*

somatic nerve roots. Blood pressure should be monitored and any hypotensive response dealt with by intravenous fluid loading and vasopressors if necessary. The patient is warned of possible postural hypotension and advised to get up slowly and with the help of an accompanying person initially.

Complications

Occasionally the aorta or inferior vena cava is punctured. The needle is withdrawn and repositioned. There is generally no harm, although the efficacy of the block may be reduced due to dilution of the neurolytic solution in a haematoma. It is important to exclude patients who are on anticoagulant therapy immediately prior to this procedure.

The most frequent complication following neurolytic lumbar sympathetic block is neuritis in the distribution of the genitofemoral nerve, with a burning pain in the anterior thigh. This may result from some spread of neurolytic solution onto the genitofemoral nerve. The condition is usually self-limiting, but if it is particularly distressing it is usually ameliorated by prescribing a small dose of amitriptyline for a few weeks.

STELLATE GANGLION BLOCK

Indications

Pain in the face and upper limb may be moderated by a sympathetic blockade of the stellate ganglia. The procedure has also been used to relieve cardiac pain.

Anatomy

The stellate ganglion is formed by fusion of the inferior cervical ganglion and the first thoracic sympathetic ganglion. It lies anteriorly to the prevertebral fascia overlying the transverse processes of the sixth and seventh cervical vertebrae. Anterior to the ganglion is the common carotid artery (Fig. 8.5).

TECHNIQUE

Before undertaking the procedure, full resuscitation facilities should be available and intravenous access secured.

The usual approach is an anterior paratracheal approach at the level of the sixth cervical vertebra. The patient lies prone with the head gently extended over a small pillow and is requested to open the mouth slightly to relax the cervical muscles and allow easier identification of the landmarks. The patient is then requested to avoid swallowing during the injection, and this may be helped by asking the patient to put out their tongue. The skin is cleansed and draped.

Identify the most prominent transverse process which is normally at C6 (Chassaignac's tubercle) by gentle palpation between the trachea (almost level with the cricoid cartilage) and the carotid sheath. Inject a small bleb of local anaesthetic subcutaneously over this point. The injection can be given with a 21 G 40 mm needle or a 23 G 25 mm needle. It is helpful to use a shallow bevel needle attached by a short fine-bore cannula to the syringe. This enables the operator to position the needle and then fix it while an assistant injects without moving the needle.

The needle is inserted vertically downwards, immediately lateral to the trachea, while the fingers of the other hand gently retract the carotid sheath laterally out of the way. The needle is advanced until the bone of the transverse process is contacted. It is then withdrawn a couple of millimetres so that it lies anteriorly to the fascia and in the same tissue plane as the sympathetic ganglia. Gentle aspiration is attempted (by the assistant if a remote needle is being used) and if this is negative, local anaesthetic (10–20 mL of 1 per cent lidocaine or 0.25 per cent bupivacaine) is injected. It is advisable to start with a small test dose of 1 mL and observe any response before completing the full volume of injection. If there is any resistance to injection, the needle should be repositioned. If there is any suspicion that CSF has been aspirated, the procedure should be discontinued. Similarly the injection should not proceed if there is any suggestion that the needle may be intravascular. Immediately following injection the patient is requested to sit up and remain so for about five minutes. A successful block usually results in the development of Horner's syndrome on the side of the injection (ptosis, myosis, enophthalmos and anhidrosis).

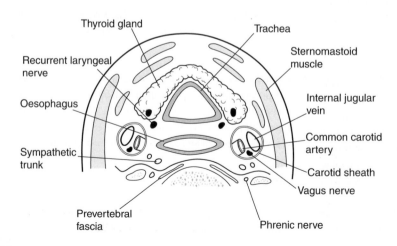

Figure 8.5 *Stellate ganglion block. Schematic diagram showing anatomical relations in transverse section of the neck*

Complications

Intravascular injection, notably of the vertebral artery, presents a major hazard. Injection should not be given without a negative aspiration test, but it is possible to obtain a false negative result, and therefore injection should start with a small test dose and then proceed with continuous observation of the patient. Even a small dose of local anaesthetic injected into the vertebral artery will produce rapid cerebral effects: dizziness, unconsciousness or convulsions.

Puncture of a cuff of dura, resulting in a subarachnoid injection, with a consequent high spinal block may not be easily detected by aspiration. The risk is reduced by injecting in small aliquots and having the necessary facilities (and skills) available to support the patient in the event of a high spinal block developing.

Blockade of a recurrent laryngeal nerve or phrenic nerve can follow stellate ganglion injection. The patient needs to be reassured about the resulting temporary hoarseness and difficult swallowing and told to avoid drinking until the effect has subsided. For this reason it is usual to avoid performing a bilateral cervical sympathetic block.

The temporary Horner's syndrome requires reassurance and advising the patient not to attempt tasks requiring accurate visual coordination, such as driving, until normal visual function has been restored. Other structures in the region of the block are vulnerable to needle trauma. This includes oesophageal puncture, pneumothorax, injection of the lymphatic duct and haematoma formation.

COELIAC PLEXUS BLOCK

Indications

Blockade of the coeliac plexus is most often indicated for relief of pain from pancreatic carcinoma; but it can be of value in managing pain from malignant disease of other viscera such as kidney, liver, spleen, stomach and colon. Destructive, neurolytic block of the coeliac plexus is rarely performed for pain relief in non-malignant disease. Its effects may be of limited duration and the procedure carries a risk of morbidity.

The injection must be carried out under radiological guidance as there is a major risk of damage to other structures, both from needle trauma and, in particular, the injection of neurolytic solutions.

Anatomy

The coeliac plexus is a collection of ganglia containing visceral afferent and efferent sympathetic fibres as well as pre-ganglionic parasympathetic fibres. It receives innervation from the greater, lesser and least splanchnic nerves and lies anterior to the first lumbar and twelfth thoracic vertebral bodies (Fig. 8.6). It is anterior and lateral to the aorta and slightly anterior to the right lie the inferior vena cava and right renal vessels. The pancreas and left renal vessels lie to the left. The plexus is surrounded by loose connective tissue so that injected solutions will normally spread freely throughout

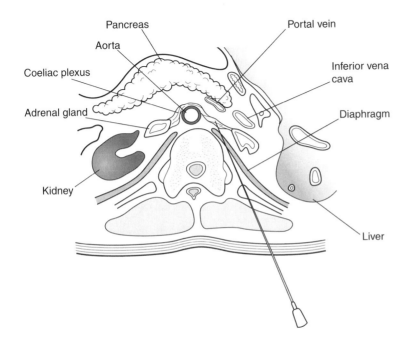

Figure 8.6 *Transverse section showing anatomical relations of coeliac plexus block*

the structure. In disease states, the presence of tumour mass or postoperative scar tissue may limit the spread of anaesthetic or neurolytic solution. It is one of the few destructive lesions which is worth performing at an early stage when pain is becoming a problem not easily controlled with opiate analgesics.

Technique

It is possible to perform a coeliac plexus block under local anaesthesia and sedation. However, it can be painful and distressing for the patient and the author usually performs the procedure with the patient under general anaesthesia. An intravenous infusion should be established prior to the block, to manage the possible resulting hypotensive response.

The patient is positioned prone on a radiolucent table, preferably with a pillow under the abdomen to straighten the lumbar spine. The position of the twelfth thoracic and first lumbar vertebrae, and the twelfth ribs, are marked. The angle which the ribs make with the spine depends to a certain extent on the build of the patient, but it should be remembered that during the injection the needle should remain inferior to the pleura. The injections are made bilaterally using a skin entry point immediately below the rib at the level of the first lumbar vertebra. A 15 cm 22 G needle is advanced with local anaesthetic infiltration in a medial, anterior and slightly cephalad direction towards the body of the first lumbar vertebra. In most patients the vertebral body will be encountered at a depth of 10–12 cm and the position on the anterolateral border of the vertebra can be confirmed radiologically. Keeping the bevel of the needle facing towards the vertebra, the needle is withdrawn slightly and redirected so that it passes anteriorly to the upper margin of L1 and comes to lie about 1 cm anterior to the upper margin of L1 and the lower margin of T12 (Fig. 8.7). Confirm the position of the needle by radiological screening in the lateral plane. At this stage, inject 0.5–1 mL of contrast medium and check the spread, which should remain anterior to the spine and in a cephalad and caudad direction (Fig. 8.8). Reposition the image intensifier screen to view again in the anteroposterior plane to check that there is no lateral spread of contrast which could indicate that the needle tip lies within the psoas sheath. During advancement of the needle, one of the great vessels may be encountered with aspiration of blood. If this is the inferior vena cava, the needle should reposition more medially. If the aorta is encountered, the needle can be redirected, or alternatively advanced to transfix the aorta and the injection made anterior to the aorta.

When a satisfactory position is achieved as judged by spread of contrast medium, a second needle is positioned on the other side in a similar manner. When both needles are correctly placed, 5 mL of 0.5 per cent bupivacaine is injected through each if the patient is awake. There should then be a pause for a few minutes to allow the local anaesthetic to

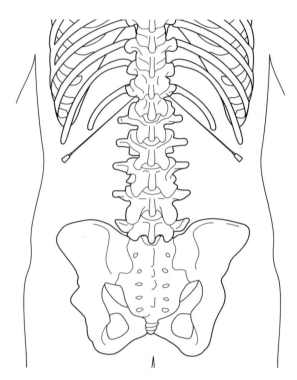

Figure 8.7 *Coeliac plexus block – direction of needle insertion*

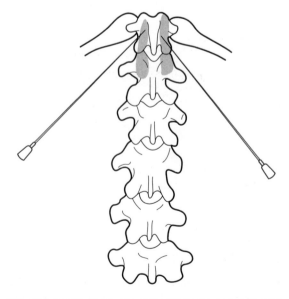

Figure 8.8 *Line drawing showing areas of contrast spread during coeliac plexus block*

take effect before injecting the neurolytic solution. In an anaesthetized patient the neurolytic solution can be injected immediately. The agent of choice is alcohol (a large volume of phenol is too toxic). Inject a mixture of 10 mL of 0.5 per cent bupivacaine with 10 mL of absolute alcohol on each side after careful aspiration. The patient should be left prone for about 20 minutes after injection so that the alcohol can fix and reduce the risk of the alcohol spreading posteriorly to involve the somatic nerves. The patient should remain in bed for the rest of the day.

Complications

The most frequent side effect of a coeliac plexus block is postural hypotension. The patient's fluid load should be maintained. The day after the block the patient is allowed to stand up under observation and with blood pressure monitoring. If postural hypotension occurs, it may be necessary to apply elasticated stockings for a while and to maintain a positive fluid balance until the blood pressure has stabilized. The loss of sympathetic activity can result in a period of gastrointestinal hypermotility with consequent diarrhoea after the procedure and this may aggravate potential hypovolaemic hypotension.

Neurological sequelae are the most serious complications. The blood supply to the spinal cord is vulnerable at this level. Damage to the artery of Adamkiewicz by direct needle trauma or vascular spasm induced by the neurolytic agent can result in severe ischaemic damage to the spinal cord with a consequent paraplegia. Damage to the great blood vessels with haematoma formation and trauma to the kidneys, pleura, adrenals are all possible sources of morbidity.

TRIGEMINAL BLOCKS

Anatomy of the trigeminal nerve

The trigeminal nerve is the largest cranial nerve arising from the ventrolateral surface of the pons (Fig. 8.9). It reaches the petrous portion of the temporal bone and expands to form the gasserian ganglion which contains the sensory nerve roots. It divides into the ophthalmic, maxillary and mandibular branches (Fig. 8.10 and Table 8.1).

Radio-frequency lesion

LANDMARKS AND METHOD

1   Locate and mark the angle between the maxilla and mandible (about two fingerbreadths lateral to the angle of the mouth at the level of the upper first molar tooth) – point A.

2   Locate the zygomatic arch and place the little finger in the ear to locate end of bone. Mark 2.5 cm (1 inch) from this point towards the face – point B.

3   Look at the pupil and put a mark on the cheek in line with it at the point of exit of the infraorbital vessels – point C.

4   Turn the patient's head 35–50° towards the side opposite to the pain.

5   Insert a radio-frequency cannula at point A directing it towards point C in the anteroposterior plane and point B in the lateral plane. The cannula is advanced until it hits bone. The beam of the image intensifier should be directed along the cannula. This should give a view of the foramen ovale. In the lateral view the tip of the electrode should lie just above the margin of the bony plate so the preganglionic fibres are destroyed. If masseteric contractions are produced the cannula is in contact with the motor nerve root. The tip should then be advanced further in. Cerebrospinal fluid in the needle means the trigeminal cistern has been entered and the cannula is in the correct place.

Complications

- Improper placement at:
  - inferior orbital fissure
  - posteromedially into the foramen lacerum (carotid artery)
  - posteroinferiorly into the jugular foramen or carotid canal
  - through the buccal mucosa (cover with antibiotics) cavernous sinus – produces eye movements and facial contractions.
- Damage to the sixth cranial nerve causing double vision – usually temporary. If large amounts of blood are seen abort the procedure.
- Thermocoagulation can cause hypertensive crisis.

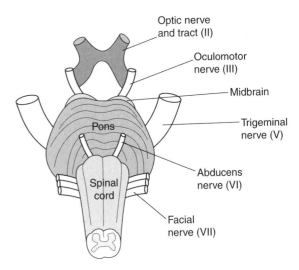

Figure 8.9 *The base of the brain*

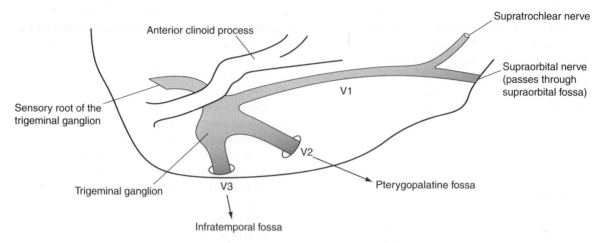

Figure 8.10 *The trigeminal nerve in the middle cranial fossa. V1, ophthalmic branch; V2, maxillary branch passing through the foramen rotundum; V3, mandibular branch passing through the foramen ovale*

Table 8.1 *Branches of the trigeminal nerve*

Branch of the nerve	Type of nerve	Distribution
Ophthalmic branch – first division (V1)	Sensory nerve	Supplies the eye. It is the uppermost and smallest branch and travels to the cavernous sinus and to the superior orbital fissure to the orbit
Maxillary branch – second division (V2)	Sensory nerve	It sends a branch to the middle meningeal artery (the middle meningeal branch) and branches to the dura
Mandibular branch – third division (V3)	Sensory and motor nerve	The motor branches supply the muscles of mastication

If CSF is seen do not inject local anaesthetic as this will cause cardiovascular collapse.

LESION

Start at 100 Hz, 60 °C for 60 seconds and increase in 5 °C increments to a maximum of 80 °C, each time testing for decreases sensitivity to pin prick. It is impossible to produce pain relief without causing numbness but by frequent testing the area of numbness will be as small as possible. Propofol and alfentanil infusions are usually used to provide sedation as they allow a rapid wake-up to assess the response to treatment.

MECHANISM OF ACTION

The mechanism of action of radio-frequency lesioning is based on (partial) nerve destruction. The undesired effects depend on the extent of the lesion. Heat destruction is probably not the only mode of action because the temperature is only measured at the electrode tip and decreases very rapidly at 1–2 mm. The tissue is also exposed to the radio-frequency field which may also explain its action. The size of the lesion depends on the temperature in the tissue, the duration of the procedure, the size of the non-insulated electrode tip and the electrode diameter. Pain relief can occur from one day afterwards and last for many months or years, but some patients get no pain relief. A second lesion should be carried out at this stage where possible.

Pulsed radio-frequency

Pulsed radio-frequency lesioning involves the use of a high generator output for a short period of time (20 ms) followed by a 'silent' period (480 ms). Heat is generated during the active burst and is eliminated during the rest period. The temperature at the electrode tip does not exceed 42 °C. Very few side effects have been reported and recent reports have been encouraging.

Balloon inflation

A balloon is inserted into the foramen ovale using a similar technique to glycerol injections and radio-frequency lesions. The balloon is then inflated for a period of time, deflated and withdrawn. The pressure exerted on the nerve during the balloon inflation causes changes within the nerve often leading to pain relief. Numbness still occurs with this technique and it is not as prolonged as with radio-frequency lesioning.

Glycerol injection

The patient is given a general anaesthetic for the procedure. A 22 G spinal needle is placed in the foramen ovale using the same landmarks as above. The patient is turned prone before injecting 0.3 mL glycerol and kept prone for 20 minutes to prevent glycerol running back into the brain. It does not cause as much numbness as radio-frequency lesioning but the effects may last only a year. Glycerol injection can be used as a diagnostic procedure. It is a much quicker procedure and can be used in those who are unfit for a prolonged anaesthetic.

COMPLICATION

Glycerol injection may lead to aseptic meningitis.

Outcome

Outcome of any treatment for trigeminal neuralgia is difficult to assess because many patients have spontaneous remission of their symptoms; also 30–75 per cent fail to obtain pain relief with medical management. If alcohol is used for injections there is often an unpleasant dysaesthesia and very high recurrent rate:

- Radio-frequency lesioning – 1 per cent – dysaesthesia; 0.8 per cent – anaesthesia dolorosa; 5.7 per cent – reduced corneal reflex.
- Glycerol – 17 per cent pain free at one year.
- Balloon inflation – 44–80 per cent are pain free at two years but there is a 10 per cent dysaesthesia rate.

PARAVERTEBRAL NERVE BLOCK

Indications

Segmental nerves can be blocked in the paravertebral space to provide relief of segmental pain, usually in the thoracic or lumbar regions. This can provide analgesia in the acute situation (e.g. chest trauma, postoperative pain) or may offer therapeutic effects in chronic pain conditions (possibly for post-herpetic neuralgia, post-thoracotomy scar pain, segmental spinal pain), when the local anaesthetic may be combined with a depot steroid preparation. For pain palliation in malignant disease it may be appropriate to use a neurolytic agent (phenol) in the paravertebral space for treating unilateral chest pain affecting several dermatomal segments due to localized tumour invasion. Although there may be resultant numbness and possible deafferentation pain, this may not be of particular consideration in patients who have a short life expectancy and where pain control is otherwise inadequate.

Anatomy

The paravertebral space in the thoracic region is bordered medially by the vertebral body, laterally by the intercostal space and costotransverse ligament, the rib and transverse process above, and the rib below. It contains the spinal nerve root which divides into the dorsal and ventral rami, and also the white and grey rami communicates and sympathetic ganglia. The paravertebral space communicates directly with the intercostal and the epidural spaces and material injected will often spread to these adjacent compartments.

Technique

In the thoracic region, the tip of the spinous process is level with the intervertebral foramen of the next lower segmental nerve root. With the patient lying in a lateral position with the side to be blocked uppermost, or sitting upright, the spinous process at the desired level is palpated. A local anaesthetic wheal is raised 2–3 cm lateral to the upper margin of the process below the nerve to be blocked. A 22 G 8 cm needle is inserted perpendicularly to the skin and advanced anteriorly until the transverse process is encountered. The needle is then slightly withdrawn and advanced in a slightly cephalad direction, so as to 'walk off' the superior margin of the transverse process, and advanced a further 0.5–1 cm. A loss of resistance should be encountered and the needle tip should now be in the paravertebral space (Fig. 8.11). If paraesthesiae are reported the needle should be withdrawn a few millimetres. An injection of 5 mL of anaesthetic solution should be sufficient to block the segmental nerve. A larger volume will spread to adjacent segments and produce a more widespread block.

Lumbar paravertebral block is performed in a similar manner to thoracic block. However, the upper border of the spinous process tends to be more on a level with the transverse

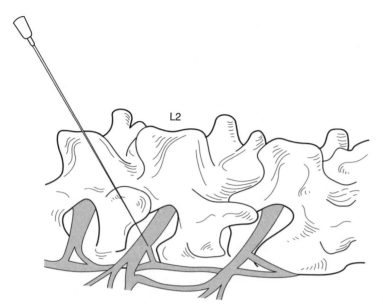

Figure 8.11 *Lumbar paravertebral injection*

process of the same vertebra. The paravertebral space lies at a greater depth in the lumbar region, so that the point of skin entry will need to be more lateral than in the thoracic region, usually about 4 cm from the midline.

Complications

It is difficult to predict the spread of paravertebral injections. Close proximity to the dura means that there is a real risk of inadvertent subarachnoid injection. Apart from the inevitable consequences of a spinal injection of local anaesthetic, the inclusion of steroid preparations or neurolytic agents could potentially cause neurological damage if the injection is subarachnoid. Probably most paravertebral injections result in some spread to the epidural space. This may be proportional to the volume and force of the injection. Small volume epidural injection may not be a problem, and might even improve the therapeutic effect of the injection, but the possibility should be considered and due precautions undertaken.

Other hazards include direct trauma to nerves and blood vessels, and the possibility of pleural puncture, with development of a pneumothorax. If the procedure is considered to be at all difficult or hazardous, it may be preferable to perform the block with the aid of an image intensifier, when the injection of contrast medium will give an indication of the expected spread of the injection. However, if adequate care and precautions are taken, the overall risk is limited, and a paravertebral block can form a simple and rapid means of pain relief for a sick patient on the ward.

A paravertebral block may be effective in relieving well-defined somatic segmental pain. If the pain is long term, consideration can be given to producing a more prolonged block. This may be produced with a neurolytic injection, but as described above, this is associated with potential morbidity and would normally be considered only for intractable pain towards the end of life. A preferable alternative would be to produce a radio-frequency thermocoagulation lesion of the dorsal root ganglion. This requires radiological imaging and the necessary facilities, and operator expertise. It also requires a patient who is able to cooperate sufficiently in positioning of the lesion. As such patients are often severely debilitated towards the later stages of a malignant disease, the procedure may not be suitable in many situations.

NERVE ROOT INJECTION

Indications

This procedure may be performed at any level of the spine, but is perhaps most frequently used in the thoracic and lumbar spine. The indications are pain along a nerve root, such as may occur when there is local compression of the root as a result of degenerative changes in the spine, or when there may be postoperative scarring or damage to the nerve root. The patient may present with pain in a single dermatome, and the pain is frequently of a neuropathic quality. A nerve root block with local anaesthetic may be used as a diagnostic procedure to confirm the level of the affected nerve root, possibly indicating that further intervention may be required at this level. The procedure is often of therapeutic value, when the local anaesthetic is combined with steroid. The steroid may reduce neuropathic pain in the nerve root directly, or it may have an effect in reducing scar tissue density and other connective tissue which may be compressing nerve tissue.

Technique

Nerve root blocks should be assisted by the use of radiological screening. The patient is being positioned prone on the radiolucent table and an anteroposterio projection on the image intensifier is viewed to establish the landmarks. After suitable skin preparation and sterile draping, a bleb of local anaesthetic is injected at about 5 cm from the mid-line at the level of the nerve root to be blocked. A 22 G 12.5 cm spinal needle is inserted through the skin bleb and, with continuing infiltration of local anaesthetic, is directed in an anteromedial direction towards the lamina overlying the intervertebral foramen of the chosen nerve root. When contact with bone is made, and the position has been checked radiologically, the needle is 'walked off' the lamina in an anterior direction until it is felt to enter the intervertebral foramen. The needle is advanced if possible to a position where the tip can be seen on a level with the mid-point of the facet joints as the point of maximum medial advancement. If paraesthesiae are reported, withdraw the needle slightly to avoid direct damage to the nerve root. At this point, change the position of the image intensifier to obtain a lateral view and confirm the position of the needle tip in the posterior part of the intervertebral foramen (Fig. 8.12). It is helpful further to confirm siting of the injection by injecting a small volume (<0.5 mL) of a radiocontrast medium. If the needle is correctly positioned, the contrast will be seen within the foramen on lateral views, and outlining the nerve root canal when seen on the anteroposterior view. For a diagnostic block, inject 1.5–2 mL of 2 per cent lidocaine or 0.5 per cent bupivacaine. If a therapeutic block is required, 0.5 mL (20 mg) of a depot steroid preparation is added to the local anaesthetic.

Following a nerve root block patients should be observed for at least one hour before discharge, or longer if there is sufficient motor block to prevent the patient from supporting their own weight when standing.

Complications

Complications include bleeding, direct trauma to nerve roots (prevent by withdrawing the needle if paraesthesiae are experienced and not injecting if injection produces sharp

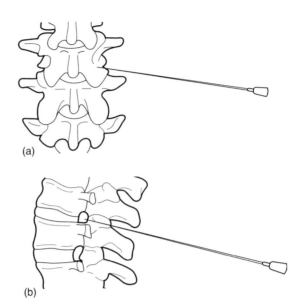

(a)

(b)

Figure 8.12 (a,b) Dorsal nerve root ganglion block

pain in the relevant nerve root distribution), aspiration of CSF and possible subarachnoid injection. In the thoracic region there is always the risk of producing a pneumothorax.

DORSAL ROOT GANGLION LESION

Pain which has been located to a specific nerve root, confirmed by diagnostic nerve root block, as described above, may be more effectively relieved by producing a lesion in the dorsal root ganglion (Fig. 8.12), usually by means of a radio-frequency lesion generator. This procedure is not without complications and can potentially result in deafferentation pain, numbness and weakness. Nerve lesioning or rhizolysis is therefore something of a last resort, when pain is intolerable and has not responded to more conservative measures. It may be more acceptable for monoradicular pain resulting from active neoplastic disease with pain from tumour which cannot be removed or decompressed in other ways.

A more recent development is the use of pulsed radio-frequency lesion generation. This technique uses radio-frequency current which is pulsed so that the tissue temperature does not rise sufficiently to cause thermocoagulation of nerve tissue. The monitored tissue temperature should not rise above 42 °C which is below the level at which tissue destruction occurs. However, subjecting the nerve tissue to this level of energy generation for three minutes is believed to result in an alteration in nerve function which may relieve pain for several months, without any long-term loss of normal function.

Technique

For a radio-frequency lesion of the dorsal root, the patient is positioned in the same way as for a nerve root block as described above. An insulated electrode (such as the Sluijter–Mehta cannula) is directed into the intervertebral foramen, with radiographic confirmation of its position in the outer posterior portion of the foramen. The stimulator of the radio-frequency generator is then used to check for paraesthesiae in the area of the patient's pain. Using a frequency of 100 Hz, aim to achieve paraesthesiae at a level of below 0.5 V. The stimulation is then checked using a frequency of 3 Hz to ensure that motor stimulation does not occur at a level below twice the sensory threshold.

When the position of the electrode is confirmed as satisfactory, inject 2 mL of 2 per cent lidocaine through the cannula and allow several minutes for this to be effective before lesioning. If a radio-frequency lesion is made, the temperature is raised to 70 °C and held for 60 seconds. For a pulsed radio-frequency lesion, a temperature of 40–42° is maintained for 180 seconds.

Complications

Patients undergoing this technique to produce a permanent lesion should be warned that the area treated may remain painful for several days. They should also be warned of the small risk of deafferentation pain and dysaesthesia, numbness and possible weakness.

CERVICAL CORDOTOMY

This procedure provides an effective means of relieving pain due to malignant disease. It is usually indicated for pain that is unilateral, which has been unrelieved by more conservative methods of pain relief and in patients who have a limited life expectancy. Although potentially very effective, cordotomy is an invasive procedure which can cause major morbidity, and is therefore rarely done for pain of benign origin.

The central nervous system is not a 'hard-wired' system and the plasticity of pain perception means that pain often returns after neurodestructive procedures. This may be pain of a different character from the original pain, but it is usually particularly unpleasant and intractable. This is the prime reason for reserving the procedure for those with a limited life expectancy.

A percutaneous technique is widely used, with reduced morbidity and mortality compared with open surgical approaches, but the technique should be learnt from an experienced operator, and written descriptions cannot be adequate for guiding the novice. The principles of the procedure will only be outlined here to enable the pain practitioner to understand the potential benefits as well as the hazards which may accompany referral of a patient for percutaneous cordotomy.

In high cordotomies there is a risk of damaging respiratory motor fibres so that if respiratory function is already compromised on one side, further loss of function would result in major difficulties. It is also important to ensure that the patient is able to cooperate well as the procedure involves lying still for perhaps an hour, with communication with the operator to enable accurate location of stimulation testing. For this reason, only minimal sedation is possible.

Anatomy

The anterolateral spinothalamic tracts lie anterior to the dentate ligament in the ventral portion of the spinal cord white matter and are arranged anatomically, representing different areas of the body (Fig. 8.13). The majority of the fibres in these tracts cross to the opposite side of the spinal cord in the upper cervical region so that a lesion at the level of C2 will normally provide analgesia on the contralateral side of the body below the level of the lesion.

Technique

The patient is positioned supine with the head supported and held in a head holder. A C-arm image intensifier is positioned at the head of the table to allow free rotation around the head and neck. The target area is visualized as the C1–C2 intervertebral space. After local anaesthetic skin infiltration, the cordotomy needle (insulated with an exposed tip) is advanced towards the cord, until the dura is penetrated and CSF obtained. The electrode can be inserted through the needle and electrical impedance measured. There will be a drop in impedance as the needle enters the CSF. It is important to identify the position of the dentate ligament, and 1–2 mL of contrast medium is injected to outline the ligament. The needle is advanced anteriorly to the ligament to enter the cord, when there will be a rise in electrical impedance. The radio-frequency generator is now used to test for sensory stimulation. At a frequency of 100 Hz test for sensory stimulation in the painful contralateral side of the body at a level of 0.2 V or less. When a satisfactory sensory threshold is obtained, use a stimulus of 2 Hz to test for motor stimulation, which should be absent below a stimulus level of 1.5 V.

When positioning of the electrode is satisfactory, a lesion is produced. It is recommended that the thermocoagulatory

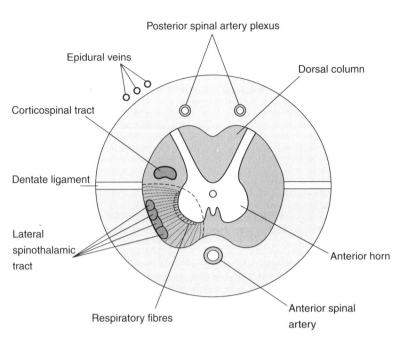

Posterior spinal artery plexus

Epidural veins

Dorsal column

Corticospinal tract

Dentate ligament

Lateral spinothalamic tract

Anterior horn

Respiratory fibres

Anterior spinal artery

Figure 8.13 *Schematic diagram showing the anatomical location of the spinothalamic tract*

lesion is produced in stages, starting with a temperature of 40 °C for five seconds, then for 10, 20, 40 and 60 seconds, testing for analgesia to pinprick in the target dermatomes after each lesion. Further lesioning is made at temperatures of 50, 60, and 70 °C if necessary, to achieve analgesia over the target area.

Complications

Cordotomy is not without potential hazards. The most common complication results from the dural puncture and CSF leak. This is managed in the usual way, with bed rest, fluid intake and analgesics. There is a risk of infection and the procedure should normally be covered by antibiotic administration.

Unwanted damage to the cord results in a number of neurological complications. Some motor weakness can occur and occasionally ataxia, dysaesthesia, urinary difficulties and impotence. Respiratory insufficiency is a possible risk in high cordotomies.

An occasional problem occurs when a cordotomy is highly effective in relieving pain in malignant disease, which has previously been managed with high doses of opiate analgesics. The consequent analgesia appears to result in a relative overdose effect of the opiate which is no longer 'antagonized' by pain. There have been reports of patients in this situation developing unexpected severe opiate-induced respiratory depression, even though the longstanding dose of opiate has not been increased. This effect should be carefully considered in the doses prescribed of any continuing opiate drugs.

FURTHER READING

Finucane B. *Complications of Regional Anesthesia*. Philadelphia: Churchill Livingstone, 1999.

Wedley JR, Gauci CA. *Handbook of Clinical Techniques in the Management of Chronic Pain*. Chur, Switzerland: Harwood Academic Publishers, 1994.

9 Treating Chronic Pain: Injection of Joints and Soft Tissues

INTRODUCTION

Injection of nerve tissue to either block or destroy neural function may be seen (often unjustifiably) as a means to reduce pain sensation even though this may not be a logical approach to treatment, or even be effective. For the injection of other tissues in the attempt to relieve pain it is perhaps even more difficult to offer a rational scientific explanation, but this practice is widespread, sometimes effective, and can at least be expected to be potentially less harmful than nerve-destroying interventions.

The procedures include:

- injection of joints
- injection of scars
- injection of trigger points.

FACET JOINTS AS A SOURCE OF PAIN

The causes of back pain are complex and there is unlikely to be a single cause in the majority of cases. There are many pain-sensitive structures in the spine and its associated tissues, as well as the behavioural and conditioning factors that influence back pain. However, the joints between the articular facets of the spine are subject to arthritic or degenerative processes, and may be damaged by strain and trauma. These joints are believed to be a source of back pain, although hard evidence for this is difficult to determine. It is a reasonable argument that pain arising in these joints will be felt in the back and also result in some referred pain in the legs because of their innervation from the posterior rami of the lumbar and upper sacral nerves. The complex of symptoms that results is often referred to as 'posterior compartment syndrome': a term which is less defining than the alternative 'facet joint syndrome'.

Patients presenting with facet joint pain usually complain of low back pain, often exacerbated by prolonged sitting or standing, and sometimes eased by limited movement. Forward flexion of the lumbar spine is typically pain free (unless other spinal structures are painful), whereas extension or lateral flexion and rotation are accompanied by increased pain. Palpation of the tissues overlying the joints usually demonstrates tenderness and there may be some protective muscle spasm. The pain often radiates to the buttocks and thighs or occasionally to the groins: it is unusual for the pain to radiate right down the leg, but it may mimic true sciatica. A common feature is that the pain is not dermatomal, to correspond with the spinal levels affected. Patients who have previously undergone a spinal fusion procedure seem prone to developing facet joint pain at the level immediately adjacent to the fusion, as would perhaps be expected where increased stress results from the immobility of the fused segments.

The techniques for treating pain which is believed to originate in the facet joints differ widely. Early techniques used a fine blade to cut the tissues surrounding the joint: this proved unreliable and resulted in excessive local trauma. As understanding of the anatomy of facet joint innervation improved, techniques to produce a lesion in the nerve supplying the facet joint using a radio-frequency generator were developed. Test injections of local anaesthetic or local anaesthetic and steroid given prior to lesioning were found to often provide pain relief which was as effective as the more destructive procedure. The nerve supply to the joint is complex, and it seems unlikely that any single lesion will result in complete denervation of the facet joint. The unpredictable and variable results of these procedures have led to widespread doubt about the value of facet joint injections or denervations. Nevertheless, the procedures are widely practised, and there is no doubt that many patients receive a useful degree of relief from their back pain.

FACET JOINT INJECTION

Pain relief may result from injection of local anaesthetic and steroid directly into the facet joint space. It may be that a good result can also be achieved by injecting the tissues immediately surrounding the joint or the nerve supply to the joint.

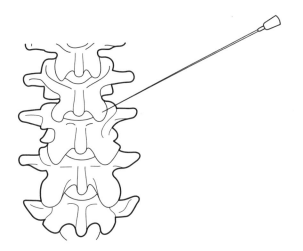

Figure 9.1 *Injection of the lumbar facet joints*

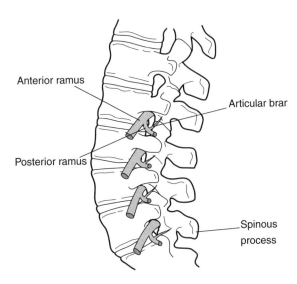

Anterior ramus

Articular brar

Posterior ramus

Spinous process

Figure 9.2 *Nerve supply to facet joints at L4/5 and L5/S1*

Facet joints are small, and accurate injection of the joints requires radiological guidance.

The patient lies prone on an X-ray table. A straight antero-posterior (AP) projection with the image intensifier should be used to identify the position of the lumbar facet joints. It is helpful to visualize the joint space of each facet, and this will usually be assisted by obtaining an oblique radiological view, either by rotating the C-arm of the image intensifier so that it projects obliquely from the side to be injected, or by rotating the patient slightly away from the side to be injected. Following local infiltration with anaesthetic, a fine spinal needle (25 or 22 SWG) with introducer, is inserted about 1 cm lateral to the point on the skin which overlies the joint in AP projection, and passed anteriorly and slightly medially to enter the joint (Fig. 9.1). The joint space is small and resistance to injection may be quite high. Sometimes it is necessary to withdraw the needle slightly until injection can be achieved. The injection usually consists of 0.5 mL of local anaesthetic (e.g. bupivacaine 0.5 per cent) mixed with about 5 mg of depot steroid, such as methylprednisolone or triamcinolone. The injection is repeated at as many of the facet joints as are considered to be contributing to the pain symptoms.

The patient is warned that following injection of facet joints, there may be period of several days when there is an increased level of pain in the low back. This resolves spontaneously and the pain relief resulting from the procedure may develop gradually over a period of up to six weeks. If pain relief results from the procedure, it may last for months, or occasionally years. If such a good result occurs then it seems justified to repeat the procedure at a later date if necessary. If the result is definite and considerable, but only lasts for a short period, then it may be considered appropriate to offer the patient facet joint denervation.

FACET JOINT DENERVATION

The innervation of the facet joint is complex, the principal supply coming from a medial branch of the posterior ramus (Fig. 9.2). There are several points of innervation of the facet joint. Some practitioners advocate the production of lesions at multiple points to include as many points of innervation as possible. Others may prefer to produce a single lesion to each joint, often with satisfactory results.

To produce a thermocoagulation lesion to the principal innervation of the lumbar facet joint, the patient is positioned on the X-ray table as for injection of the joints (see above). The facet joint and the transverse process at that level are identified. The target lies at the junction of the transverse process with the inferior articular process of the facet joint, where the medial branch of the posterior ramus lies in a depression along the base of the articular process.

Following local anaesthetic infiltration of the superficial tissues, a 100 mm insulated needle/cannula is introduced just lateral to a point overlying the target. The connulae is then guided to the target area at the base of the articular process at the point where it meets the medial end of the transverse process (Fig. 9.3). It is often helpful to use an oblique projection with the image intensifier to view the target area satisfactorily. The radiological view of the facet joints when viewed obliquely is often described as looking like a Scotty dog (with a little imagination!), and the target area is likened to the eye of the Scotty dog.

The electrode is inserted into the cannula which has been positioned near the target area. Using the radio-frequency generator in stimulation mode, stimulation is applied to the electrode at a frequency of 100 Hz. While gradually increasing

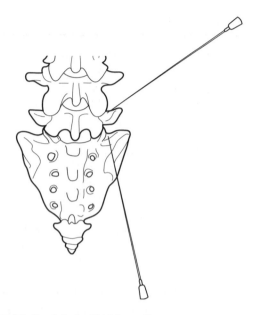

Figure 9.3 *Targets for facet joint denervation*

the amplitude of the stimulation the patient is requested to report the onset of sensory stimulation. The threshold for stimulation is ideally between 0.2 and 0.5 V. If this is not achieved, the position of the electrode can be adjusted with further testing until the required threshold is obtained. The frequency of the stimulatory signal is now changed to 3 Hz and the motor stimulation threshold determined. There should be no motor response below a stimulus level which is twice the amplitude of the sensory threshold.

When the electrode is in the optimal position, 2 mL of local anaesthetic is injected through the cannula before the thermal lesion is produced. Using the radio-frequency generator, the temperature of the electrode tip is raised to 80 °C and held for 60 seconds. The procedure is then repeated at other joints as is considered appropriate.

The configuration of the L5/S1 joint is rather different from the other lumbar levels (see Fig. 9.3). The principal target lies in a depression between the medial end of the sacral ala and the sacral superior articular process. The entry point for this level lies slightly inferior to the lumbosacral articulation.

INJECTION OF ABDOMINAL CUTANEOUS NERVES

Patients can present with persistent abdominal pain which has been thoroughly investigated but where no visceral cause for pain has been identified. Some of these will be identified as 'abdominal cutaneous nerve entrapment'. The concept of 'a trapped nerve' seems to be quite common among the lay population. It provides a neat and easy explanation for painful symptoms: the medical evidence for the

existence of such an entity is less convincing. However, such patients often have localized abdominal pain which can be provoked by applying pressure over a well-defined point in the abdominal wall, and it may be that this represents a point where the cutaneous nerves to the abdominal wall are under pressure or traction.

There is often a history of abdominal surgery, and the pain may be related to scar tissue which contracts and applies either direct compression on the cutaneous nerves or a degree of traction on the abdominal fascia with resulting compression of cutaneous nerves as they pass through the fascia at the edge of the rectus abdominis muscle. This effect may occur without previous surgery and the reason for apparent compression of cutaneous nerves is unclear.

Examine the abdominal wall, checking for intra-abdominal masses and for scars on the surface. Detailed examination of the painful region may reveal a trigger point in the scar, or commonly along the lateral margin of the rectus muscle (more easily identified by requesting the patient to raise their head and so tense the abdominal muscles). Pressure on the trigger point should reproduce the pain of which the patient complains. Testing of cutaneous sensory function to pin-prick will often reveal an area of altered sensitivity in the region of the pain trigger.

Treatment of an abdominal 'nerve entrapment' is usually by injection. Once a well-defined trigger point has been identified, pass a bevelled needle down until the deep fascia is felt or the needle is deep to the scar tissue. Inject 2 mL of local anaesthetic mixed with steroid (e.g. depot methylprednisolone) at this point. This procedure may result in relief of pain for a few weeks or sometimes indefinitely. Possibly the effect of the steroid is to break down connective tissue, relieving pressure on the cutaneous nerves, but this remains speculative.

If pain is relieved by injection but recurs, the procedure can be repeated at intervals of six weeks, when a gradual increase in effect and period of relief may result. Alternatively a more permanent effect can be achieved by injecting 0.5–1 mL of 6 per cent aqueous phenol at the trigger point. Another technique is to use the radio-frequency generator to produce a low-temperature pulsed radio-frequency lesion at the point.

TRIGGER POINT INJECTIONS

Myofascial pain syndrome is a common presentation of musculoskeletal pain of obscure aetiology (see Chapter 13). Common practice is to treat this condition by repeated injection of the trigger points. The trigger points may represent areas of taut muscle or motor points, and they frequently correspond to classically described acupuncture points. Trigger points are usually predictable from the pattern of pain referral and they are reproducible such that maps of trigger points can be consulted to determine the most likely location of the points in a described condition. Treatment may include dry needling of the points, injection of local anaesthetic (with or without steroid), or injection of botulinum toxin. All of these techniques usually need repeating at frequent intervals to maintain beneficial effects. Treatment with botulinum toxin may provide relief for three months, but occasionally injection of anaesthetic and steroid will produce similar results.

The patient should be positioned in as relaxed and comfortable a manner as possible. Identify the trigger point (which may be in muscle, fascia or even subcutaneous tissues) by gentle palpation. The trigger point is often felt as an area of increased tension or bulk in the muscle tissue, or direct pressure will reproduce the patient's pain, sometimes accompanied by a slight twitch response in the local muscle fibres. A fine needle is then introduced into the trigger point and either manipulated gently to produce an acupuncture-type effect from dry needling, or a small volume (about 0.1–0.2 mL) of the chosen injection is made. If botulinum toxin is being injected, the dose at each injection is in the order of 10 units in 0.1 mL.

PAINFUL SCARS

Painful scar tissue resulting from trauma or surgery presents a frequent problem. The incidence of painful scars is generally underestimated and contributes to the general incidence of chronic post-traumatic pain. Pain may arise from dysfunction of mechanical structures (joints), damage or compression of nerve tissue, or as part of a general reaction to trauma forming a complex regional pain syndrome (causalgia, sympathetic dystrophy, algodystrophy and all the other multiple terms which have been used to describe this syndrome). Scars can be painful without fitting clearly into any of these more defined syndromes. Painful scar tissue can be infiltrated with local anaesthetic and depot steroid (methylprednisolone or triamcinolone) which is often effective in relieving pain. The process may need to be repeated several times at intervals of about four to six weeks to achieve an accumulating effect. Injection of steroid to subcutaneous tissue should not be continued indefinitely at this frequency as there can be cumulative systemic effects of chronic steroid administration as well as localized tissue atrophy.

10 Treating Chronic Pain: Stimulation and Physical Techniques

PHYSICAL METHODS OF NEUROSTIMULATION

Neurostimulation

The physiology of pain perception is complex and there is little resemblance to the 'hard-wired' system (as proposed by Descartes, Chapter 1) where a stimulus will produce a predictable and reproducible pain experience. The pain perceived by the sufferer is the result of a complex integrated function of the nervous system in which there is an interaction between afferent stimuli conducted along nerve tracts which differ structurally and functionally, with information from other parts of the sensory system and activity within the central nervous system which may be excitatory or inhibitory. The 'gate theory' of pain attempts to describe in a basic model one of the lowest levels of this integrated activity. Sensory input to the central nervous system is subject to a continuing central modulation. It follows from this concept that destruction of one part of the nervous system may result in impairment of these modulatory processes so that normal physiological sensation is perceived as painful, or existing painful stimuli may become more severe and difficult to control. It also leads to the possibility of modulating pain by stimulation of the inhibitory functions of the nervous system. On the basis of the model of the gate theory (see Chapter 1), the concept of transcutaneous electrical nerve stimulation (TENS) developed and was found to be a practical and effective means of controlling pain.

Transcutaneous electrical nerve stimulation

Transcutaneous electrical nerve stimulation is used to provide segmental stimulation of Aβ fibres to block input from C fibres. Presynaptic inhibition of C fibres occurs with release of inhibitory neurotransmitters. Stimulation of Aβ fibres may also activate descending inhibitory pathways within the central nervous system (CNS) via 5-hydroxytryptamine (5-HT) transmission. Polysegmental inhibitory circuits probably require recruitment of C fibres as well as Aβ fibres. This is believed

to be one of the mechanisms involved in acupuncture-produced analgesia and highlights the differences between the two techniques. Transcutaneous electrical nerve stimulation produces a low threshold segmental stimulation whereas acupuncture causes a high intensity extrasegmental stimulation. Differences in the basic mechanisms of analgesia between the two systems are further illustrated by the observation that acupuncture analgesia, unlike TENS, may show some sensitivity to naloxone.

APPLICATION OF TENS

The aim of TENS is to stimulate large myelinated sensory fibres, without causing muscle contraction or unpleasant sensory stimuli. It requires a pulse generator, an amplifier and electrodes.

PULSE FORM

The nature of the pulse can be varied. It may be delivered as a continual train of pulses, or sometimes in a series of bursts or a modulated waveform of intensity. Both of the latter two modes are claimed to reduce the fade of stimulus with repetition. The wave form of the pulse is variable, square, sinus or biphasic. A square wave form is the most commonly used, possibly producing less painful stimulation than the alternatives. With continuing use, skin impedance can change and the amplifier may need adjustment to maintain a constant stimulus. The aim is to activate large sensory myelinated fibres without causing muscle contraction or unpleasant sensory stimuli.

Generally, the greater the pulse width used for stimulation, the lower the required current for TENS to be effective. If the pulse width is too short, there will be no effective stimulation. High intensity, low frequency stimulation may cause painful muscle contractions, and should be avoided.

FREQUENCY

Stimulation of Aβ fibres may be achieved with pulse widths of 100–200 ms to produce a tingling sensation. Pulse widths greater than 500 ms recruit smaller nerve fibres resulting in a painful stimulus. A pulse rate of 75–150 Hz is usually achieved with a current of 10–30 mA.

ELECTRODES

The electrodes used for TENS need to be able to deliver an adequate current density to excite fibres in adjacent nerves in a controllable manner and without causing skin damage. Pads of carbon-impregnated silicone rubber are commonly used, applied to the skin using an adhesive conductive gel or with a simple conductive gel and adhesive tape. An alternative is to use self-adhesive gum electrodes which contain a conductive medium and can be applied directly to skin without additional adhesive. The latter are more convenient to use and are less likely to cause local skin irritation, but are more costly. Electrodes used without an adequate conductive medium will produce a pricking painful sensation and increase the risk of thermal damage.

PRACTICAL USE OF TENS

Placement of TENS electrodes is to some extent empirical. It is common to place the electrodes over the course of the nerve which may be innervating the painful region, ideally proximal to the pain. This is not always possible and other points may be stimulated with effect. Knowledge of acupuncture points is helpful in planning electrode placement as stimulation over acupuncture points which are local to the pain is often helpful. There is an element of trial and error and patients should be encouraged to vary the site of electrode placement within the distribution of the pain to achieve the optimum effect. Patients are also instructed to experiment with waveform, variations of stimulus frequency, pulse width and amplitude.

An important precondition for TENS to be effective is the presence of some normal skin sensation. Transcutaneous electrical nerve stimulation will have no effect when applied to anaesthetic skin or where there is severely abnormal sensory function as it requires an intact nerve supply.

Patients are instructed to apply TENS stimulation for several hours a day. The short periods (20 minutes) sometimes recommended by commercial suppliers of TENS devices are generally ineffectual; in some individuals it can take up to 20 minutes for an analgesic effect to develop with TENS. As patients become used to using the device in the most effective way, use can be extended to cover most of the day if required. Other patients will find it most useful for selected shorter periods, for instance when they know that certain activities or times of day are associated with more pain.

CONTRAINDICATIONS

It is generally recommended that TENS units are not used in bed, in the bath or while driving. The use of TENS in the presence of a cardiac pacemaker is usually contraindicated and manufacturers of the devices often state this. This is probably not an absolute contraindication, depending on the type and function of a particular pacemaker. However, caution is advised and if necessary specialist cardiological advice should be sought before using TENS in such situations.

INDICATIONS

- Back pain
- Neck and shoulder pain
- Large peripheral joint pain
- Segmental thoracic/intercostal pain
- Complex regional pain syndrome (CRPS)
- Scar pain

Dubious benefits for:

- Post-herpetic neuralgia
- Radiculopathy
- Peripheral neuropathy

Unlikely to be any help for:

- Fibromyalgia
- Headache
- Trigeminal neuralgia
- Acute incident pain, e.g. pain when weight bearing on arthritic hip or fracture

EFFICACY

There is undoubtedly a strong placebo effect in the use of TENS (not that placebo effect should be regarded as invalid if the patient experiences pain relief), but generally its effect is superior to placebo. There is often a fall-off effect with time, and one study has shown that 68 per cent of patients experienced short-term relief with TENS, whereas only about 30 per cent were still experiencing beneficial pain relief after one year of use. Placebo effect tends to diminish rapidly, whereas therapeutic effect seems to decline more slowly. There is a higher rate of beneficial effect when patients are given regular support and advice in the use of TENS and there is greater attention to detail. Patients who purchase their own TENS device with no advice or back-up, or who are given a machine with no help or following support and advice, are less likely to achieve satisfactory results.

COMPLICATIONS

- Local skin allergy or irritation
- Stimulation to anterior of the neck may adversely stimulate carotid sinus

- Potential interference with cardiac pacemakers
- Difficulty of use for patients with learning difficulties or immobility of limbs

Acupuncture

AN ANCIENT PRACTICE ADAPTED TO MODERN USE

Acupuncture is part of an ancient system of medicine which probably originated in China more than 2000 years ago. Traditional acupuncture is based on complex theories of health and disease, in which the balance of certain life forces can be used to diagnose and treat many ailments. Two vital energies which occur universally, 'Yin' and 'Yang' are represented in the organ systems of living creatures; the balance between these forces is essential for good health and is dependent on the flow of energy, or 'chi', in channels throughout the body. Diagnosis of disease involves detection of energy balance which includes a complex analysis of different pulses. Balance can be restored and the flow of 'chi' promoted by stimulating the body at recognized points which lie along the channels, or 'meridians', in order to treat symptoms and restore health.

This system of medicine does not fit in any way with the scientific concepts which have formed the basis of modern western medicine and is difficult to explain in terms of our own knowledge of anatomy and physiology. However, there is clearly some basis for the widely observed effect of acupuncture and even if the traditional theory and explanations seem to be incompatible with our scientific knowledge, this should not necessarily invalidate the observed clinical effects of acupuncture. Over the past four centuries there has become an increasing awareness of and interest in the claims made for acupuncture, and over the past four decades it has become a popular form of 'alternative' medicine in the West.

Research in China and the West has started to show some of the mechanisms that may help to explain the action of acupuncture and its use has gradually evolved from being a fringe practice regarded with scepticism by conventional medical practitioners to being widely accepted by many Western-trained medical practitioners as a useful tool in the therapeutic armamentarium.

MECHANISMS OF ACTION

Acupuncture stimulation has been shown to increase the level of encephalins in cerebrospinal fluid, and different modes of stimulation may alter the pattern of different encephalins released. Intense acupuncture analgesia shows some sensitivity to naloxone and it seems likely that endogenous opioids are involved in some of the effects of acupuncture. Electrical stimulation of areas of the mid-brain such as the periaqueductal grey matter can produce profound analgesia which is probably mediated by endogenous opioids and this could be one way in which acupuncture stimulation could produce analgesia. It seems likely that descending inhibitory tracts in the spinal cord are involved in acupuncture analgesia and, interestingly, the effects of acupuncture are often bilateral, following stimulation of one side of the body. Acupuncture can produce prolonged analgesia, and it has been suggested that there may be continuing activation of endogenous inhibitory systems.

Acupuncture has developed along two paths. Traditional acupuncturists practise diagnostic techniques and believe that good results can only be achieved by accurate stimulation of acupuncture points lying along the mapped meridians. However, many practitioners of modern acupuncture do not subscribe to the full system of traditional acupuncture and use acupuncture needling to stimulate palpable trigger points or tender points in the painful area. Effective pain relief seems to be possible by both methods, and there are probably some advantages in using a combination – stimulation of both recognized trigger points and a number of points along meridians which pass through the painful area.

Acupuncture is frequently recommended for the following indications:

- soft-tissue pain associated with palpable trigger points, as in myofascial pain syndrome
- back and neck pain with tender tense muscles
- large joint pain
- headache
- epicondylitis ('tennis elbow').

There are many other painful conditions where acupuncture may be helpful.

PRACTICE OF ACUPUNCTURE

Simple 'Western-style' acupuncture is usually practised by physicians, physiotherapists and nurses who have had some basic training in the use of acupuncture techniques. Patients are given a course of acupuncture consisting of four to six treatments at regular intervals of about one week. Sterile disposable acupuncture needles (fine round-tipped atraumatic) are inserted into the chosen tender trigger points and/or traditional acupuncture points and stimulated. The stimulation is most often manually performed by rotating and oscillating the needles for about 10 minutes. Stimulation is sometimes produced electrically by connecting a square wave generating electrical source to the needles and using a low frequency (4–20 Hz) stimulation. A more traditional approach is to attach a burning herbal mixture to the needles (moxibustion) to produce a thermal stimulus. Correct stimulation of acupuncture points is usually associated with a warm tight sensation around the needle, which in traditional acupuncture is called 'chi'.

PRECAUTIONS

Acupuncture treatment must be conducted with strict attention to sterility to avoid transmission of needle-borne infection. Care should be taken to avoid damage to nerves and blood vessels or puncture of internal organs by the needle. Puncture of the pleura with production of a pneumothorax is a specific hazard to be avoided. After acupuncture treatment patients may experience a pleasant period of relaxation or even somnolence, about which they should be warned. Perhaps this is an effect of encephalin release.

PHYSICAL THERAPY

The role of physiotherapy in the management of chronic pain has developed a broader remit in recent years. The traditional role of restoration of function and mobility of damaged muscles and joints continues to provide a valuable form of treatment. The use of exercise, manipulation, postural training, ultrasound and the other physical therapeutic techniques can be helpful in restoring mobility and relieving pain in stiff joints, painful backs, and limbs affected by CRPS, but a broader view of pain management has involved physiotherapists in the multidisciplinary rehabilitation of patients with chronic pain. From passive treatment of disease and disability, the physiotherapist now frequently forms part of a team whose role is to educate the patient in the active participation in management of their pain – overcoming the physical and psychological obstacles to restoration of function and the development of a positive approach to achieving goals in physical and social activity.

Although physiotherapy may not be directly responsible for pain relief, it may be that the restoration of function has an effect on pain by the stimulation of normal afferent activity in the central nervous system, and it certainly has important psychological benefits for the patient coping with chronic pain.

The body with chronic pain usually functions poorly. Activity is associated with pain, and increasing inactivity results in deconditioning of the musculoskeletal system. The physiological deterioration associated with deconditioning results in a reduced resilience to activity, with pain being perceived at ever lower thresholds. The perceived inability to be active, the fear of damage being caused by activity, and the exhaustion of coping with pain and deconditioning result in further distress, disability and despair.

The rehabilitation programme is planned to give an individual a graded fitness schedule which must be within their capacity to achieve. It is important to have goals which can be realistically achieved so that the effects of pain can be placed in a related context without becoming overwhelming and preventing further activity. Patients are taught how to effectively pace their activities: many people alternate between driving themselves to excess activity with prolonged periods of pain, exhaustion and rest. Appropriate pacing skills aim to smooth out these cycles of activity and rest which are pain driven, so that a more patient controlled level of moderated activity can be maintained. The physiotherapist can also enable the patient to identify situations which cause exacerbations or relapses of pain, identify and reduce such challenges, and cope with them when they occur so that they are not seen as a complete failure of the rehabilitation process.

11 Treating Chronic Pain: Implantation of Devices to Modify Pain

INTRODUCTION

Multiple surgical procedures have been attempted over the years to relieve intractable pain. Destructive lesioning produces short-term pain relief but in the long term, pain returns, which can be as bad as or even worse than the original condition. This is the reason why neuromodulatory techniques have been explored.

Under 3 per cent of patients referred to a pain clinic for other than malignant disease are treated by neurosurgical intervention. All available treatments for neuropathic pain (anticonvulsants, tricyclic antidepressants, local blocks, etc.) must have been tried and any anatomical correction complete before considering stimulation techniques or intrathecal pumps. The available techniques are:

- **Modulative** or **neuroaugmentation** techniques using stimulation directed to the peripheral nerves, the spinal cord, the thalamus or the precentral cortex. Stimulation procedures depend on inhibition of stimulatory pathways or by stimulation of inhibitory pathways. It is a reversible process – the stimulator can be removed.
- Implantation of delivery systems (programmable pumps) to infuse analgesic drugs intrathecally.

SPINAL CORD STIMULATION

Historical background

Spinal cord stimulation (SCS) was developed in the 1960s and the first system was implanted by Shealy in 1967 for malignant pain. Since then neurostimulation technology has improved significantly, including refinements in patient selection criteria, equipment design, flexibility, reliability and the lifespan of the components.

How does it work?

The concept of SCS developed from the gate control theory of pain. The greatest concentration of Aβ fibres lies in the dorsal columns, therefore, stimulation of these should provoke inhibition of the C fibres and produce pain relief.

The basic neurophysiological mechanisms of SCS are still poorly understood and the mechanism of action has not yet been fully explained. Some of the effects are difficult to explain by this theory alone, particularly the action in angina and the increased blood flow that occurs with the use of stimulation in peripheral vascular disease. Although the mechanism is thought to be similar to transcutaneous electrical nerve stimulation (TENS) there is no correlation between the response to TENS and the response to stimulation. It is known that SCS:

- activates inhibitory interneurones in the dorsal horn
- inhibits spinothalamic neurones that respond specifically to pain due to enhanced release of γ-aminobutyric acid (GABA) from the dorsal horn interneurones
- decreases glutamate and aspartate release from the dorsal horn
- attenuates wide dynamic range (WDR) neurone activity
- may abolish tactile and thermal allodynia, but it has no effect on acute nociceptive pain.

Indications for spinal cord stimulation

The British Pain Society (2004) has drawn up a list of recommended uses for SCS.

GOOD INDICATIONS (LIKELY TO RESPOND)

- Neuropathic pain in the leg or arm following lumbar or cervical spine surgery sometimes called failed back surgery syndrome (FBSS)
- Complex regional pain syndrome
- Neuropathic pain secondary to peripheral nerve damage
- Pain associated with peripheral vascular disease
- Refractory angina
- Brachial plexopathy (partial, not avulsion), post-irradiation

INTERMEDIATE INDICATIONS (MAY RESPOND)

- Amputation pain (stump pain responds better than phantom pain)
- Axial pain following spinal surgery
- Intercostal neuralgia (e.g. post-herpetic neuralgia, or post-thoracotomy pain)
- Pain associated with spinal cord damage
- Other peripheral neuropathic pain syndromes

POOR INDICATIONS

- Central pain of non-spinal origin
- Spinal cord injury with complete loss of posterior column function
- Perineal/anorectal pain
- Phantom limb pain
- Cancer pain
- Cauda equina syndrome
- Primary bone and joint disease

UNRESPONSIVE

- Complete cord transaction
- Non-ischaemic nociceptive pain
- Nerve root avulsion

Spinal cord stimulation can only be effective if the dorsal columns retain sufficient function. If interruption of the pathway is central and total it cannot be effective, because of degeneration of axons of the dorsal root ganglia all along the spinal cord, up to their brain stem relay nuclei.

When pain is due to spinal cord lesions and the territory below the lesion is totally anaesthetic, SCS will not work. When pain is in the territory corresponding to the (injured) lesioned segments of the spinal cord, SCS may be effective on that pain, but only if the segmental primary afferents of large calibre (i.e. the lemniscal fibres) are still – at least partially – functional.

Patient selection criteria

Adherence to the following patient selection criteria is critical to long-term success:

- conservative therapies have failed
- further surgical intervention is not indicated
- no serious untreated drug habituation exists
- psychological evaluation is complete
- where possible, trial stimulation has been successful
- no contraindications to implantation are present
- the patient has been fully informed about the technique, about short-, medium- and long-term effects, side effects and complications.

Psychological assessment

Psychological assessment is a valuable part of pain management in patients being considered for implantation of a spinal cord stimulator. Information collected from the psychological assessment:

- exposes psychological factors that should be addressed in treatment
- suggests specific treatments that may help resolve psychological risk factors
- may help to evaluate the patient's response to a screening test or treatment.

Education and expectations

Before insertion of the stimulator the patient must:

- have realistic expectations about pain relief
- understand the process and recovery
- understand that it may not help the pain at all, or that they may find the sensation that replaces the pain more unpleasant than the pain itself.

The spinal cord stimulation system

The SCS system consists of:

- a lead that delivers electrical stimulation to the spinal cord
- an extension wire that conducts electrical stimulation from the power source to the lead
- a power source that generates electrical stimulation.

Also required are:

- a test stimulator (screener) – an external power supply for the trial stage
- a programmer – allows setting of the parameters and modes. This can either be a large machine which communicates coded information with the patient's stimulator via telemetry, or a hand-held programmer that is given to the patient
- a magnet – to turn the system on and off when a hand-held programmer is not provided.

THE LEADS

The electrodes can be inserted percutaneously or they can be placed under direct vision surgically. The percutaneous leads are usually quadripolar or octapolar with cylindrical electrodes. The surgical leads are all quadripolar with four plate electrodes to create multiple stimulation combinations and a broad area of stimulation.

The top electrode should lie neurologically rostral to the area of pain. Evoked paraesthesia must cover at least the majority of the area. There is more position specificity with the percutaneous electrodes than with surgically placed electrodes, and in the majority of cases it is best to use the percutaneously implanted leads while the patient is awake to optimize positioning.

EXTENSIONS

Temporary (for the trial stage) or permanent (for the implanted stage).

POWER SOURCE

There are two types of power source. The first is a self-powered neurostimulator with non-invasive programmability. The implantable pulse generator contains a lithium battery and is activated or controlled by transcutaneous telemetry and turned on and off by a magnet. The second type is a radio-frequency power source. A transmitter is worn externally with an antenna applied to the skin to correspond to the receiver. The patient needs to wear the external components and this can be inconvenient, but it allows for greater control.

STIMULATION WAVEFORM

Amplitude (V)

The strength of the paraesthesia = 0–12 V.

Pulse width (μs)

The pulse width is the duration of the pulse. The wider the pulse width, the larger the area of tissue stimulation and the stronger the paraesthesia produced. It is usually about 210 μs.

Rate

The rate is the number of times per second that the pulse is delivered (Hz). It is usually 30–80 Hz (TENS = 180 Hz).

ELECTRODE SELECTION

All electrodes can be selected to have either negative or positive polarity, providing there is at least one positive and one negative electrode.

STIMULATION OPTIONS

Stimulation can be continuous or cyclical to preserve battery life.

PERCUTANEOUS LEAD INSERTION

The placement of the system must take place in a sterile environment. Prophylactic antibiotics are recommended in accordance with local hospital policy, but teicoplanin is the drug of choice.

MRSA-POSITIVE PATIENTS

Where practical the patient should be screened for methicillin-resistant *Staphylococcus aureus* (MRSA) no longer than four weeks before the procedure. MRSA-positive patients should be given 48 hours of nasal mupirocin or topical triclosan before insertion and gentamicin or a cephalosporin 30 minutes prior to the procedure according to local policy.

The patient is positioned prone on the operating table and intravenous access secured. The epidural space is located under local anaesthesia using a specially designed epidural needle and a loss of resistance technique. A guidewire is passed through the needle and the position is checked using an image intensifier. The tip of the wire should lie in the midline or on the side of the pain.

POSITION OF ELECTRODE (FIG. 11.1)

- Cervical stimulation
  - C2–3 – for upper neck
  - C3–5 – for upper limb pain

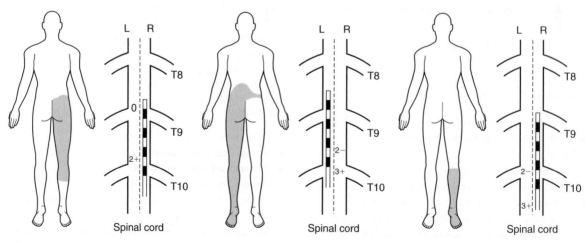

Figure 11.1 *Areas stimulated in spinal cord stimulation and the electrode settings that may produce such stimulation*

- – C4–5 – for radial nerve
- – Just below C5 – for median nerve
- – C6–7 – for ulnar nerve.
- ■ Lumbar stimulation
  - – T11 for foot pain
  - – T9–10 – for lower leg and hip/back
  - – T1–T2 – for upper chest wall
- ■ Midline placement is recommended for bilateral pain but two leads, one on either side, are usually necessary.

Problems of insertion at this stage include:

- ■ the wire crosses the midline to lie on the side opposite the pain
- ■ the wire lies too anterior (seen on lateral view) and motor nerves are stimulated
- ■ epidural fat or fibrous tissue or scar tissue prevents the wire threading up into the epidural space.

The guidewire is removed and replaced with the electrode. The electrode is positioned to produce stimulation in the region of the pain (see list above). The electrode is then connected to the temporary power source and the waveform altered to produce stimulation in the area of the pain. As the lead is positioned and electrode selections are changed, the patient provides feedback about the location and intensity of paraesthesia. The electrode position may need to be adjusted at this stage. When stimulation has been achieved in the correct area the procedure may continue in one of two ways:

1 The patient finds the sensation pleasant and the permanent system is implanted immediately under local or general anaesthetic. The electrode is connected to an extension wire that is then tunnelled subcutaneously around to the abdomen. The wire is connected to the battery and the battery is inserted into a subcutaneous pocket in the abdominal wall.

2 The patient is uncertain whether the sensation is helping the pain so the system is trialled for a period. The electrode is attached to the extension wire as before and tunnelled subcutaneously, but the extension wire is then brought out onto the surface and attached to an external power source. A trial stage is often used for up to four weeks to allow the patient to decide if the sensation is pleasant, whether there is any improvement in pain or quality of life, and whether drug use is reduced. A successful trial does not assure success, and an unsuccessful trial does not preclude benefit from a permanent system.

The stimulator can either be removed at the end of the trial period or converted to a permanent system by attaching the electrode to a new extension lead and completing the technique as before. If there is difficulty placing the electrode percutaneously, it can be sited under direct vision under general anaesthesia. The disadvantage of this technique is that the position of the electrode cannot be checked as the patient is asleep. However, because the electrode is bigger and the area of stimulation is wider it is easier to achieve stimulation in the correct area. The system can be trialled in the same way before implanting the battery.

Determining the implant site

The neurostimulator pocket site should be determined prior to surgery:

- ■ It should be placed where the skin will not be irritated by restrictive clothing and/or the sides of a wheelchair.
- ■ It should not be placed at the belt line.
- ■ It should not be placed near the pelvic bone or rib cage.

Guidelines for the patient after insertion of the system

The patient must avoid bending, twisting, stretching or lifting for five to six weeks after implantation of the trial and permanent stage, especially if the leads have been placed in the cervical region, because they can move. Maintaining a neutral position helps to reduce lead migration. Motor vehicles should not be driven while the stimulator is on. As fibrous tissue forms around the electrode it is less likely to migrate and the patient can resume normal activities.

Contraindications to stimulation

- ■ Active psychosis
- ■ Major uncontrolled depression or anxiety
- ■ Active suicidal behaviour
- ■ Serious alcohol or drug addiction
- ■ Serious cognitive defects
- ■ Serious sleep disturbances
- ■ Difficulty with fine motor skills
- ■ Inability to read
- ■ Coagulopathy
- ■ Systemic or local sepsis
- ■ Demand pacemaker or implanted defibrillator
- ■ Immunosuppression (relative)

Assessment of outcome

When a patient undergoes a trial of stimulation, agreed criteria should be met prior to proceeding with insertion of the permanent system. The criteria may differ among centres but should include the following:

- Subjective and objective
- A specified and meaningful reduction in pain (visual analogue scale (VAS) score)
- Patient satisfaction
- Change in analgesic consumption
- Level of daily activity achieved.

The outcome of all patients having both trial systems and permanent systems should be assessed against agreed criteria to audit the benefits and complications of the procedure.

COMPLICATIONS

The overall rate of complications is 34.3 per cent (range 0–81 per cent).

Complications of the procedure

- Dural tap (2.5 per cent) – usually the needle but the wire and electrode can pierce the dura. The 14 G cannula causes significant cerebrospinal fluid (CSF) loss and severe headache.
- Infection – the major limiting factor in trial length:
  - trial lead at exit site 0.5–15 per cent
  - superficial infection – 4.5 per cent
  - deep infection – 0.1 per cent
  - the commonest organisms causing infection are *Staphylococcus aureus* or *Staphylococcus epidermidis*.
- Intraoperative nerve damage and paralysis.
- Wound related pain (5.8 per cent).
- Postoperative bleeding.
- Epidural haemorrhage and haematoma.
- Seroma at the neurostimulator or receiver site (seen in 80 per cent of patients but usually resolves over four to eight weeks).
- Hygroma.
- Wound dehiscence.
- Abscess/meningitis.

Complications of the hardware

- Equipment failure (10.2 per cent)
- Lack of effect
- Lead/extension fracture
- Erosion of electrode, receiver or generator through skin
- Lead/extension disconnection

- Receiver damage/rotation/failure
- Electrical leakage
- Undesirable change in stimulation described by some patients as uncomfortable, 'jolting' or 'shocking'

Other

- Removal (11–17 per cent)
- Stimulator revision – up to 60 per cent of patients need revision in the first six months, usually to reposition the electrode for an inappropriate area of stimulation
- Fibrosis around the electrode
- Migration of electrode, receiver or generator. Cervical leads migrate more than lumbar
- Short circuit
- Radicular chest wall stimulation
- Allergic or immune system response to the implanted materials
- Loss of pain relief
- Loss of stimulation
- Pain over the receiver site

OUTCOME

- 10 per cent patients stop using it.
- 25 per cent patients will not do it again.
- 50 per cent of patients benefit for the first two years but this falls to 25 per cent in the long term.
- Only 30 per cent of patients return to work.
- Average hours of use per day – 14.4 hours.
- At 30 months – 72 per cent patients still using SCS and 80 per cent would do it again.
- At 48 months – 37 per cent patients still using SCS and 30 per cent would do it again.
- FBSS – 50–60 per cent report >50 per cent pain relief but there are no blinded trials and there may be significant placebo response.

It seems that the effect of stimulation may fall over time, but large numbers of patients have many years of pain relief. The analgesia of SCS even if temporary may be sufficient to break the pain–stiffness–immobility–inflammation–pain cycle and after using the stimulator for a while they may no longer require it.

REASONS FOR DECREASING LACK OF EFFECT

- Fibrotic changes isolating the tip of the electrode from the dura and interfering with the spread of current.
- Plasticity and consequent alteration of the ascending afferent nociceptive pathways allowing pain perception after initially successful interruption of primary pathways.

Spinal cord stimulation for peripheral vascular disease

MECHANISM OF ACTION

A reversible functional sympathectomy is the probable method of pain relief in peripheral vascular disease. There is an increase in blood flow and a measurable increase in oxygen supply to the limb.

OUTCOMES

- Pain relief
- Improved microcirculatory occlusion
- Healing of ulcers
- Prevention of amputation – there may be a reduced amputation rate

Spinal cord stimulation for angina

GUIDELINES FOR THE MANAGEMENT OF ANGINA

Many patients continue to experience severe angina despite maximum medical and surgical treatment – chronic refractory angina – and they are severely restricted in daily activities. Management of refractory angina is unusually complex and none of the multiple refractory angina therapies in use has been compared directly; when treatments have been adequately studied different disciplines tend to measure different endpoints thus rendering standardized comparison between treatments difficult. The primary objective of treatment is the improvement of quality of life but none of the treatments has been evaluated in a randomized placebo controlled trial. The British Pain Society has produced guidelines on best practice for the management of chronic refractory angina.

DIAGNOSIS

- Requires a cardiological and cardiothoracic surgical opinion that the patient has angina of ischaemic origin and that revascularization is unfeasible. Regular angiographic review is recommended to exclude the development of 'new' revascularizable disease.
- Outpatient assessment should include review of pain history, drug history and physical exam. It is essential to ensure that the patient has failed to respond to maximum tolerable medication. Poor compliance should be considered and the need for compliance explained. Simplification of the drug regimen is recommended.
- Exclude non-cardiac causes, e.g. costochondritis, intercostal neuralgia, anaemia, thyrotoxicosis, reflux oesophagitis (consider trial of proton pump inhibitors).
- It is important to consider the possibility that depressive disease may contribute a significant component to their total

pain experience. The Hospital Anxiety and Depression questionnaire is a simple screening tool that can help to identify patients who might benefit from psychiatric or psychological assessment.

MANAGEMENT

Outpatient counselling should include explanation of management plan, lifestyle advice (diet, smoking, physical activity).

- Rehabilitation based on recommended guidelines – involving exercise programme, lifestyle advice, relaxation training.
- Multidisciplinary cognitive behavioural pain management programme can be of value.
- TENS.
- Temporary sympathectomy – stellate ganglion block, T3/4 paravertebral block or high thoracic epidural.
- SCS.
- Opioids – there is limited evidence of the effectiveness of opioids in refractory angina but oral and transdermal opioids can be helpful. A trial of epidural followed by intrathecal opioids might be beneficial if oral therapy fails.
- Destructive sympathectomy – thoracoscopic, surgical, phenol – depending on local expertise.
- Myocardial laser (percutaneous or transmyocardial) – there are insufficient data to support this therapy outside clinical research. These therapies should only be undertaken as part of a formal clinical trial.

Spinal cord stimulation for angina was first described in 1987. The stimulator is positioned for stimulation to occur in the area where the pain is perceived, usually between C7 and T2. If used when the patient experiences angina, there is:

- improvement in symptoms in terms of severity and frequency of attacks
- reduced use of nitrates
- reduced degree and duration of ST depression
- increase in exercise capacity
- a reduced rate of hospital admission
- overall a 75–85 per cent improvement in symptoms.

No increase in mortality is seen, and myocardial infarction pain is still obvious. Coronary artery bypass grafting (CABG) and SCS are equal in terms of symptom relief. When used for the treatment of angina SCS increases myocardial blood flow and reduces sympathetic tone. This reduces myocardial oxygen consumption and improves myocardial microcirculatory blood flow. Positron emission tomography (PET) scans show a redistribution of myocardial blood flow in favour of ischaemic parts of the myocardium. An increase in coronary flow velocity is also seen when TENS is used, and TENS can reduce anginal pain.

Further management of the patient with a spinal cord stimulator

- Unipolar diathermy should not be used in patients with a stimulator *in situ*. Short-wave diathermy is hazardous.
- If a patient requires a magnetic resonance imaging (MRI) scan the procedure must be discussed with a radiologist. The following must be documented:
  - details of the manufacturer
  - type and serial number of the SCS
  - date of manufacture.
- Security systems may be activated by stimulation – the patient should carry details of the SCS.
- The patient does not require prophylactic antibiotics for other procedures.

Questions about spinal cord stimulation that remain unanswered

- What are the effects of SCS on pain and functioning among patients with different chronic pain conditions compared with other treatments?
- Among injured workers with chronic pain, what is the impact of SCS on work status?
- Do certain SCS parameters result in significantly different patient outcomes or a lower complication rate?

The literature on SCS remains inadequate and further research is needed.

PERIPHERAL NERVE STIMULATION

Peripheral nerve stimulation (PNS) has been used since 1965 but there are very few published studies on its use. The mechanism of action is unclear but it may be based on the gate control theory. The most appropriate candidates suffer from pain secondary to damage to a single nerve.

Prior to implantation the patient should:

- show complete relief after diagnostic block with local anaesthetic
- have failed to respond to all other therapy
- be free of any major personality disorders
- be free from depression
- have no alcohol or drug addiction.

The commonest upper extremity nerves treated with PNS are:

- ulnar nerve
- median nerve
- radial nerve.

The commonest lower extremity nerves treated with PNS are:

- tibial nerve
- common peroneal nerve
- sciatic
- femoral
- lateral cutaneous nerve of thigh.

Others are:

- intercostal nerves
- occipital nerves.

The electrodes are inserted under general anaesthetic and attached proximal to the site of injury. They are tunnelled under the skin and attached to a receiver that is implanted subcutaneously in the abdominal wall for lower extremities and the chest wall for upper extremities, chest wall and head. Seventy-eight per cent of patients have a good outcome, 22 per cent a poor outcome. Selection of patients remains difficult as there do not seem to be well-established factors for predicting outcome.

The technique has been used to produce long-term pain relief and has a relatively low complication rate and although costs remain high it may be worth considering the technique in patients where all other therapy has failed.

MOTOR CORTEX STIMULATION

It has been shown that stimulation of the prefrontal cortex of the rat can produce pain relief. Epidural motor cortex stimulation (MCS) was introduced in 1991 as a treatment for deafferentation pain. A number of patients with thalamic pain have been treated with epidural MCS since 1991 with good to excellent pain relief. Other techniques involving stimulation of areas within the brain including thalamus and internal capsule have been developed that also produce pain relief.

The scientific basis for this method of pain relief is not well understood. At least part of the effect of MCS may be via inhibition of the thalamic pathways or projections to the brainstem nuclei.

Mechanisms of central pain

Central pain is pain initiated or caused by a primary lesion or dysfunction in the central nervous system. There may be several mechanisms interacting.

THEORIES

- The cause of the pain may be an imbalance of transmission between the sensory cortical domain and the sensory thalamus. Patients with pain derived from spinal cord injury have thalamic neurones that are hyperactive compared with similar neurones in control patients.
- If patients with central pain and symptoms of hyperpathia or allodynia undergo intraoperative stimulation of the lateral thalamus, painful sensations are elucidated. Control patients do not experience such pain.
- The thalamus is known to play an established role in central deafferentation pain.
- Prefrontal cortical stimulation, when applied simultaneously with a noxious stimulus, abolishes mid-brain neuronal response to pain.
- Stimulation reduces allodynia, dysaesthesia and hyperaesthesia.

STIMULATION AND CEREBRAL BLOOD FLOW

Cortical stimulation increases cerebral blood flow in the ipsilateral thalamus, cingulate gyrus, orbitofrontal cortex and brainstem. There is a correlation between the extent of pain relief and the increase in cingulate blood flow. This suggests that stimulation improves the suffering component of chronic pain. Although an intact somatosensory system is not required for successful treatment, the presence of an intact corticospinal tract neuronal system originating from the motor cortex is required for pain relief to be effective.

Clinical indications

There is no obvious clear-cut indication for MCS but it has been tried for the management of many neuropathic pains resistant to other forms of treatment. It should always be tried as a last resort. Indications include:

- Central neuropathic pain syndromes that have failed to respond to conventional therapy
- Facial and arm phantom pain syndromes may respond the best. Facial representation is so much larger than other areas of the brain that it is easier to identify and this may be why this technique is more successful for facial neuropathic pain. The leg motor cortex is difficult to target
- Anaesthesia dolorosa
- Central pain secondary to stroke
- Post-herpetic neuralgia
- Spinal cord injury.

Post-stroke pain in the presence of severe motor deficits should be considered a contraindication. Patients who also suffer dense weakness in the painful area are less likely to benefit.

Technique

Preoperative screening should be done in the way as for SCS. A preoperative MRI scan will identify the contralateral central sulcus, the sylvian fissure and the inferior and superior frontal sulci.

The procedure is carried out under general anaesthesia. It can be done through a craniotomy incision. A two burr-hole method is much less invasive but may have more morbidity (e.g. epidural haemorrhage). The epidural electrodes are placed over the motor cortex subdurally perpendicular to the central sulcus.

POSITION OF THE ELECTRODES

For facial pain the target is anterior to the central sulcus adjacent to or below the inferior frontal sulcus. For upper limb pain the target is anterior to the central sulcus in the mid-precentral region.

The two central electrodes cross the identified target. The electrodes are sutured to the outer layer of the dura and the lead is tunnelled under the skin. A trial period should be used to ascertain whether the stimulation is useful. Only small numbers of patients may respond. Fits may occur if the stimulation is too strong. Testing can cover several days and stimulation should ideally reduce the pain by 50 per cent.

A permanent pulse generator is positioned in a pocket in the upper chest wall. All patients must receive long-term anticonvulsant medication.

Complications

- Intraoperative seizures
- Stimulator pocket infection
- Aphasia and dysphasia
- Upper limb extremity fatigue
- Burning sensation in the area of stimulation
- Presence of a left-sided supernumerary arm
- Epidural haematoma and clots
- Subdural effusion
- Gradual reduction of pain relief with time
- Dehiscence of the stimulator pocket
- Lead fractures, migration and insulation fractures (8–65 per cent)

Outcomes

- Cortical and thalamic blood flow is increased.
- Temperature in the region of the pain is raised.
- There is more than 50 per cent pain relief in trigeminal neuralgia.

MCS is now being used in the treatment of post-stroke pain. About 50 per cent of patients achieve good pain relief and a smaller percentage achieve excellent or complete relief. Benefit occurs within minutes and may last after stimulation is turned off.

Studies have found it is impossible to predict which patients will respond to the treatment – outcome is not condition-specific. Motor cortex stimulation has been effective in some patients but careful patient selection is important and there may be a diminished response with time. Further investigation of the technique is warranted, and since long-term outcome is not yet known it may affect use of the technique if its benefits are not long term.

DEEP BRAIN STIMULATION

What is it?

Deep brain stimulation (DBS) involves stereotactic positioning of stimulator electrodes in a specific area of the thalamus (usually the ventral posterolateral nucleus (VPL)). The advantage of DBS is that the patient can remain awake.

Central post-stroke pain (CPSP) or thalamic pain syndrome can be very difficult to manage and DBS may have a role to play. It has been shown to provide some measure of pain relief for at least 50 per cent of patients, with some achieving excellent relief of pain. The results appear to be comparable to motor cortex stimulation, with about 50 per cent of patients achieving good pain relief and a smaller percentage achieving excellent or complete relief. The selection of DBS versus MCS depends on the character and distribution of the pain, as well as the extent of the stroke and other factors.

As with all chronic pain syndromes, psychological factors play a major role in the intensity of the pain. It is recommended that all patients with post-stroke pain are evaluated by a pain management psychologist prior to invasive therapy.

Indications

Thalamic stimulation may produce or abolish pain depending on the electrode site. A stroke involving the inhibitory portion of the thalamus may cause the thalamic syndrome – hemi-anaesthesia at the onset contralateral to the lesion, followed by diffuse, burning exacerbated by the touch of clothing. The results of drug therapy are poor and stimulation may help but it may also increase the sensory deficit. Indications include:

- Post-stroke pain
- Pain associated with spinal cord injury
- Nerve injury
- Phantom limb pain
- Post-herpetic neuralgia
- Cancer pain.

Technique

Patient selection and trial procedures are the same as for SCS. The surgical procedure is performed under local anaesthesia in the operating room. Computer assisted imaging techniques known as stereotaxy are employed to identify the targets of stimulation. An electrode is carefully guided through a small hole made in the skull and passed to specific brain areas, which may be the periventricular or periaqueductal grey matter or the thalamic sensory nuclei. The usual targets are the internal capsule and the VPL complex. The other end of the stimulating electrode is connected to a battery-powered programmable device that is implanted under the skin below the clavicle.

One potential drawback to this treatment modality is the development of tolerance, or diminished effectiveness over time. This possibility is diminished by avoiding the use of continuous stimulation.

INTRATHECAL INFUSIONS

Opioids

Intrathecal and epidural opioids relieve pain by stimulation of opiate receptors in the spinal cord and brainstem. They affect primarily the presynaptic and postsynaptic receptors in the substantia gelatinosa of the posterior horn of the spinal cord. Pain is relieved without affecting any other sensation. The drug is delivered using an implantable drug infusion system via a catheter positioned in the intrathecal space to deliver small amounts of medication directly into the CSF.

Since the opioid is administered directly it produces analgesia at lower doses than those used orally and therefore there are fewer side effects. Intrathecal doses can be 1/300 the oral dose.

Most patients can manage oral medication but a small proportion cannot tolerate the necessary doses. Administration of the drug intrathecally or via the epidural route allows smaller doses to be used to provide better pain relief. This route of administration is highly effective in selected cases but there is a lack of comparative trials to assess its effectiveness against other measures. There are different types of pump available. In patients with non-malignant pain and a long life expectancy, a totally implantable system is usually selected with a reasonably large reservoir that requires refilling every three months or so depending on rate of delivery. This minimizes the infection risk.

Selection criteria

Intrathecal opioids should be considered a therapy of last resort. The selection criteria include:

- failure of all other conservative treatment either from lack of efficacy or intolerable side effects
- analgesia induced by preoperative trial
- no allergy to the drug being used.

These should not be used in the presence of:

- drug seeking behaviour
- rapid escalation in opioid dose
- evidence of excessive alcohol intake
- litigation/compensation problems that have not been resolved or where there is evidence of other secondary gain
- unreasonable goals and expectations
- unmotivated characteristics
- pain unresponsive to opioids
- cognitive deficits – psychosis, suicide, and major depression, hypochondria, somatization, and lack of social support.

Psychological evaluation

No standards have been established for intrathecal therapy but the patient should have appropriate tests before proceeding with intrathecal therapy such as:

- McGill pain questionnaire
- Beck Depression Inventory
- Oswestry Disability Score.

Benefits

- Improved activity
- Better quality of life
- Programmable for flexibility
- Non-destructive

The system

THE TRIAL

The patient should be on a stable dose of oral morphine. He or she is admitted to hospital and an intrathecal catheter is implanted percutaneously. Either a single shot of the test drug is injected into the CSF or an infusion of morphine is started at 0.5–1 mg/24 h. If the first injection does not relieve symptoms the procedure should be repeated with a larger dose or the infusion rate is increased by 1 mg/day until a minimum 50 per cent reduction in the VAS score is achieved. It may take up to three weeks to screen the patient adequately. Antiemetics and laxatives should be prescribed and the dose of oral morphine should be reduced by 50 per cent the day after the intrathecal dose. This dose should be maintained for three days and then stopped. If morphine is unsuccessful buprenorphine can be tried at a dose of 0.1 mg/day.

Positive trial

During the trial there should be either a 50 per cent reduction in pain or a 50 per cent reduction in analgesic intake per 24 hours.

PERMANENT SYSTEM

Intrathecal pumps are implantable, battery-powered devices that store and dispense drugs according to instructions received from the programmer. The system is implanted under general anaesthesia. An intrathecal catheter is inserted percutaneously. The catheter is a flexible, silicone tube. A small cut is made in the back to sew the catheter to the fascia around the muscles to secure it from movement. A pocket is made in the lower abdomen to place the pump. The tubing is tunnelled under the skin from the back to the front and the pieces are connected. It takes several months following the implantation of the pump to adjust the level of morphine to control pain adequately and safely. The patient must remain in hospital overnight and woken hourly for monitoring:

- blood pressure
- pulse
- SaO_2
- respiratory rate.

THE PUMP (FIG. 11.2)

The system is connected to and driven by a subcutaneous pump. The pump is a round metal (titanium) device about 2.5 cm thick, 8.5 cm in diameter and about 205 g in weight. The reservoir is the space (18 or 10 mL) within the pump that holds the medication. There is a fill port in the centre portion of the pump through which the pump is refilled.

The pump is driven by compressed inert gas and is programmed by telemetry. This is controlled by a mechanism powered by a lithium battery that needs to be replaced on average every four years depending on the flow rate. Information about individual prescriptions is stored in the

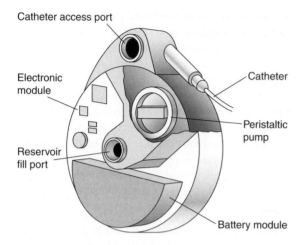

Figure 11.2 *Internal components of an intrathecal pump*

pump's memory and it can be reviewed and altered using the programmer that communicates with the pump by radio signals.

To fill the pump, medication is injected through the reservoir fill port, and into the expandable reservoir. An inert gas puts pressure on the reservoir. The pressure forces the medication through a bacteria-retentive filter and into the pump chamber. From the pump chamber, the medication is pumped out of the device and into the catheter. A microprocessor controls the rate at which the pump delivers medication.

Reservoir

The reservoir is the cavity inside the pump where the medication is stored. The volume is 10 or 18 mL.

Reservoir fill port

In the centre of the pump is a raised area (called a 'port') that is used for filling and emptying the pump. In the middle of this port is a self-sealing, silicone septum that is used during the pump refilling procedure.

Refilling

Pumps need to be refilled before being empty. An alarm will sound when a small amount of fluid is left. A refill kit is supplied containing sterile needles and syringes and also a template that is placed over the pump to help locate the port position.

The pump is refilled by placing a needle into the pump through the skin about every three months. The pump will need to be replaced about every five years.

Catheter access port

Most pumps feature a catheter access port. The catheter access port allows bypass of the pump reservoir to send medications directly into the implanted catheter. The catheter access port may also be used for diagnostic purposes, such as testing to ensure medication is able to flow through the length of the catheter.

Programmer

Attached to the programmer is a component known as the 'programming head'. This head looks similar to a computer mouse. Instructions for rate and dose adjustments are transmitted through the programming head to the pump by radio signals (telemetry). The two-way radio-frequency link also allows the programmer to receive information from the pump.

Complications

SURGICAL

- Infection (0.77/1000)
- CSF leak
- Neural damage
- Meningitis
- Epidural abscess
- Bleeding
- Pump pocket seroma
- CSF hygroma
- Post-spinal headache
- Improper pocket placement

MECHANICAL

- Catheter kinking
- Catheter obstruction
- Catheter dislodgement
- Catheter disconnection
- Pump failure
- Pump battery depletion

Drugs used

- Usually morphine.
- Diamorphine to be used but has now been withdrawn because it used to crystallize in the pump, causing damage.
- Buprenorphine.

PAIN RELIEF WITH OPIOID

- Pain relief is better overall in terminal disease than in chronic pain

Table 11.1 *Hormonal changes with intrathecal infusions*

Abnormality	Percentage of patients affected
↓ Testosterone	85.7 (men)
↓ Lutenizing hormone	60.9 (men)
Anovulation	28.5 (premenopausal women)
Amenorrhoea	43 (premenopausal women)
↓ Growth hormone	20
↓ 24-hour urine cortisol	19.4
↓ 24-hour urine aldosterone	56

- 50 per cent have 90 per cent pain relief
- 30 per cent have 75 per cent pain relief
- 20 per cent have fair (40 per cent) pain relief

PHARMACOLOGICAL SIDE EFFECTS

Intrathecal morphine infusion has a large number of side effects. Those which occur most frequently are:

- memory impairment (68 per cent)
- constipation (66 per cent)
- excess sweating (56 per cent)
- urinary retention (51 per cent – via inhibition of micturition reflex – usually self limiting, males > females and commoner in the elderly)
- loss of libido (48 per cent) and ejaculatory failure
- dry mouth (39 per cent)
- swollen legs (37 per cent)
- nausea and vomiting (30 per cent)
- hair loss
- weight gain, especially in young women.

Abnormal hormonal changes seen with intrathecal morphine are given in Table 11.1.

Serum androgens, oestrogens, insulin-like growth factor (IGF)-1 and 24-hour urinary cortisol levels should be checked when treatment is commenced and corrected as necessary. The hormonal changes may be related to impotence which may occasionally occur with intrathecal morphine.

OTHER DRUGS USED INTRATHECALLY

Local anaesthetics

Bupivacaine can be used for nociceptive and neuropathic pain and is started at 3–5 mg/day and increased slowly. The dose can be increased by 20 per cent every week. The average dose is 11 mg/day using 40 mg/mL solution (4 per cent).

No neurological side effects have been seen with doses up to 25 mg/day. Bupivacaine <15 mg/day is associated with few side effects but above this the patient may experience urinary retention and weak limbs.

Midazolam

Midazolam increases the affinity of opioids for their receptor sites but it is only useful for a few weeks or months.

Baclofen

Baclofen (4-amino-3-(p-chlorophenyl) butyric acid) binds to presynaptic GABA$_B$ receptors in the central nervous system and reduces the release of excitatory neurotransmitters. It inhibits calcium uptake so impeding the release of excitatory neurotransmitters. It is useful for relaxing muscle when spasm is responsible for pain and can be very effective and safe. The oral dose is 30–100 mg/day in divided doses but this dose is often associated with unacceptable side effects. It has poor lipid solubility so even at large oral doses only small amounts are found in the CSF (the site of action). Thus direct delivery to the spinal cord reduces dosage and side effects. Given intrathecally it acts directly on the GABA receptor sites.

Indications

- Side effects with oral dosing.
- Reduction of spasticity associated with:
  - multiple sclerosis
  - cerebovascular incidents
  - spinal cord injuries
  - cerebral palsy.

There is little evidence available on the beneficial effects and in whom they are useful. Spasm is caused by an imbalance of excitatory and inhibitory input in the spinal cord leading to hyperactive stretch reflexes, increased muscle tone and involuntary spasms. Baclofen restores the balance of excitatory and inhibitory input to reduce muscle hyperactivity.

Indications

- Chronic stable disease
- Severe disabling spasticity interfering with activity or nursing care
- Spasticity refractory to oral drugs or oral treatment not tolerated
- Painful spasms
- Consent
- Multidisciplinary evaluation
- Positive response to trial

Trial stage

A 50–100 mg intrathecal bolus of baclofen should produce a benefit for at least four hours.

Side effects

These are usually dose related and include:

- Dizziness
- Drowsiness
- Headaches
- Nausea
- Weakness
- Fainting light-headedness
- Buzzing in the ears, visual disturbance
- Clumsiness
- Unsteadiness
- Dry mouth.

Treatment of severe side effects is with physostigmine.

Clonidine

There are both $\alpha 1$ and $\alpha 2$ receptors in the dorsal horn (70 per cent postsynaptic and 30 per cent presynaptic). Analgesia comes from the $\alpha 2$ actions in the dorsal horn. Clonidine acts on the postsynaptic receptors to produce hyperpolarization of the synaptic membrane and activates the noradrenergic inhibitory descending pathways. It also acts on the presynaptic receptors by modulating the release of neurotransmitters involved in pain. It is usually given with morphine or bupivacaine because opioids and $\alpha 2$ adrenergic agents are synergistic.

Dose

- Intrathecal
  - Variable but usually about 75–170 μg/day but occasionally up to 700 μg/day.
  - It can cause hypotension and bradycardia at 25 μg/hour or more.
  - There is no tolerance.
- Epidural
  - 30 μg/h

Somatostatin analogues

Octreotide 5–20 μg/h has been used intrathecally with success.

SUMMARY

Chronic pain often responds poorly to management with medication. This has led to development of techniques to modulate the pain centrally to try to improve the outcome of patients with long-term pain. The majority of these techniques are complex and expensive and are designed to be used when all other therapy has failed. The numbers of patients who will be treated will be small and it will take time to identify those patients who will benefit most and establish guidelines for good clinical practice.

CASE SCENARIO

A 47-year-old woman underwent a microdiscectomy for cauda equina syndrome six months ago. Preoperatively she had pain in her left leg down to her big toe. This pain persisted into the postoperative period and although all the abnormal neurology resolved the pain has now become very severe. She describes the pain as burning in nature and it is associated with pins and needles. It keeps her awake at night and prevents her being as active as prior to the surgery. She has managed to return to work but finds it difficult to cope. She takes regular paracetamol 1 g four times daily, ibuprofen 400 mg three times daily and amitriptyline 30 mg at night. Occasionally when the pain is bad she takes codeine with the paracetamol. She has been unable to tolerate any anticonvulsants because of severe side effects and does not find that stronger analgesia helps. She uses a TENS machine for the back pain she has had since surgery.

On examination, she has hyperaesthesia in the L5 dermatome with some mild allodynia. She has a brief response to caudal injections with local anaesthetic and steroid.

It is felt that she would be a good candidate for SCS. She attends a pain management programme to improve coping skills and to improve her activity levels as far as possible and responds well to the course. However, she is unhappy about continuing with her tablets long term because they do make her tired, and she is keen to proceed with SCS.

The stimulator is inserted with the patient awake and good stimulation is achieved in the L5 dermatome. After a trial period of four weeks she is delighted with the improvement and has been able to reduce her analgesia. A permanent system is implanted and at the 2-month follow-up she has stopped her amitriptyline and takes analgesia only when necessary. After a period of two years her life is very active and she uses analgesia only intermittently when the pain flares up.

12 Psychological Aspects of Pain Management

INTRODUCTION

Chronic pain can persist for extended periods despite all efforts to treat any underlying physical pathology. This may be due to the disease process or a physical injury and the pain may be proportional to objective measures of the severity of the disease (e.g. rheumatoid arthritis). However, the pain may be disproportional to objective measures of the severity of the disease, or there may be no obvious underlying disease or injury to account for the pain.

Increases in the intensity of the pain do not correlate with disease progression. Persistent pain is associated with physical decline, physical impairment, disability and emotional distress. There is no correlation between the severity of chronic pain and the magnitude of underlying physical problems. Medical, pharmacological and surgical interventions used effectively for acute pain often fail to provide patients with longlasting relief from chronic pain.

Pain is complex and multidimensional. Once it has become persistent, seldom can any one intervention return an individual to the pre-pain state. The selection of interventions depends on accurate assessment of the patient's psychological reactions to their pain and the previous treatments received.

The International Association for the Study of Pain definition of pain highlights that it is a 'sensory and emotional response'. It is not measurable on the basis of traditional physical, tissue-oriented medical disease models but is a complex physical, mental, social and behavioural process that compromises quality of life. Pain begins as a noxious process where signals are transmitted to the brain and interpreted. Emotional and psychological factors affect the way the person perceives and reacts to the signals. Pain is more of a perception than a simple sensation and is affected by sensory, psychological, cognitive, emotional, behavioural, interpersonal, environmental and situational factors.

Many people believe avoiding thinking about pain avoids pain, but pain grabs attention and it is important what the individual thinks and does next – which differentiates those who are preoccupied with pain from those who continue despite it. Minor pains are very frequent, and each time they occur it may lead to the thought processes of 'What is the cause?' and 'What can I do to get rid of it?'. When action taken for minor pain succeeds in reducing that pain, patients become puzzled and confused when these processes no longer help in more severe and persistent pain.

Emotional and psychological factors affect the way a person interprets or perceives a noxious stimulus. The pain experience is influenced by beliefs about the meaning of pain, memories of the past and expectations of the future. Perception of pain at different points in time is likely to vary as a function of psychological and situational circumstances. It can be very difficult for a patient to accept the chronicity of pain and that life will not be the same again. Many continue to seek a cure for many years and continue to suffer increasing disability. Only when the patient has come to accept the situation, and requests help with managing the pain, is a psychological approach going to be helpful.

ATTENTION AND PAIN

It has always been difficult to explain why there are so many variations in people's experience of pain and why pain intensity varies with time in the same person. It is becoming clear that behavioural models of attention may provide the key to understanding some of these questions. Behavioural models may also help to explain why and how nociception emerges into awareness as pain, and how other concerns displace pain from awareness (distraction). Box 12.1 lists the factors to be considered in a patient with pain.

Relation between pain beliefs, negative thoughts and psychosocial functioning in chronic pain

Psychological factors influence why and how people respond to their pain and their subsequent demands for analgesia (Box 12.2). These factors also influence the response to

> **BOX 12.1 Factors important when attending to pain**
>
> **Characteristics of the stimulus**
> - Novelty
> - Predictability
> - Intensity
> - Threat value
>
> **Characteristics of the person**
> - Negative affect
> - Vigilance
> - Pain-related fear
> - Pain catastrophizing
>
> **Characteristics of the environment**
> - Escape or avoidance benefit of pain
> - Emotional value

> **BOX 12.2 Psychological effects of chronic pain**
>
> - Negative thinking
> - Stress
> - Disability
> - Loss of control
> - Impaired mental and physical performance

treatment and the outcome of pain and disability. Beliefs come from our social environment and this environment also reinforces behaviour. A caring spouse taking over as carer may reinforce the idea that the patient is disabled and needs to be cared for. Negative belief predicts:

- more pain, disability and distress
- a greater use of healthcare resources
- greater use of pain medication.

Beliefs about the nature of reality shape our perceptions of our environment and ourselves. Changes in pain-related beliefs are correlated with improvement in depressive symptoms and physical function and reduced use of healthcare provision.

Even after controlling for demographics, work status, pain severity and pain beliefs, the use of negative self-statements such as 'I am useless', 'I am going to become an invalid', is positively associated with affective distress and interference of pain in daily activity and a lower activity level. It is the disability that pain causes, rather than the pain itself, that has a greater negative effect on the quality of life and sense of self.

Learned behaviour in response to pain leads to acquired patterns of response. Children of patients with chronic pain have more pain-related responses during stressful times and exhibit greater illness behaviour, indicating that it is not just personal experience that is important in the development of chronic pain but also one's upbringing.

Secondary gain

When physical or psychological disability results from chronic pain, there may also be an interaction with factors that have the potential to produce secondary gains. These include:

- financial compensation or disability payment. This alone is not normally a predictor of persistent pain but litigation (principally work-related) is strongly associated with higher levels of pain related disability even after taking other variables into account
- time off work
- attention of others provided by the response to the pain behaviour.

Pain and suffering

Pain is a perceived threat to one's biological integrity and is crucial to survival. Suffering is a 'state of severe distress associated with events that threaten the intactness of the person'. Patients suffer when they are unable to continue normal physical, psychological, occupational and social activity because of pain. Pain intensity is only one of the issues that needs to be addressed in the management of patients with chronic pain. Therapy that addresses only one component of the pain experience is destined to fail.

Factors influencing pain perception

COPING MECHANISMS

Coping strategies alter perception and ability to manage pain and continue everyday activities. Different strategies are appropriate for different people at different times with different levels of severity. **Active coping** means maintaining activity and ignoring the pain. **Passive coping** means restricting activities, depending on others and this leads to increased pain and depression.

PERCEPTION OF CONTROL

The degree to which an individual believes that their health or severity of pain is determined by factors of chance, by the powerful actions of others (e.g. family, doctor etc.) or as a consequence of their own actions and behaviour can have a powerful effect on that individual's experience of pain. Those who see others as responsible for causing or treating their pain are said to have an external locus of control and this tends to be associated with more self-reported pain, higher levels of depression and the use of maladaptive coping strategies such as catastrophizing. Those who emphasize their own actions (internal locus of control) have lower pain intensity, better coping strategies and better compliance with treatment protocols.

CATASTROPHIZING ('FEARING THE WORST')

Catastrophizing can be described as 'dwelling on and magnifying the negative aspects of a situation'. This is one of the most significant predictors of poor coping and adjustment to living with pain. Patients who expect the worst cope poorly and fare poorly, report more pain and have poorer outcomes. They are more aware of pain (hyper-vigilance). Studies show that activity in the brain is increased when attention is paid to a stimulus and decreases when the patient is distracted. Hyper-vigilance may be an autonomic process and not under conscious control. Distraction only works when patients do not catastrophize and in those who have a low level of health anxiety.

ANGER AND PAIN

Anger is often self-directed and relates to the perceived interference of pain in an individual's life. It is a particularly powerful predictor of pain following spinal cord injury. Others may be angry with someone who they perceive as responsible for causing their pain, e.g. after an injury at work, or after surgery.

HISTORY OF ABUSE

A history of physical or sexual abuse is commonly elicited in patients with chronic pain. Patients with pelvic pain often report a history of sexual abuse. Abuse leads to depressive symptoms, low self-esteem and a sense of powerlessness.

Dependent individuals who have low self-esteem with poor tolerance for and lack of ability to deal with stress appear to be more likely to become a victim of an accident. They are often dissatisfied with a stressful job and may experience family and interpersonal tensions. A disability absolves an individual of responsibility and avoids a situation. The onus for recovery is placed on the doctor. When reinforced by social acceptance (the illness is not their fault) and financial factors (disability payment) attention (sympathy) dysfunction can rapidly become an entrenched way of life.

WORK

Injured patients with low back pain who are not back at work one year after the injury are unlikely to return to their original job. This is due mainly to the degree of perceived control over the work situation and the degree of job satisfaction. These patients often use more medication and health services. The single most important factor in returning to work for a back injury is fear of re-injury.

Work-related disability has increased exponentially over the past few years. The significance and meaning to an individual of commonly experienced symptoms is influence by what is going on in the world and the following all add to the occurrence of work-related disability:

- Doctors are too willing to apply spurious pathological labels to symptoms.
- The law is fixated that medical diagnoses are an arbiter of the truth about the severity of symptoms and disability.
- There is a persisting belief that managing a workplace symptom like arm pain (repetitive strain injury or RSI) or back pain such as a disease, independent of social and psychological circumstances, will make the problem go away.
- Symptoms like pain do not become trivial in the absence of physical diagnosis. Symptoms are not simple reflections of the prevalence of a disease in a population. Their expression and significance depend on how we as a society define ill health, approach disability in the workplace or compensate for symptoms.
- The encouragement to seek compensation for injury may produce justice for ill people but may turn symptoms into illness and make ill people more ill.

Stress and pain

Pain both produces and is exacerbated by stress. A stressor is any experience, physiological or psychological that disrupts homoeostasis. Negative psychological stressors include loss of control over one's circumstances and lack of predictability of the environment. Negative beliefs and expectations can also act as stressors. Noxious stimuli elicit the stress response, which is enhanced by negative thinking.

PHYSIOLOGICAL MANIFESTATIONS OF STRESS

- Extensive and extended sympathetic nervous system arousal producing neuroendocrine secretion.
- Immune system activation resulting in the release of interleukin (IL)-1, IL-6 and cytokines, producing fever, leucocytosis, increased slow wave sleep, reduced activity,

muscular soreness, and diminished sexual interest and reduced cognitive abilities.

Common manifestations of the sustained stress response in chronic pain include:

- Disrupted sleep – patients who have their sleep disturbed by pain suffer more than those who sleep well
- Fatigue
- Dysphoria
- Muscular aches and pains
- Reduced appetite
- Relationship problems and reduced libido
- Impaired physical function
- Impaired concentration.

Malingering

Malingering is the conscious and purposeful faking of a symptom to achieve benefit (usually financial). It is uncommon to see these patients in a pain clinic.

Gender and pain

Women tend to report more pain and more negative responses to pain than men. They report more recurrent pain and more severe pain, and more frequent and longerlasting pain than men.

Culture and pain

Pain assessment and management can be difficult because of health beliefs and practices in different populations especially when different cultures are involved. There are also educational, occupational and economic factors to consider in the different ways that pain is expressed, the way a patient behaves and in their coping mechanisms.

Race: initially biologically oriented, it is a social construct and there are no biological criteria that can be applied to assign persons to specific racial groups.

Ethnicity: This term is derived from the Greek word *ethnos* meaning 'tribe'. A tribe is a group of people who share a common ancestral origin or social background, culture and traditions. They usually have a common language and religious tradition. Self-identification is the most valid method to consign ethnic identity.

Culture: This term refers to behavioural and attitudinal norms. These attitudes shape illness, beliefs and behaviours, healthcare practices, help-seeking activities and receptivity

to medical care and interventions. Cultural factors related to a pain experience include:

- pain expression
- pain language
- lay remedies for pain
- social roles and expectations
- perceptions of the medical care system.

It is important to remember that during the psychological assessment that cultural, ethnic and linguistic patterns may influence how pain is expressed and interpreted.

PAIN BEHAVIOUR

The term 'pain behaviour' refers to a habitual maladaptive behavioural reaction resulting from the pain experience. If physical activity causes pain, then eventually the fear of causing pain may lead to avoidance of physical activity. This is one of the commonest coping activities, but over a period of time more and more physical activity is avoided causing the patient to become considerably disabled. The underlying fear also causes muscle tension, which in turn produces altered posture, which then exacerbates the pain. Inactivity and help-seeking behaviour often initially improve pain and this reinforces the idea that rest will help.

Pain behaviour includes overt expressions that communicate pain and distress to others (Box 12.3). They initially result from reflexive avoidance of the aversive experience and may at first serve to protect against exacerbating tissue damage. Some pain behaviours may be reinforced by the environment, for example, if the grimacing produces attention, the attention received may reinforce this action. Once the behaviour has become established, it no longer needs the pain to maintain it. Maintenance of maladaptive behaviour will contribute to disability. Learned pain behaviour is unintended. The patient is usually not aware of displaying this behaviour or that there are positive benefits.

It is important to assess the pain behaviour prior to starting treatment and it is necessary to obtain the patient's perceptions of his or her own behavioural responses to pain. Failure to reduce pain behaviour is usually associated with failure to restore function in the patient.

Avoidance behaviour

It still remains unclear why some patients go on to develop chronic musculoskeletal pain after an apparently healed injury whereas others do not. The idea that fear of pain and

BOX 12.3 Different kinds of pain behaviour

Non-verbal pain behaviour

- Limping
- Grimacing
- Moaning
- Anxiety
- Sighs
- Rigid or unstable posture
- Seeking medical help
- Excessively slow or laboured movement
- Use of protective device, e.g. cane, collar
- Seeking and using pain medicine

Verbal pain behaviour

- Statements of helplessness
- Crying
- Hostility
- Sighs
- Screaming
- Excessive requests for assistance
- Complaining

Self-defeating behaviour

- Sleeping excessively
- Avoiding activity
- Forgetfulness
- Not working
- Resting
- Decreased activity

BOX 12.4 Factors contributing to:

A negative outlook

- Put on light duties at work or made redundant – feel it is their fault
- Feel unappreciated
- Worry about future employment
- Feel useless
- Ashamed because unable to support the family
- Feel miserable
- Withdraws

A positive outlook

- Feel their employer is in the wrong if they are forced out of work
- Feel they still have much to offer
- See the positive side of the situation, e.g. spending more time with the family
- Feel it is an opportunity to try something new
- Willing to take risks

the pain problem. Many studies have shown that fear of pain is one of the most potent predictors of observable physical performance and self-reported disability levels, and it appears to be an essential feature of the development of a chronic problem for at least some patients. The more fearful the patient, the more disability they suffer.

Pain and depression

Of patients with chronic pain 40–50 per cent suffer from depression, and it is those who feel the pain is outside their control who experience more depressive symptoms. Those who continue to function despite pain and maintain control do not become depressed. See Box 12.4 for factors influencing a patient's attitude towards pain.

It is not easy to start to question these assumptions when one is depressed. One begins to notice only failures or short-comings, feels miserable and withdraws from everything. It is possible to slowly change these feelings but it does involve taking risks and re-entering the social world. Doing something is likely to be better than doing nothing. Punishing oneself will make the individual feel more miserable and is unlikely to help them change. One needs to see how to do things differently with positive thoughts, not negative ones. It is an individual approach as everyone is different but the underlying principles apply to everyone. Formal certification of disability may lead to further deterioration.

(re)injury may be more disabling than pain itself refutes the notion that the lowered ability to accomplish tasks of daily living in chronic pain patients is merely the consequence of pain severity. The 'fear avoidance' model may help to explain this process. Fear avoidance relates to the avoidance of movements or an activity based on fear of damage or exacerbation of pain. Individuals learn that the avoidance of pain-provoking or pain-increasing situations reduces the likelihood of a new pain episode so they avoid particular activities. For example, a patient with back pain may develop a fear of lifting after experiencing pain while lifting. Avoiding the threatening situation is reinforced by reductions in pain, tension and anxiety. Avoidance behaviours occur in anticipation of pain, rather than as a response to pain. Once established, avoidance behaviour is extremely difficult to reverse. There continues a downward spiral of increasing avoidance, disability and pain and avoidance of daily activities results in functional disability. Longstanding avoidance of activity reduces musculoskeletal function. This leads to the 'disuse syndrome', which worsens

PAIN IN DEPRESSION

Among the somatic symptoms of major depressive illness, pain ranks second only to insomnia. Headache, facial pain, neck and back pain, thoracic, abdominal and pelvic pain occur in >50 per cent of major depressive disorders. Treatment of the depression may relieve some of the pain.

DEPRESSION IN PAIN

Among patients with chronic pain, 40–50 per cent suffer from depression, but usually as a consequence of the pain. Depression worsens the effect of pain on social and occupational functioning. Depressed patients are less active than their non-depressed counterparts and there is a reduced likelihood of response to pain treatment. There is increased use of medical services.

Causes of depression in pain

- Childhood hospitalization – risk for depressive illness and chronic pain in adults.
- Childhood neglect and illness cause inwardly directed aggression and pain.
- Perceived life interference and reduced self-control.
- Previous episodes of depression predispose some individuals to a depressive episode after the onset of pain.

ROLE OF THE PSYCHOLOGIST

It is understood that although patients will continue to have pain, quality of life can be improved despite this. Understanding and accepting this can be more difficult for the patient. One assumes that the patient would prefer to be without pain and the associated difficulties that accompany the pain. It is unlikely therefore that the patient attending the pain clinic is likely to understand or believe what we have to say. It can also be difficult to know what it is the patient wants to achieve. It is important early on in pain management to ask the patient what outcome he or she is aiming to get from the visit. If 100 per cent pain relief is the aim then a psychological input may not be helpful at this stage.

The input of a clinical psychologist can improve quality of life significantly when the patient has accepted that further medical treatment is not possible, and is not pursuing further intervention. Acceptance of the pain can be manifested by:

- an increased focus on solving the problems of the consequences of pain rather than the pain itself
- giving up unproductive ways to control the pain.

Patients who can adopt an accepting attitude towards pain show:

- lower pain-related distress and disability than those who persevere in their attempts to solve the problem of pain
- engagement in normal life activities
- recognition that pain may not change.

It is a shift away from pain and non-pain aspects and from a search for a cure with an acknowledgement that pain may not change. Psychology-based treatment approaches do not aim to relieve pain but they can:

- help people feel more sense of control
- reduce depression and worry
- improve memory
- improve concentration
- increase self-esteem
- improve coping skills
- help with reconditioning and activity.

No longer viewing reduced pain intensity as a primary goal may enable patients to focus on aspects of pain that may be partly controlled.

PSYCHOLOGICAL EVALUATION

This is indicated when:

- a patient with acute or chronic pain does not seem to be progressing with medical treatment
- there is a negative, emotional or behavioural reaction to the pain
- treatments are only partially effective, leaving the patient with the need to cope with substantial pain

PSYCHOLOGICAL ASSESSMENT

Methods used in the assessment of patients with chronic pain are mainly for evaluating the outcome of treatment. They are not necessary for planning a treatment programme, but instead indicate whether a patient has made progress during the programme.

The assessment and management of a patient with chronic pain is complex and requires a wide range of skills. Assessment is a multidisciplinary process and includes input by doctors, clinical psychologists, physiotherapists and occupational therapists. Assessment should take place at the first visit, at the end of the programme and if possible follow up should be arranged for six months after the end of the programme. The purpose of the psychological assessment is to identify:

- the pain experience in the context of the patient's life
- beliefs about their pain
- the expectations of the patient
- the impact of pain on function
- the effect of the pain on current relationships
- the role of the patient's financial situation
- the role of other factors that may influence the patient's reaction to pain
- the patient's mood
- the patient's fears
- the coping responses
- level of anxiety
- level of depression
- the effect of prior life experiences on the pain experience.

The assessment should include:

- Severity of distress – sickness impact profile
- Level of suffering
- Interference of the pain with activities – (short form (SF)-36, Oswestry Disability Score)
- Level of depression – Beck's Depression Inventory
- Alienation and maladjustment
- Psychological motivation for treatment
- General psychological assessment
- Self-efficacy
- Psychological and behavioural coping strategies.

Methods for assessment are discussed in Chapter 2.

PAIN MANAGEMENT PROGRAMMES

There is good evidence that pain management programmes are effective in improving quality of life. The aim is to bring about understanding of pain and an alteration of beliefs. The pain management programme is a structured, goal-oriented, educative, short-term programme. The aims are to:

- teach coping skills
- teach skills for identifying, evaluating and responding to their self-defeating thoughts
- developing techniques for changing beliefs, thinking, mood and behaviour
- reduce disability and distress caused by chronic pain by teaching physical, psychological and practical techniques to improve quality of life
- restoring physical conditioning and increasing activity levels

- decrease frequency of flare-ups
- change habits, behaviours and attitudes that are maintaining maladaptive behaviour.

These goals are only reasonable and achievable if the patient agrees they are reasonable, desirable and possible. The underlying philosophy is that patients can do something on their own to control their pain. This may mean changing attitudes, feelings or behaviours associated with pain, or understanding how forces and past events have contributed to the present painful predicament.

Role of cognition in pain control

Patients who feel helpless and out of control have poor coping skills and they feel everything that happens to them is a matter of luck. Patients who feel in control of their success and failure are better able to cope. Those patients who confront their fears and difficulties have better coping skills than those who avoid their difficulties. The aim is to encourage patients to deal with their stress, to divert their attention from their pain and to improve their coping skills through education. In a recent study patients were scanned before and after cognitive behavioural therapy (CBT). The results showed significant metabolic changes in the brain, with increased activity in the hippocampus and dorsal cingulate regions and decreased cortical activity.

Positive emotional states such as pleasant involvement, absorption in an activity, the drive to accomplish something, satisfaction in an accomplishment, dedication, etc. can inadvertently ward off pain or decrease its intensity. Thoughts and attitudes affect a person's mood rather than external events. Therapy helps to create more positive and realistic attitudes to negative thoughts and emotions.

Cognitive behavioural therapy

We cannot change our negative emotions to positive just by wishing it, but we can examine what we believe and how we describe to ourselves the world as it impinges on us.

In a group of patients with apparently similar clinical examination and diagnostic findings, individuals with chronic pain differ considerably in their levels of psychological and physical dysfunction. Cognitive means the way in which a patient perceives, interprets and relates to the pain. Cognitive behavioural therapy holds that individual's beliefs and coping behaviours related to their pain play important roles in their adjustment. Therapies that aim to identify and modify maladaptive beliefs and increase the use of adaptive cognitive and behavioural coping skills have been shown to improve physical and psychological functioning. The aim is to change negative patterns of thinking and expand resources for coping by:

- education
- skills acquisition
- cognitive and behavioural reversal
- generalization and maintenance.

Unless a patient's attention is directly focused on these abnormal behaviours they may be unaware of them. They may not be under conscious control. The therapist helps the patient learn to identify and correct erroneous beliefs to try to enhance their efforts to cope. Return to work is not an aim of most pain management programmes, but the trial programmes that have recently been set up with the aim of returning people to work have so far been very successful.

Groups of up to 12 people meet for a half-day a week for about eight weeks with a follow-up session at six months. Patients are asked to practise the skills and approaches to managing pain that are discussed in the group.

Learning to manage pain is very individual – what works well for one person will not necessarily work for another, so some aspects of the programme help some more than others. Some inpatient programmes last for three to four weeks, but the majority are outpatient programmes because the patient has to learn to cope within the community and at home.

The patient must be willing to cooperate fully with the programme and have the support of family members to be successful. The patient must be rewarded with praise and attention for positive efforts, but rewards must be withheld following negative, demanding or dependent behaviour. Before inclusion in a programme the patient is given a full assessment following which a care plan is developed according to the individual needs of the patient.

Pain management programme sessions include:

- education to aid understanding of the pain system
- learning to pace activities. There is a need for pain sufferers to regulate and remain in control of the frequency, intensity and duration of their activities. Pain is not constant and many patients have days when lower pain levels lead to over-activity. Patients with chronic pain often waver between inactivity and over-exertion and this leads to exhaustion, flare-ups and re-injury. They need to be coached in setting baseline activity and pacing activity. It is better to build up endurance gradually than to overdo an activity – small increases in pain are to be expected, a large increase in pain is a sign of over-exertion
- focus on achieving measurable treatment goals established with the patient. Goals must fit with a patient's abilities and

expectations and it is important to discuss that complete cure and return of full function is unlikely
- developing relaxation skills
- learning ways to manage feelings of frustration, depression and worry
- a gentle exercise programme. The type of exercise is less important than actually doing more exercise
- managing pain-killing medication. In patients with continuous or frequently occurring pain, pain medication should be administered on a fixed time-interval dosing basis. This maximizes continuous blood levels and dampens pain if it flares up. Also, if pain intensity is responsible for the patient taking analgesia, the amount of drug taken may escalate to unacceptable levels. However if pain relief is taken on a time contingent basis, drug intake tends to remain more constant
- managing sleep difficulties:
  - establish regular wake up time
  - only sleep in bed
  - stop trying to fall asleep
  - relaxation techniques and tapes
  - amitriptyline
  - exercise
  - no sleeping during the day
- communicating with others about living with pain, and involving partners
- dealing with flare-ups – they will happen so it is important to have a plan for when they do
- how to progress in the future
- understanding the role of health professionals and long-term relationships with doctors.

REALISTIC GOALS

- Improved physical functioning
- Improved mood
- Improved sleep
- Development of active coping skills
- Return to work.

A reduction in suffering usually occurs as a result of all the above.

Methods for reducing anxiety

RELAXATION AND MEDITATION THERAPY

This form of training allows people to relax tense muscles, reduce anxiety and alter the mental state. Both physical and mental tension can make pain worse. Some techniques of relaxation that may be used are:

- Breathing relaxation
- Progressive relaxation

- Autogenic relaxation
- Guided imagery
- Meditation.

HYPNOSIS

Franz Mesmer introduced a technique into Western medicine in the eighteenth century and the technique became known as mesmerizing. About 20 per cent of people are highly hypnotizable, 30 per cent are not hypnotizable at all and the remainder lie somewhere between. Hypnosis can be self-induced or induced by another person with the hypnotist acting as a guide or assistant. The aim is to relax the subject by directing their attention with verbal, rhythmic, repetitive monotonous instruction. By using a self-induced technique, some patients are able to control the impending attacks of pain in migraine and other tension-like states producing pain.

The role of hypnosis in chronic pain is uncertain and long-term benefit has not been proved. About 15–20 per cent of hypnotizable patients report pain relief. Its role, when used, is usually seen as part of a multidisciplinary approach to pain management.

BIOFEEDBACK

The word 'biofeedback' was coined in the late 1960s to describe laboratory procedures being used to train experimental research subjects to alter brain activity, blood pressure, heart rate and other bodily functions that normally are not controlled voluntarily. Biofeedback is a process in which a person is trained to influence physiological responses by using signals from their own bodies. Research has demonstrated that biofeedback can help in the treatment of many diseases and painful conditions. The intention is to regain control of neuromuscular and neurovascular aspects of painful disease states.

Electrical devices are used to detect, record and amplify the neuromuscular and vascular response and convert visual and auditory responses into a form recognized by the patient, e.g. a louder sound meaning an increase in muscle tension.

Some individuals can learn voluntary control over certain body activities if they are provided with information about how the system is working – how fast their heart is beating, how tense are their head or neck muscles, how cold are their hands. How people use this 'biofeedback' to learn control is not understood, but some masters of the art report that imagery helps, e.g. when a patient wants to raise the temperature of their hands they may think of a warm tropical beach.

The technique of biofeedback is predominantly indicated in tension or vascular (migraine) headaches and fibromyositic conditions. It has been used in the treatment of complex regional pain syndromes when some patients can raise the temperature of a limb by several degrees and get relief of pain. It is unknown how the mechanism works and the results of several studies have been mixed.

Self-help groups and the expert patient programme

Self-help groups can often be a way of providing a bridge back to social activity because they offer some understanding of how difficult life can be, especially when constrained by pain. The expert patient programme is a new idea that involves patients themselves running groups for patients. Patients are trained to provide help for other patients in a way similar to the pain management programme but professionals will not be involved to the same extent in the running of the programme. It is too early at the present time to be certain of the effect of these programmes on the overall functioning of patients in pain, but it may prove an effective way of helping patients with chronic pain to cope with their difficulties.

Outcome of pain management programmes

There is evidence to show that after attending a programme:

- fewer people take analgesic or psychotropic drugs
- fewer people seek additional medical advice in the following year
- walking distance improves
- people suffer less depression.

Patient selection and patient cooperation are all-important. Analysis of individuals who have improved dramatically with one or another of these approaches is helping to pinpoint what factors are likely to lead to successful treatment.

OVERALL CLINICAL RECOMMENDATIONS FOR PAIN MANAGEMENT

- A multicomponent programme including stress management, coping skills training, cognitive restructuring and relaxation therapy are useful for chronic back pain.
- Multimodal cognitive behavioural/mind–body therapies and an educational/informational component (self-management programme) may be helpful in rheumatoid arthritis and osteoarthritis.
- Relaxation and thermal biofeedback may help recurrent migraines and relaxation ± electromyographic muscle biofeedback may help with recurrent tension headaches.
- Relaxation, imagery, etc. are helpful for procedural pain.

SUMMARY

Effective management of chronic pain depends on patients assuming an active, responsible collaborative role in their treatment. They must:

- take a responsibility for managing their pain
- make an effort
- become aware of their needs
- know their limitations
- take an active part in their recovery
- follow advice.

A patient must be ready for this approach – a patient who is not ready to contemplate learning self-management skills for pain control is unlikely to respond favourably to training in pain management skills. It is important to acknowledge that it takes a lot of ongoing motivation, strength, courage and regularly reviewed confidence to cope well with chronic pain.

Things do not change, we do

Henry David Thoreau

CASE SCENARIO

A 30-year-old woman is referred to the pain clinic by her general practitioner with severe upper thoracic pain. She has been seen by the orthopaedic surgeons and does have a thoracic kyphoscoliosis but they are not keen to operate. She has four children under the age of 6 years and the youngest is 9 months old. She has a long history of back pain, but it is much more severe than in the past. She is taking paracetamol, diclofenac, slow release morphine (MST) 60 mg twice daily and Oramorph 20 mg for breakthrough pain about four times a day. She is spending most of the day lying on her side in bed. She is unable to care for her children and is only able to read to them on her bed. Her husband has given up his job to look after the family. She has also had acupuncture and uses a transcutaneous electrical nerve stimulation (TENS) machine. Lumbar facet joint injections made her symptoms worse. She is worried about reducing her medication because it may exacerbate the pain but she has pinpoint pupils and is drowsy. She is also very tearful and does not see how anything can be improved. Physiotherapy at home has not improved the situation. It is painful and the patient does not cooperate with passive movements and finds it difficult to stand and walk at all.

It is important that this patient is assessed by a clinical psychologist and a pain management physiotherapist. She needs to begin a programme of rehabilitation and a gradual reduction of her analgesia but there are many factors preventing her doing this including the fear of pain on movement. There may be other factors involved in this flare-up of pain following the birth of her fourth child and it will take some time to sort out all her underlying difficulties.

13 Chronic Pain: The Common Problems

HEADACHES

Migraine and vascular headaches

CAUSES

The pathogenesis of migraine is still poorly understood. Most of the brain is insensate and as far as we know pain can arise from only the:

- large cranial vessels
- proximal intracranial vessels
- dura mater.

The vessels are innervated by branches of the ophthalmic division of the trigeminal nerve. Thus there must be an abnormality somewhere in one or all of the following:

- blood vessels
- trigeminal innervation of the blood vessels
- reflex connections to the trigeminal system with the cranial parasympathetic outflow.

The mechanism of generation of the pain is unclear but may result from any of the following:

- **Extracranial arterial vasodilatation**: Migraine headaches are of the vascular type, associated with throbbing pain on one side of the head. Predominantly the frontal branch of the superficial temporal artery is involved, giving rise to pain in the temple. There is much indirect evidence that the nerve growth factor (NGF) may regulate the presentation of vascular headache.
- **Extracranial neurogenic inflammation**: Inflammation of peripheral tissue caused by release of chemicals from the primary sensory nerve fibres involved in nociception. Nerve fibres are coiled around the blood vessels and when the blood vessel dilates the nerves are stretched, depolarized and activated.
  Nerve supply to the cerebral blood vessels is via sympathetic fibres containing noradrenaline and neuropeptide Y, and sensory fibres containing substance P and calcitonin gene-related peptide (CGRP), which act as vasodilators.
- **Decreased inhibition of central pain transmission**: Genetic factors play a role in determining who will be a victim of migraine, but many other factors are important as well.

INCIDENCE

Migraine occurs in 6 per cent of men and 18 per cent of women. Most have the first attack <30 years of age. About 30 per cent occur before the age of 10 years. Migraine can be associated with:

- chocolate
- cheese
- positive family history
- motion sickness.

Migraine attacks can vary in intensity from mild to excruciating among the population of sufferers and within individuals. Box 13.1 lists the diagnostic criteria for migraine.

AURAS

The aura is thought to be caused by a wave of short lasting neuronal excitation that travels over the cortex, followed by a prolonged period of depression of cortical neuronal activity. Visual auras are the commonest. They often appear in one field as a moving, expanding bright, curved saw-toothed line with obscured vision. Some of these figures are strikingly colourful whereas others are dull and monochromatic. Some bright-coloured figures have shapes that are not zigzag lines. Visual auras consisting of absent or blurred vision in one or a part of one visual field are also common. Spreading numbness, in one side of the face or upper limb, or both, is the next most common aura. Mild hemiparesis and speech disturbances (dysphasia) are not rare.

MIGRAINE AND THE MENSTRUAL CYCLE

Many women state that they are more likely to have migraines close to or during their menstrual period. Headaches are

BOX 13.1 International Headache Society diagnostic criteria (1988)

Migraine without aura (common migraine)
At least five attacks
Headache attacks lasting 4–72 hours
Headache has at least two of the following four characteristics:

- unilateral location
- pulsating quality
- moderate or severe intensity (inhibits or prohibits daily activities)
- aggravated by walking stairs or similar routine physical activity

During the headache at least one of the following accompaniments:

- nausea and/or vomiting
- photophobia and phonophobia

Relatives of migraine sufferers have the same abnormalities and there is a 40 per cent chance of first-degree relatives developing migraine.

Migraine with aura (classic migraine)
At least two attacks lasting 4–72 hours fulfilling at least three of the following:

- one or more fully reversible aura symptoms indicating focal cerebral cortical and/or brainstem function
- at least one aura symptom develops gradually over more than four minutes, or two or more symptoms occur in succession
- no aura symptom lasts >60 minutes, if more than one aura symptom is present, the accepted duration is proportionally increased
- headache follows aura with free interval of at least 60 minutes (it may occur simultaneously with the aura)

At least one of the following aura features establishes a diagnosis of migraine with typical aura:

- homonymous visual disturbance
- unilateral paraesthesias and/or numbness
- unilateral weakness
- aphasia or unclassifiable speech difficulty.

significantly more likely to occur in the two days before the onset of menses and the first five days following the onset of menses. So-called true menstrual migraine (migraine occurring on the first day of menstruation or two days before or

after and at no other time) occurred in 7.2 per cent of a series of patients.

TREATMENT

Non-pharmacological

Education about the disorder and lifestyle changes that may help include:

- regular sleep
- regular meals
- stress reduction
- exercise
- discontinuation of an oral contraceptive
- avoidance of certain foods or beverages, especially red wine.

Pharmacological

The drugs fall into two main classes:

1 Those that alleviate or abort the pain. These drugs affect the headache, but not the neurological symptoms.
2 Those that prevent the pain. These drugs decrease the frequency of migraine attacks whether they occur with or without neurological symptoms (auras).

Analgesic agents
- Non-specific

These drugs should be taken as soon as the attack is recognized. Non-steroidal anti-inflammatory drugs (NSAIDs) are more effective than paracetamol. The addition of an antiemetic or a drug that speeds gastric emptying may help because gastric emptying can be delayed during an attack of migraine. These drugs should not be taken more than two to three times a week. The response to treatment may vary as may the severity of the migraine attack. The following are of proved benefit:

- paracetamol 1 g has an NNT (number needed to treat) 7.8 (4.8–21) for migraine
- aspirin and metoclopramide – NNT 3.2 (2.6–4.0)
- ibuprofen – NNT 2.0
- rectal ketoprofen
- naproxen.

Opioids can be used to alleviate migraine attacks in patients poorly responsive to the above drugs, but their use should be limited to a dose or two no more than two days a week and it is better to avoid them if at all possible as they do not often have any better effect than paracetamol and NSAIDs.

- The triptans

The triptans are selective 5-hydroxytryptamine (5-HT, serotonin) agonists at 5-HT_{1B} receptors on intracranial arteries and $5-HT_{1D}$ receptors on the trigeminal nerve terminals of these arteries. All are very effective in alleviating or aborting migraine headaches. In general, they are the preferred drugs for migraine. The possible mechanisms of action include:

- cranial vasoconstriction
- peripheral neuronal inhibition
- inhibition of transmission through second-order neurones of the trigeminal complex.

- Drugs available
    - sumatriptan 6 mg subcutaneously (NNT 2.0), 50 mg oral (NNT 4.1), nasal spray (NNT 3.4)
    - naratriptan
    - rizatriptan
    - zolmitriptan 5 mg orally NNT 3.1
    - almotriptan
    - eletriptan.

Rizatriptan and eletriptan are more effective than sumatriptan. Some benefit in two-thirds of attacks will occur in 67 per cent of patients, but the drugs may be ineffective in some patients.

Side effects
- Serious side effects are rare
- Mild, brief, odd sensations (especially pressure in the chest or throat) are common after sumatriptan injections but less frequent after the other administration routes
- Tingling
- Paraesthesias
- Sensations of warmth
- Flushing

Contraindications
- $5-HT_{1B}$ receptors are also found in the coronary circulation. They can cause vasoconstriction, chest pain and very rarely myocardial infarction.
- Ischaemic heart disease (angina pectoris, history of myocardial infarction, or documented silent ischaemia) or Prinzmetal's angina.
- Poorly controlled hypertension. Sumatriptan can give rise to increases in blood pressure (usually small).
- Cerebrovascular disease.
- It should not be used concomitantly with ergotamine.

When the first triptan tried is not effective, one or two others should be tried before giving up on this drug class for any patient because individual responses to the triptans vary. Treatment should be undertaken in a stepwise manner, e.g. starting with aspirin and metoclopramide and two hours later if there is no response using zolmitriptan and so on until relief is obtained.

Lidocaine nose drops
Instillation of 0.5 mL of 4 per cent topical lidocaine nose drops into the nostril on the side of the headache with the head hyperextended 45° and turned 30° towards the side of the headache. For bilateral headaches, the drops should be instilled into both nostrils. A repeat dose should be given when the headache is more than mild two minutes after the first instillation.

Other
Feverfew (a herbal remedy) may provide some benefit. Treatments of no proved benefit so far include acupuncture, chiropractic treatments, homoeopathy, verapamil and the serotonin selective reuptake inhibitors (SSRIs).

Prophylactic treatment
Preventive medicines should be offered to patients whose quality of life is diminished by frequent migraine attacks. The following should be taken into consideration:

- frequency (minimum three times a month)
- duration
- severity
- tractability
- preference of patient
- unresponsiveness to acute attack medication.

It is not clear how the preventive medicines work but it may be by modifying the sensitivity of the brain.

Propranolol
If the small initial dose of propranolol (generally 20 mg orally twice daily) is ineffective after several weeks, the dose should be slowly increased while monitoring the pulse and side effects, such as tiredness and depression. Doses larger than 60 mg twice daily are seldom needed. Propranolol is a particularly good choice for anxious patients. There is a 34 per cent reduction in frequency of attacks.

Antidepressants
Amitriptyline or nortriptyline – 25–75 mg nocte.

Anticonvulsants
- Sodium valproate – NNT 3.5 (2.6–5.3); 400–600 mg twice daily
- Gabapentin – 900–2400 mg/day
- Topiramate – 25–200 mg/day

Pizotifen

Pizotifen is an antihistamine and serotonin antagonist structurally related to the tricyclic antidepressants. The dose is 0.5–3 mg nocte.

New developments

- Selective A1 adenosine receptor agonists
- CGRP antagonists
- Drugs that block nitric oxide synthesis

Chronic tension-type headache

Chronic tension-type headaches are one of the commonest forms of headache. They are recurrent episodes of headache lasting minutes to days that involve continued contractions of the head and neck muscles.

INCIDENCE

The 1-year prevalence of all tension-type headaches is about 74 per cent. The female/male ratio for tension-type headache is approximately 1.4/1.

SYMPTOMS

At least two of the following pain characteristics must be present:

- the pain is typically pressing (non-pulsating) or tightening in quality
- mild to moderate intensity
- bilateral in location
- photophobia or phonophobia may occur
- no aggravation by walking stairs or similar routine physical activity.

TREATMENT

Medication

Simple analgesics, such as paracetamol or NSAIDs, are the commonest form of treatment. There is some evidence that the addition of caffeine (roughly 100 mg, the amount in a strong cup of coffee) enhances the effect of the analgesics. They may not work well and when taken daily or almost daily, they may add a degree of analgesic-abuse headache to the primary headache. To avoid this the patient should be encouraged to use analgesic agents as infrequently as possible and to try to restrict their use to particularly severe episodes of pain. A recent retrospective study of venlafaxine suggests some efficacy in a dose of 150 mg daily.

Other treatments

Heat and cold may provide temporary relief. Reports of benefit from **cognitive behavioural therapy** and **biofeedback therapy** have been appearing for many years. Combined antidepressant/stress management therapy may have advantages over either alone.

ANALGESIA-INDUCED CHRONIC DAILY HEADACHE

People who frequently take any type of drug to alleviate migraines or episodic tension-type headaches for several consecutive weeks risk inducing a chronic daily headache. In general, the more potent the drug, the less often it need be taken to induce such a headache state. Opioids including codeine may be used only three times a week for several weeks before the headache occurs daily, whereas paracetamol may need to be taken almost daily to induce such a state. Headache is more likely to develop or flare up when the medication level in the body is waning (hence the term 'rebound headache'), but it can also occur despite heavy medication levels. When doses are missed or delayed, the headache generally flares up, since the headache mechanism is no longer suppressed by medication.

Cluster headache

Cluster headaches are attacks of severe unilateral pain in the orbit and/or surrounding areas, lasting between 15 and 180 minutes, recurring from once every other day to eight times per day, and accompanied on the ipsilateral (headache) side by one or more of the following symptoms:

- conjunctival injection (reddened eyeball)
- lacrimation (excessive tears from the eye)
- nasal congestion (stuffy nose)
- ptosis (lowered upper eyelid)
- miosis (smaller pupil)
- facial sweating.

Attacks occur in series lasting for weeks or months separated by remissions lasting for months or years – hence the name **cluster headache**.

TREATMENT

Subcutaneously injected sumatriptan (6 mg in 0.5 mL) is the most effective, reliable and rapid abortive therapy for cluster headache attacks. In the majority of patients the headache diminishes or is eliminated by 100 per cent oxygen delivered by a tight-fitting mask at a flow rate of 7 L per minute for about 15 minutes; however, oxygen is less effective and reliable than sumatriptan injections and is difficult to use outside the home, although small, portable oxygen tanks are available.

Verapamil

Verapamil 40–120 mg three times daily is an effective preventive agent for cluster headaches.

Acute and chronic post-traumatic headaches

Roughly 50 per cent of patients who are stunned or knocked out by a blow to the head experience headache soon afterwards. These headaches disappear within a few weeks in about 70 per cent of the sufferers, but the other 30 per cent continue to have headaches for years. No correlation exists between the severity of the trauma and the chance of developing a chronic post-traumatic headache. The headache is not caused by brain damage but is most likely related to a person's reaction to the traumatic event. The main therapy should be psychological.

DRUG THERAPY

- Analgesics
- Antidepressants, e.g. amitriptyline

Cervicogenic headaches

Some headaches may be associated with neck pain. The attacks may be provoked by head and neck movements. The pain is nearly always unilateral, particularly in the orbit or temple and in the upper posterior neck, and throbbing in nature. The pain is sometimes prolonged and can be induced by firm manual pressure on the neck especially over the upper cervical or occipital region.

There is often a restricted range of motion in the neck. The headaches can be accompanied by ipsilateral neck, shoulder or arm pain of a rather vague non-radicular nature or, occasionally, arm pain of a radicular nature. They are not accompanied by nausea/vomiting. Photophobia and phonophobia can occur rarely.

Diagnostic anaesthetic blockades of cervical nerves and joints, such as blocks of the C2 and C3 nerves, may reduce pain.

FACIAL PAIN

Trigeminal neuralgia

See Table 8.1 (page 156) for the branches of the trigeminal nerve and their distribution.

INCIDENCE

Little is known about the natural history of trigeminal neuralgia, but it appears suddenly and spontaneously. The incidence is unknown. It may be about three to five cases per year per 100 000 population and increases with age. The disease is commoner in patients with multiple sclerosis (MS), and MS also increases risk of bilateral disease. It is commonest in patients over 50 years (median age 67 years) but can occur in young adults. The pain is usually unilateral.

SYMPTOMS

- The pain can be due to involvement of the gasserian ganglion or the peripheral branches.
- Character – shooting, sharp, electrical paroxysms of pain. Pain is not a problem during sleep.
- Severity – moderate to most severe.
- Periodicity – relapsing/remitting.
- Site – the pain is in the distribution of the trigeminal nerve. It is commoner in the mandibular and maxillary areas.
- Provocation – innocuous stimuli such as light touch, eating, washing, and talking stimulate the 'trigger zone' which is found around the chin, cheeks, lips and tongue for the second and third divisions and around the eye when the first division is involved.
- Duration – usually less than two minutes but there may be many attacks.
- Occasionally the pain radiates outside the trigeminal distribution.
- There may be some quantitative sensory changes in up to 50 per cent, and some patients with involvement of the first division of the nerve have a reduced corneal reflex.
- The first division of the nerve is involved in 30 per cent, and in less than 4 per cent only the first division is involved.

DIAGNOSIS

The diagnosis depends strictly on clinical criteria as there are no tests to prove the diagnosis. The pain is usually brief and followed by long pain-free periods, but the pain can be extremely severe. Patients become hesitant about eating, drinking, washing and brushing their teeth. There may be mild numbness in the painful area but little else to find. There must be a 'trigger' and paroxysmal pain in the distribution of the trigeminal nerve.

DIFFERENTIAL DIAGNOSIS

The diagnosis of trigeminal neuralgia should be made on the specific symptoms and on the distribution of the pain. It can still sometimes be difficult to distinguish the symptoms from atypical facial pain.

AETIOLOGY

It has been suggested from clinical observations that vascular compression of the central axons of the trigeminal nerve at the root entry zone near the pons results in focal demyelination of the trigeminal nerve which alters the electrical activity of the trigeminal neurones. Many patients with trigeminal neuralgia have an aberrant blood vessel (usually an artery but sometimes a vein), found on magnetic resonance imaging (MRI) that appears to be pressing on the nerve. Decompression of the nerve results in almost immediate pain relief in many patients but not all, and the pain may return despite successful surgery. Aberrant vessels are not seen in 100 per cent of patients. Generally, about 6–32 per cent of individuals also have the vascular contact but without any symptoms.

It is difficult to understand how a vessel would compress nerves sufficiently to produce such a well-defined syndrome. There remain many doubts about this theory that have yet to be explored. There are profound gaps in our knowledge about trigeminal neuralgia and much more research is needed into mechanisms and treatment.

PROBLEMS WITH TREATMENT

- Assessing outcome of treatment is difficult because of the possibility of spontaneous remission.
- It is impossible to compare treatment with placebo because the severity of the pain requires that some treatment be given.
- There are no randomized controlled trials that compare the relative safety of surgical procedures.

DRUG TREATMENT

Analgesia

Analgesia should be prescribed following the World Health Organization (WHO) ladder (see Chapter 4) but often these drugs will have little effect.

Anticonvulsants

- Carbamazepine has for years been the treatment of choice but the NNT is 2.2. This means that only 50 per cent of patients will get more than 50 per cent pain relief. The others may get some pain relief and it may be meaningful but we do not know to what extent this occurs. Side effects of carbamazepine and loss of efficacy have prompted the search for another drug.
- Oxcarbazepine has a safer side effect profile and works in some patients whose pain is refractory to carbamazepine.
- There is weak evidence for an effect from gabapentin but the clinical effects are often disappointing.
- Phenytoin is less effective but may help with refractory pain and may be used in combination with carbamazepine.
- Lamotrigine has been subjected to controlled trials and has proved beneficial especially when combined with carbamazepine.

Local anaesthetics

Tocainide, mexiletine and intravenous lidocaine are all worth trying in refractory pain.

Antidepressants

Amitriptyline has not proved so useful in trigeminal neuralgia as the anticonvulsants.

Other drugs

Baclofen and pimozide have proved helpful particularly in pain refractory to carbamazepine.

Additional measures

- Alcohol or local anaesthetic injections into the trigger points have been used successfully but often only last up to a year at the most.
- General support and information about the disease.
- Attention to nutritional and hydration support when the pain is bad.

SURGICAL TREATMENT

Surgery generates a very powerful placebo response and so comparison with medical treatment can be difficult. There are no randomized controlled studies comparing the outcome between the various procedures. Radio-frequency lesion, balloon inflation and glycerol injection are all carried out using a similar approach and the techniques are discussed further in Chapter 8.

Microvascular decompression

Microvascular decompression (MVD) was first described by Janetta in 1967. It is the commonest open procedure used for treatment of trigeminal neuralgia. A small incision is made behind the ear in the mastoid area and the trigeminal nerve is freed from the compressive/pulsating artery by a piece of Teflon. It is a major intervention and there is a serious risk of complications (see Table 13.1). About 75 per cent of patients will have immediate pain relief following surgery but it does sometimes recur. The results are poorer if the patient has had previous ablative procedures.

Table 13.1 *Complications of microvascular decompression*

Complication	Incidence (%)
Cerebrospinal fluid leak	1.6
Hearing loss	2–13 (lower rate if use evoked response monitoring)
Cranial nerve palsy	5
Permanent disability	1
Mortality	0.5

Major predictors of recurrence after MVD

- Female sex
- Symptoms >8 years
- Venous compression of trigeminal root entry zone (rather than arterial compression)

Gamma knife treatment

The area for treatment is located stereotactically and radiation beams are targeted with high precision to the base of the nerve. The procedure is pain free, non-invasive and carried out with the patient awake so there is no need for a general anaesthetic.

Outcome

- The outcome is similar to MVD but is worse in patients who have failed previous interventions.
- 73 per cent have an excellent outcome. They are free from pain and off all other treatment.
- 20 per cent have a fair result (>50 per cent pain relief).
- 7 per cent have a poor outcome with little or no pain relief.
- It is more effective as a primary treatment.

THE PROBLEM WITH THE HYPOTHESIS OF THE PATHOPHYSIOLOGY

It is not really understood how a normally innocuous input such as a blood vessel can activate severe paroxysmal pain. There is no comparable situation where light touch initiates paroxysmal pain. It is unknown whether low threshold Aβ fibre input activates peripheral hyper-excitable C fibres or if the Aβ fibre input activates hyper-excitable neurones in the spinal trigeminal nucleus in the medulla. It is also unknown why it increases with age and why it occurs more in women.

Atypical facial pain

Atypical facial pain is a label encompassing a wide group of facial pain problems. There may be many different causes but the symptoms are all similar. Facial pain, often described as burning, aching or cramping, occurs on one side of the face, often in the region of the trigeminal nerve and can extend into the upper neck or back of the scalp. Although rarely as severe as trigeminal neuralgia, facial pain is continuous, with few, if any, periods of remission.

POSSIBLE CAUSES

- Infections of the sinuses or teeth. A low-grade infectious and inflammatory process occurring over a long period can result in nerve damage and be the triggering factor.
- Trauma
  - dental
  - physical.

DIAGNOSIS

The diagnosis of atypical facial pain is not an easy task. Patients often have numerous dental procedures, see multiple doctors and have many medical tests before the diagnosis is made usually by eliminating all other possible causes of pain. Only after tests rule out other factors can a diagnosis of atypical facial pain be made.

TREATMENT

Treatment is difficult and frequently unsuccessful. It is usually worth trying medication as some patients may respond.

Medication

- Amitriptyline and other antidepressants
- Gabapentin and other anticonvulsants

Other treatments

- Hot and cold compresses
- Acupuncture
- Biofeedback
- Dental splints

Surgical procedures generally are not successful.

ARM PAIN

There are many causes of arm pain including:

- pain referred from the neck
- shoulder pain
- complex regional pain syndrome
- brachial plexus lesions usually due to traumatic avulsion and tumours.

Pain secondary to trauma is usually immediate but if delayed it always starts within six weeks. The pain usually presents as burning in the hand, a feeling like being hit with a hammer or the arm feels as if it is in a vice.

Treatment includes analgesia, anticonvulsants and antidepressants. For those with brachial plexus lesions who do not respond to medical treatment dorsal root entry zone (DREZ) lesions can produce good pain relief. The management of complex regional pain syndrome is discussed later in the chapter.

LEG PAIN

Restless legs syndrome (Ekbom's syndrome)

Symptoms in the legs begin immediately on sitting or lying down and are worse during the early evening and at night.

They can be relieved by moving the legs but the relief is only brief. The syndrome can severely disturb sleep and impair the quality of daily life.

CAUSE

It is an idiopathic condition but there is some evidence that it may be due to altered dopaminergic function in the central nervous system (CNS) resulting in a decreased threshold for the spinal flexor reflex and/or to reduced iron acquisition in the brain.

INCIDENCE

- 1:7 people.
- It may be seen in pregnancy – 19 per cent of women in the third trimester experience restless legs. The symptoms are relieved by the birth.
- There is an increased incidence in patients with diabetes mellitus and hypothyroidism.
- It can occur at any age but is commoner with increasing age.
- It is more common in women than in men.
- Up to 92 per cent of patients have a family history.
- It can be the initial manifestation of iron-deficiency anaemia.

DIAGNOSTIC CRITERIA

- An overwhelming desire to move the limbs (akathisia) which may be associated with paraesthesia or dysaesthesia (burning, tickling, crawling, etc.).
- Symptoms are worse or exclusively present at rest and relieved by activity.
- Motor restlessness. There is a build up of discomfort and involuntary jerking if the legs remain still.
- Symptoms are worse in the evening or at night.
- Symptoms are usually bilateral but can be unilateral and can affect the arms.

DIFFERENTIAL DIAGNOSIS

- Nocturnal leg cramps
- Peripheral neuropathy
- Vascular disease
- Parkinson's disease
- Anaemia
- Diabetes

TREATMENT

- Explanation and reassurance
- Self-help measures
  - Avoid caffeine before bedtime
  - Keep cool
  - Avoid standing or sitting for long periods
  - Avoid CNS stimulants, diuretics, tricyclic antidepressants, calcium antagonists, phenytoin
  - Walking, stretching, bathing, relaxation and massage can help
- Drug treatment
  - Analgesic agents
  - Antidepressants
  - Anticonvulsants
    - Gabapentin up to 1800 mg/day
    - Carbamazepine
  - Benzodiazepines
    - Clonazepam 1 mg nocte has been used but the evidence for its effect is weak
  - Other
    - Opioids, particularly oxycodone, may help
    - Clonidine 0.5 mg day
  - Dopamine receptor antagonists
    - The usual dose of levodopa for restless legs is 100–500 mg per day but occasionally patients need 1000–1500 mg per day. Use levodopa/carbidopa 100/25 mg immediate or slow release increasing as required
    - Pergolide 0.05–0.75 mg daily
    - Bromocriptine up to 7.5 mg day
    - Pramipexole up to 1.5 mg day
    - Ropinirole 0.5 mg day
    - Cabergoline 2.1 mg day

The clinical benefits and the safety of these drugs need confirmation because all studies that have been conducted have been small.

Side effects of the dopamine receptor antagonists

- Augmentation of symptoms
- Pulmonary, retroperitoneal and pericardial fibrosis
- Sleepiness

SPINAL CORD INJURY

Pain follows 7.5–100 per cent of spinal cord lesions with an average of 65 per cent and in one-third of these it is severe. The pain has a direct bearing on the ability to regain an optimal level of activity. There is no significant relation between the presence or severity of pain and level or completeness of the spinal cord injury (SCI). Trauma is the commonest cause but onset of the pain can be delayed and the pain may change over time:

- Neuropathic pain from incomplete lesions is commoner.
- Pain may occur without sensory loss.

- The pain is often aggravated by movement.
- Patients may experience phantom movement.
- Injuries to the lower cord tend to produce more pain.
- Gunshot wounds cause more pain.

Pain is increased with:

- changes in the weather
- smoking
- fatigue
- emotions
- bowel or bladder problems.

Types of pain associated with spinal cord injury

- Nociceptive pain – due to mechanical instability of the spine and damage to bones or ligaments. It occurs in the region of the spine and may radiate towards the extremities but it is not radicular. It is related to posture, increased with activity and relieved by immobilization. Treatment includes NSAIDs, opioids and fusion of the spine.
- Muscle spasm pain – involuntary muscle spasm occurs in areas that have lost motor function particularly when muscles or joints are stretched.
- Secondary overuse pain or pressure syndromes – occur in normally innervated regions like the proximal muscles. This pain may occur months or years after the injury.
- Lancinating and burning pain – caused by nerve root entrapment that may be bilateral. It occurs at or just below the level of spinal trauma at a point where normal feeling stops. It is usually present from time of injury, but may not occur for days or weeks after injury and may worsen with time. Treatment is with NSAIDs, neuropathic drugs, opioids and surgery.
- Burning pain – produced by damage to cauda equina and occurring in the legs, feet, perineum, genitals and rectum.
- Nerve compression pain.
- Segmental deafferentation pain – neuropathic pain often occurs at the border of normal sensation and anaesthetic skin. It occurs within a band of two to four segments and can be bilateral, unilateral or circumferential. Allodynia or hyperaesthesia may be present. This pain develops in first few months post injury. All the drugs used for the treatment of neuropathic pain can be tried as well as epidural injections with local anaesthetic and steroid, nerve root blocks, DREZ lesion, dorsal rhizotomy, spinal cord stimulation or cordotomy.
- Spinal cord injury pain – diffuse pain in anaesthetic regions below level of injury. It is usually bilateral and can be burning, tingling, numb or aching in nature. It is usually constant and unrelated to activity. This pain is very difficult to manage but treatment should include neuropathic medication and sometimes responds to intrathecal opioid and/or clonidine. It rarely responds to stimulation techniques.
- Visceral pain – often delayed in onset. It is a burning, cramping and constant pain in the abdomen. It is poorly defined, as with most visceral pain.

Syringomyelia is an abnormal cavity in the spinal cord that may develop years after the original injury. It causes ascending neurological deficits and pain with reduced pain and temperature sensation above level of lesion. Pain can occur from overuse injury, e.g. tendonitis of rotator cuff as a result of pushing a wheelchair. Cognitive, affective and environmental factors are important to the way the patient copes with the difficulties caused by an SCI.

Classification of pain related to spinal cord injuries

See Table 13.2.

CENTRAL PAIN

Central pain arises secondary to incomplete lesions of the brain, brainstem and spinal cord, e.g. strokes, MS and brain and spinal cord injuries. The pain may be generated in the cortex or nociceptive transmission may be abnormal all the way up to the cortex. The lesion is always contralateral to the pain. The exact cause of the pain is not yet clear.

Central post-stroke pain or thalamic pain syndrome

- This occurs after a stroke or cerebrovascular accident (CVA). A stroke implies there has been infarction and cell death in part of the CNS, caused by either lack of blood flow (thrombosis) or lack of oxygen (ischaemia).
- As well as the usual features of stroke caused by infarction in the cerebral hemispheres (weakness, numbness, paralysis, speech difficulties, confusion), up to 10 per cent of people develop central post-stroke pain (CPSP) when the infarction also involves the thalamus (brainstem sensory processing area).
- Minor CPSP symptoms are reported by 50 per cent of stroke victims. The full blown syndrome is less common.
- CPSP occurs more commonly when the right side of the brain becomes infarcted (left-sided stroke). The onset time for symptoms to develop is variable, ranging from days to

Table 13.2 *Pain related to spinal cord injuries*

Pain		Distinguishing features	Specific structures/pathology
Nociceptive	Musculoskeletal	Dull aching, movement related, eased by rest, responsive to opioids and NSAIDs	Bone, joint, muscle inflammation, mechanical instability, muscle spasm, secondary overuse syndrome
	Visceral	Dull, cramping, located in abdominal region with preserved innervation	Renal calculus, bowel sphincter dysfunction, dysreflexic headache
		Also includes dysreflexic headache (vascular)	
Neuropathic		Sharp, shooting, burning, electrical abnormal responsiveness (hyperaesthesias, hyperalgesia)	
	Above level	Located in the region of sensory preservation	Compressive mononeuropathies, CRPS
	At level	Located in segmental pattern at level of injury	Nerve root compression (including cauda equina)
			Syringomyelia, spinal cord trauma/ischaemia, dual level cord and root trauma
	Below level	Located diffusely below the level of injury	Spinal cord trauma/ischaemia (central dysaesthesia syndrome, etc.)

NSAID, non-steroidal anti-inflammatory drug; CRPS, complex regional pain syndrome

years. Pain can be felt in the face, arm, leg and/or the trunk on the stroke side. Symptoms may affect the whole of one side of the body.

FEATURES OF CENTRAL POST-STROKE PAIN

- Pain may occur without sensory loss or sensory abnormalities may be incomplete.
- The pain is usually worse distally and in the centre of the face but it may affect half the body or may be focal such as a limb or the face.
- The pain is usually poorly localized, constant and unrelenting, with a tendency to increase in intensity over time.
- There is often a bizarre burning pain with light touch which may be very difficult for the patient to describe and can be highly variable. The patient is usually numb in areas affected by burning pain.
- Movement, changes in temperature, or other unrelated stimuli may aggravate the symptoms. Patients often seek an ambient temperature.
- Poorly localized dysaesthetic pain is most prominent and most frequent.
- The pain is usually unresponsive to opioids.
- Pain can be spontaneous or continuous.
- There are abnormalities in superficial touch, temperature or pain.
- There is usually a time delay from onset of touch to the increase in burning pain. This is a characteristic that distinguishes central pain from peripheral neuropathy where the pain of light touch is instant.
- All pain modalities are affected in different proportions.
- Symptoms may vary in degree in any given patient.

It is very important to differentiate between CPSP and other forms of musculoskeletal pain that commonly occur in stroke victims, for example, a frozen shoulder or tight muscles. These musculoskeletal problems often resolve with physiotherapy and injections.

ORAL MEDICATIONS

Generally central pain responds poorly to medication and CPSP is a difficult condition to treat. The combination of low-dose amitriptyline (10–50 mg at night) plus gabapentin (between 300 mg/day and 1800 mg/day) produces the best pain relief with the lowest incidence of side effects. Intravenous lidocaine infusions are useful for some patients.

Pain in multiple sclerosis

About 2.5 million people worldwide are affected by MS, and over 60 per cent of patients experience moderate to severe pain.

CHARACTERISTICS OF PAIN IN MULTIPLE SCLEROSIS

- It is often diffuse, affecting several areas of the body at a time.
- It often changes over time, getting worse or better for no apparent reason.
- MS-related pain may be directly related to the disease itself and characterized as central pain (pain associated with optic neuritis and neuralgia), or it may develop secondary to the protracted symptoms of MS (pain caused by painful muscle contractures and stiffened joints).

ACUTE MS PAIN

- Burning, tingling, shooting or stabbing – these symptoms come on suddenly and may go away suddenly. They are often intense but can be brief in duration.
- Lhermitte's sign – a brief, stabbing, electric-shock-like sensation that runs from the back of the head down the spine, brought on by bending the neck forward.
- Painful optic neuritis.
- Painful limb spasms.
- Deep, aching leg pain.
- Uncomfortable buzzing sensations derived from spinal cord involvement.

CHRONIC MS PAIN (LASTING FOR MORE THAN A MONTH)

- Pain from spasticity that can lead to muscle cramps
- Tight and aching joints
- Back or musculoskeletal pain
- Trigeminal neuralgia
- Burning, aching, or 'girdling' around the body, dysaesthesia or a very intense sensation of pressure.

The commonest acute pain conditions are neuralgia, Lhermitte's sign, pain associated with optic neuritis, and brief painful tonic spasms. The most frequent chronic pain syndromes are pain associated with tonic spasms, tension, and painful sensations in the limbs, dysaesthesias and low back pain.

SITE OF PAIN

- Head – 53 per cent
- Arm – 58 per cent
- Leg – 73 per cent
- Trunk – 49 per cent
- More than one site – pain is commonly reported to occur in more than one site (76 per cent)

Although pain may be one of the worst symptoms of MS little information is available about the intensity of pain experienced by those reporting MS-related pain. Pain severity is unrelated to the duration of the disease or symptom severity, number of painful sites, age or gender.

EFFECTS OF PAIN ON MENTAL AND PHYSICAL FUNCTIONING

MS patients with pain report poorer mental health and greater deficits in social functioning relative with a comparison group of individuals with MS who report no pain. As many as 50 per cent of individuals with MS-related pain may have clinical depression, and 40 per cent report that pain affects their daily life.

MANAGEMENT OF MS-RELATED PAIN

Under-management of pain conditions in MS is widespread. Paracetamol is used by 83 per cent of patients using pain medications. Medications usually used to treat neuropathic pain are used by 65 per cent of patients treated for pain. Antidepressants such as amitriptyline may help. Regarding anticonvulsants:

- Carbamazepine may be effective in the early stages of neuralgia, but it may lose its effectiveness over time and alternative medications may need to be added.
- Gabapentin 900 mg three times daily improves spasticity and may improve pins and needles, throbbing and cramping pain but has little effect on aching pains.
- Levetiracetam (Keppra®) 500–4500 mg/day. Some studies show up to 50 per cent of patients improve.

Side effects of the anticonvulsants include fatigue and disorientation and seem to affect patients with MS more than other patients. Botulinum toxin is used to manage spasticity and bladder problems and it also has an effect on pain. Many patients with MS use cannabis to relieve their pain with some success although available research does not support this. Currently available cannabinoids include nabilone and dronabinol and both have been found to have a limited effect on pain in MS.

About 1 to 2 per cent of patients have extremely refractory pain that is very hard to manage and even aggressive efforts to manage pain can fail. Management of chronic pain is particularly complicated, and there are no clear guidelines for its pharmacological treatment.

Physical therapy

- Rehabilitation approaches may also be helpful in the management of MS-related pain.
- Soft collars might help diminish symptoms of Lhermitte's syndrome.
- Physical and occupational therapies that emphasize body mechanics and reconditioning are frequently offered, but little work has been done to confirm the efficacy of these approaches for reducing pain.
- Transcutaneous electrical nerve stimulation (TENS) may have some benefit.

PSYCHOSOCIAL IMPACT OF PAIN IN MS

Individuals with MS:

- Retire from employment early
- Are more likely to experience clinical depression
- Are at increased risk for suicide

- Experience low self-esteem
- Have lowered perceptions of social support
- Have lowered levels of marital satisfaction.

The specific and incremental effects of pain on psychosocial functioning and emotional wellbeing have only recently become a focus of investigation. Fifty-seven per cent of those persons reporting pain indicated that their ability to work had been reduced by 50 per cent or more because of pain. Compared with persons without pain, those acknowledging pain reported significantly poorer overall mental functioning.

Although it is likely that pain significantly influences physical and psychosocial functioning, limitations in this area of research preclude substantive conclusions at this time. Elicitation of a pain complaint should indicate a more comprehensive assessment of pain, as well as an assessment of potential pain-related interference with social-role functioning and compromised emotional wellbeing.

PSYCHOLOGICAL TREATMENT

There have been limited efforts to examine the efficacy of psychological interventions, particularly cognitive–behavioural therapy for pain in MS. No controlled studies have been done of psychological interventions for pain in MS. Self-hypnosis may contribute to pain relief in the short term, but longer-term benefits may be confounded with the progression of the disease and other rehabilitation efforts.

PELVIC PAIN

Incidence

In the UK about 38 women in every 1000 have chronic pelvic pain. Pelvic pain is responsible for:

- 10 per cent of all gynaecology consultations
- 20 per cent of laparoscopies (a third of all laparoscopies are normal)
- 10–12 per cent of hysterectomies.

The nerve supply to the pelvic contents involves the:

- pudendal nerve (S2–4)
- thoracolumbar sympathetic nerves
- uterovaginal and inferior hypogastric plexus.

Causes of pelvic pain

- Endometriosis
- Adhesions
- Ovarian remnant syndrome

- Pelvic congestion
- Gastrointestinal disease
- Urological disease
- Musculoskeletal conditions

Other causes are:

- Nerve entrapment pain can follow surgery or can be secondary to trigger points on the abdominal wall, in the vagina and sacral area. Ilioinguinal and iliohypogastric nerve entrapment may also cause pelvic pain.
- Psychological factors – women with pelvic pain with or without pathology have a higher lifetime incidence of major depressive illness, drug abuse and adult sexual dysfunction than controls.
- Increased incidence of childhood sexual abuse and physical abuse.
- Visceral hyperalgesia – the visceral structures are sensitive to distension and inflammation. Inflammation may make a viscus sensitive and non-painful stimuli are then perceived as painful.

CHRONIC UROGENITAL PAIN SYNDROMES

The aetiology of these focal pain syndromes is not known. Patients presenting with these pain syndromes are best assessed and treated using a multidisciplinary approach. The pain syndromes include:

- Vulvodynia
- Orchialgia
- Urethral syndrome
- Penile pain
- Prostatodynia
- Coccydynia
- Perineal pain
- Proctodynia
- Proctalgia fugax

Coccydynia

Pain in coccydynia occurs in the area of the coccyx. It can be anything from discomfort to acute pain, varying among people and varying with time in any individual. The name describes a pattern of symptoms (pain brought on or aggravated by sitting), so it is really a collection of conditions which can have different causes and need different treatments.

Coccydynia can follow after falls, childbirth, repetitive strain or surgery. In some cases the cause is unknown. The pain can disappear by itself or with treatment, or it can continue for years, and may get worse. It is five times more common in women than men, probably because the female pelvis leaves the coccyx more exposed.

Treatment

- Analgesia
- Antidepressants/anticonvulsants

Local infiltration around the coccyx can relieve the pain in some people. Caudal epidural injections with local anaesthetic and steroid are often successful. When the above treatments have not helped, TENS may relieve some of the pain, as may avoiding trauma to the coccyx, for example sitting on a ring cushion can relieve some symptoms.

Chronic pelvic pain

Chronic pelvic pain is a common and debilitating problem that can significantly impair quality of life. Patients with chronic pelvic pain are usually evaluated and treated by gynaecologists, gastroenterologists and urologists. Often the examination and work-up remain unrevealing and no specific cause of the pain can be identified.

Pudendal nerve neuropathy

Pudendal neuropathy is a complicated condition that mimics other conditions and is often diagnosed as vulvodynia, vulvar vestibulitis, levator ani syndrome, coccydynia, pelvic floor myalgia, interstitial cystitis, urethral syndrome, dyspareunia and pelvic floor dysfunction. It may occasionally be caused by a compression neuropathy or mechanical and/or inflammatory damage to the pudendal nerve (PNE). Compression or stretching of the pudendal nerve in the Alcock's canal can also induce the so called 'pudendal canal syndrome' (PCS).

Pudendal nerve neuropathy is a rare condition. Patients with PNE typically present with symptoms typical of an entrapment neuropathy:

- pain in the penis, scrotum, labia, perineum, or anorectal region
- may be unilateral or bilateral
- aggravated by sitting
- relieved by standing
- absent when recumbent
- absent when sitting on a toilet seat.

Pain occurs in the territory of the pudendal nerve (S2, 3, 4) and this syndrome is a clinical diagnosis in patients with the typical history:

- may often begin as light pain or itching on one side of the perineum without visible disease
- burning, searing, stabbing pain, pin pricking, cold sensation, pulling sensation
- foreign body sensation
- allodynia
- proctalgia – repetitive acute anal pain of short duration
- difficulty voiding or opening the bowels
- sexual intercourse may be very painful.

The pain associated with this condition is frequently quite intense and does not lend itself to treatment with conventional analgesics, and opiates provide some/minimal relief for only a few. After a night of sleep, a patient may notice some improvement in their condition, owing to the prolonged assumption of the supine position which allows for a marked lessening of pressure on the affected nerve(s).

Treatment

All treatments for chronic pain may be tried but the outcome with any one treatment is poor. Conservative measures are important such as:

- sitting on a ring cushion to avoid further trauma
- avoid sitting for long periods
- limiting exertional activities.

Therapeutic blocks

Computed tomography (CT)-guided infiltration of the pudendal nerve with local anaesthetic and steroid either at the ischial spine or the sacrotuberous ligament (Alcock's canal) has eased the pain in a few patients. If the pain goes away with local anaesthetic the nerve can be suspected of being a source of pain. The steroids may lead to more prolonged pain relief but this can take days or weeks. Long-term relief usually requires two or three injections, and usually the pain does not go but is reduced. These injections cannot be considered a cure for the pain and are carried out only rarely.

Interstitial cystitis

Interstitial cystitis is a chronic, painful and often debilitating disease, whose aetiology and pathophysiology is largely unknown. It is characterized by pelvic and suprapubic pain, urinary symptoms such as frequency and urgency, and in females often by dyspareunia that may be relieved by voiding. Interstitial cystitis has been considered to belong to the category of chronic pelvic pain syndromes. Current epidemiological studies show that this disease is commoner in women than in men.

Prostatitis-like urogenital pain

Of the men whose conditions are diagnosed as chronic prostatitis, 95 per cent have no evidence of bacterial infection or inflammatory cells in the prostatic fluid.

Vulvodynia

Vulvodynia is defined as burning, aching and soreness of the vulval area. Nerve fibres of the vulva are irritated or damaged and fire abnormal nerve signals back to the spinal cord resulting in pain. This can occur even when the painful area of skin involved is not touched.

The intensity of pain can vary from a mild discomfort to a severe, constant pain which can even prevent sitting down comfortably. The pain is usually continuous and can interfere with sleep. There are good days and bad days. Itching is not usually a feature of the condition. The pain in vulvodynia is not always restricted to the vulval area. It can be around the inside of the thighs, upper legs and even around the back passage and the urethra. Some women also have pain when they empty their bowels. It can have an effect on sexual activity, and is associated with pain during foreplay and on penetration. The condition usually affects women from the mid-forties onwards. Usually there is nothing to see on examination.

CAUSE

- In the majority of cases the precise cause of the nerve damage or irritation remains unknown.
- Back problems, e.g. slipped discs, can cause spinal nerve compression and cause referred pain to the vulval area.

TREATMENT

- Simple analgesia.
- 5 per cent lidocaine gel.
- Tricyclic antidepressants.
- Some women do gain some benefit from different types of creams and lotions applied to the vulval area which act as soothing agents.
- Vaginal lubricants can help during intercourse.
- Complementary treatments are widely used by women with vulval pain and can be more successful than prescription-based treatments. *Aloe vera* gel and *Calendula* are alternative homoeopathic treatments useful for treating sore and painful skin. Aqueous cream is a very bland plain emollient. It is

perfume free and is therefore less likely to irritate than the steroid creams. Many women gain benefit from the use of this cream as it soothes and rehydrates the skin. Some women keep the cream in the fridge and this can help even further with inflamed skin. It can be used indefinitely and frequently. For severe attacks of pain oatmeal baths are an alternative treatment available from most health shops without prescription.
- Acupuncture has been shown to benefit women with vulvodynia.

Testicular pain

Testicular pain is a fairly common condition treated by urologists. Frequent causes include:

- Infection of the testicle (orchitis)
- Epididymis (epididymitis)
- Post-surgical pain
- Trauma
- Tumours
- Hernia
- Torsion (twisting of the testicle)
- Varicocoele
- Hydrocoele
- Spermatocoele

Most of these conditions are easily diagnosed and treated. Chronic testicular pain is defined as continuous or intermittent unilateral or bilateral testicular discomfort of at least three months' duration compromising the patient's daily activities and prompting him to consult for medical advice. In up to 25 per cent of patients with chronic testicular pain, no cause can be found. In many men the co-existence of a physical abnormality and pain are not linked.

Testicular pain is commoner in men who have had prior surgery or trauma to the scrotum. Although no tests give a specific diagnosis, ultrasound will help in reassuring that there is no underlying abnormality, since anxiety over this often plays a part. After exclusion this can be a difficult condition to treat. Surgical treatment options include orchiectomy or epididymectomy but these radical approaches do not relieve the pain in a substantial number of patients. The average success rate of conservative therapeutic approaches varies between 27 and 90 per cent; the success rate of surgical interventions is as low as 10–50 per cent.

Management of chronic pelvic pain

Most pelvic pain does not respond well to any available treatment. Some pain relief can be provided to almost all patients using a multidisciplinary approach including pain medications, local treatment regimens, physical therapy and psychological support, while exercising caution towards invasive and irreversible therapeutic procedures. Treatment should be directed towards symptomatic pain management. Treatment modalities are available to lessen the impact of pain and improve functional status. Usually it is best managed by a multidisciplinary approach including cognitive behavioural therapy.

FIBROMYALGIA

Fibromyalgia is a painful, non-articular condition predominantly involving the muscles. It is the commonest cause of widespread musculoskeletal pain and hyperalgesia. Approximately 2 per cent of the population is believed to suffer from the condition, with females outnumbering males in the ratio of 9:1. It impairs quality of life and is associated with excessive use of healthcare.

The pain tends to be felt as diffuse aching or burning, often described as head to toe. It may be worse at some times than at others. It may also change location, usually becoming more severe in parts of the body that are used the most. The associated fatigue ranges from feeling tired, to the exhaustion of a 'flu-like' illness that may come and go.

SYMPTOMS

The cardinal feature of fibromyalgia is generalized allodynia and hyperalgesia with diminished pain thresholds most likely to be due to abnormal central pain processing at the level of the spinal cord and brain. It has been shown that patients mobilize diffuse noxious inhibitory control less effectively than normal subjects in response to experimental pain. Fibromyalgia is known as a syndrome because it is a collection of symptoms rather than a specific disease process that is well understood. Besides pain and fatigue, symptoms often include:

- unrefreshing sleep – waking up tired and stiff
- headaches – ranging from 'ordinary' types of headache to migraine
- irritable bowel
- cognitive dysfunction
- temporomandibular joint dysfunction
- anxiety and depression in 14–71 per cent of patients with fibromyalgia, but it does not cause or maintain the symptoms.

DIAGNOSIS

Fibromyalgia syndrome can be difficult to diagnose partly because it cannot be identified by standard laboratory tests or in radiographs. Many of its signs and symptoms are found in other conditions as well especially in chronic fatigue syndrome (CFS). The American College of Rheumatology has defined diagnostic criteria. Once other medical conditions have been ruled out through tests and the patient's history, diagnosis depends on two main symptoms:

- widespread pain for more than three months. The pain is present on both sides of the body and above and below the waist. In addition axial skeletal pain (cervical spine, anterior chest, thoracic spine or low back pain) must be present
- pain in at least 11 of 18 specified tender point sites when they are pressed (Fig. 13.1). Digital palpation of the tender points should be performed with an approximate force of 4 kg (using an algometer) and should be classed as painful on palpation (tender is not considered painful).

PATHOLOGY

The actual cause of fibromyalgia syndrome has not yet been found. It often develops after some sort of trauma that seems to act as a trigger, such as a fall or a car accident, a viral infection, childbirth or an operation. Sometimes the condition begins without any obvious trigger. The following may be found:

- a disturbance of deep delta sleep by the intrusion of alpha waves, leading to a decrease in the secretion of growth hormone and insulin-like growth factor (IGF)-1 during sleep
- elevated levels of substance P in the cerebrospinal fluid (CSF) leading to central sensitization and a decreased pain threshold
- a central metabolic disturbance causing a decline in the production of ATP and altered muscle physiology
- a disturbance of the hypothalamus–pituitary-adrenal axis causing an exaggerated response of adrenocorticotrophic hormone and decreased levels of 24-hour free cortisol
- decrease in serotonin, neuropeptide V and calcitonin and elevated levels of prolactin and angiotensin-converting enzyme
- genetic causes may be relevant.

It is impossible to determine whether the biochemical changes are a cause of or a result of the distressing symptoms of this syndrome.

MANAGEMENT

Current treatment modalities are successful in less than 50 per cent of patients. Although patients present with similar symptoms there may be many different mechanisms underlying these symptoms requiring different types of input.

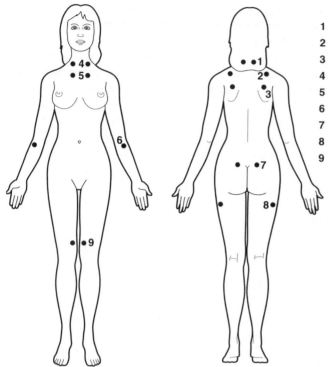

1 Insertion of nuchal muscles into occiput
2 Upper border of trapezius – mid-portion
3 Muscle attachments to upper medial border of scapula
4 Anterior aspects of the C5, C7 intertransverse spaces
5 Second rib space – about 3 cm lateral to the sternal bor
6 Muscle attachments to the lateral epicondyle
7 Upper outer quadrant of the gluteal muscle
8 Muscle attachments just posterior to the greater trochar
9 Medial fat pad of knee proximal to joint line

Figure 13.1 *Tender points in fibromyalgia*

Treatment for fibromyalgia aims at reducing pain and improving sleep. In other words, the symptoms are being treated, rather than the condition itself.

- Analgesia
    - NSAIDs are ineffective
    - Tramadol has a limited effect
    - 15–20 per cent patients prescribed opioids but their long-term effects are unknown.
- Hypnotics/sedatives have no effect.
- Tricyclics have a variable effect (about 36 per cent response rate).
- SSRIs are not helpful in the management of fibromyalgia.
- Trigger point injections – there is no good evidence to support their use.
- Muscle relaxants such as baclofen have been tried.
- Pain management programmes are the best hope providing a multidisciplinary approach but patients often do not engage.
- Exercise – most patients are physically deconditioned and functionally impaired. Aerobic exercises should be the low impact type. Aerobic exercise and strength training reduce hyperalgesia and improve functional ability but the therapeutic effects depend on level of exertion and compliance. The rate of compliance is low, often declining to 22 per cent.
- Self-management programmes including sessions of swimming-pool-based exercise, relaxation and advice on

daily living as well as education and discussion. Patients report feeling less fatigued, depressed or anxious with greater vitality. Patients do not experience an improvement in pain levels after these programmes. They are only designed to improve activity and coping skills.
- Chiropractic treatment has no benefit.
- Relaxation has only a minor effect if used alone.

Heat is important. Heating a hot water bottle and hot baths or showers will help reduce pain and banish morning stiffness. Exercise is the most common prescription for fibromyalgia. Two kinds of exercise are beneficial: stretching and aerobic. Effects are still modest due to patient passivity and lack of compliance.

Learning to manage the condition seems, so far, to be the most successful way of dealing with fibromyalgia. A combination of heat, rest, exercise and reduction of stress can enable a person with fibromyalgia syndrome to maintain a productive life.

MYOFASCIAL PAIN

Myofascial pain is defined as acute or chronic pain with sensory or motor autonomic symptoms, referred from active myofascial triggering points with associated dysfunction.

Myofascial pain is caused by trigger points that cause taut bands that constrict muscles and cause pain. Its aetiology and pathogenesis are not understood but there are several theories relating to the causes including:

- Peripheral sensitization hypothesis
- Ischaemic muscle spasm
- Neuromuscular dysfunction
- Motor end plate hyperactivity
- Central sensitization with referred hyperalgesia

There is probably involvement of some or all these mechanisms but muscle spasm plays a fundamental role. A myofascial trigger point is a localized area starved of oxygen. It creates an increased local energy demand. This local energy crisis releases neuro-reactive chemicals that sensitize nearby nerves. The sensitized nerves initiate the motor, sensory and autonomic effects of myofascial trigger points by acting on the CNS.

Incidence

It is a common condition occurring more frequently in women than men. Trigger points are usually found in the trapezius muscles and the upper back but can occur in any muscle.

Treatment

The aim of treatment is to desensitize areas that are sensitive and to restore function and mobility. Anti-inflammatory drugs are used frequently. Trigger point injections (injections into the tender spots) are commonly used to relax the remaining points of muscle contraction. A dry needle can be used or saline and local anaesthetic injected. The injections usually have permanent effects and can be effective after one treatment, or can be done multiple times if symptoms return.

Botulinum toxin can be used for resistant cases. It is a muscle relaxant which will last for about three months. Treatment can be repeated as necessary. The toxin may act directly on the muscle end plate, inhibiting muscle contraction, or another mechanism may be involved but it appears to be better than most other available treatments so far. Other treatments include:

- Ibuprofen topical gel
- Acupuncture
- TENS
- Osteopathy
- Physiotherapy

POST-HERPETIC NEURALGIA

Incidence

The incidence of post-herpetic neuralgia (PHN) is between 2.2 and 3.4 per 1000 persons/year. It occurs in 9–34 per cent of all patients with herpes zoster with a similar incidence in men and women. Pain of the acute episode usually resolves in three to four weeks but it may become chronic and continue for many years. The most important factors in long-term pain are age, severity of the acute pain and inflammation. The incidence increases with age:

- 66 per cent of patients are over 50 years.
- Less than 2 per cent are under 50 years.
- 20 per cent of patients with herpes zoster over 50 years will develop long-term pain.
- 35 per cent of patients with herpes zoster over 80 years will develop long-term pain.
- There is an increased incidence in immunosuppressed patients.

Site

- Thoracic – 55 per cent
- Cervical – 12–20 per cent
- Trigeminal – 17–25 per cent
- Lumbosacral – 11–17 per cent

Symptoms

- Burning
- Paraesthesia
- Hyperalgesia
- Lancinating pain
- Sensory loss

Pathophysiology

Chicken pox is due to infection with the varicella zoster virus. The virus settles in the dorsal horns of the sensory ganglia as the infection wanes. The virus lies dormant until there is a recrudescence, often during an episode of immunosuppression.

Acute pain of post-herpetic neuralgia

Reactivation of the virus produces inflammation in the peripheral nerve which causes pain in the distribution of that nerve. Inflammation of the nerve leads to oedema of the nerve and a corresponding increase in intrafascicular pressure, impairing endoneural blood flow. Inflammation also produces sympathetic stimulation and vasoconstriction, adding to the reduction in endoneural blood flow and tissue hypoxia. Activation of the sympathetic nervous system amplifies the activity of the primary afferent neurone and increases pain.

Chronic pain associated with post-herpetic neuralgia

The viral activity in the dorsal root ganglia and inflammation cause neural destruction. Loss of afferent neurones produces spontaneous activity in deafferentated central neurones generating constant pain in an area of marked sensory loss and minimal allodynia. Sprouting of spinal terminals of Aβ mechanoreceptors which contact receptors formerly occupied by C fibres produces hyperalgesia and allodynia. Regeneration of damaged axons produces sub- or intracutaneous neuromas and ectopic impulse activity of injured cell bodies.

The multiple clinical presentations of PHN may be due to the different extents to which the various pathophysiological mechanisms contribute to its development.

Treatment in the acute phase

Treatment is generally poor and all efforts should be aimed at preventing the development of PHN. An important factor in the development of chronic pain is good early pain control which may reduce the incidence of chronic pain. Famciclovir and valaciclovir reduce the duration of PHN and should be given as soon as the first symptoms are felt. Oral steroids reduce the severity of the acute herpes zoster pain but not PHN. Indications are that early epidural/intrapleural local anaesthetic/steroid may be helpful.

Treatment of post-herpetic neuralgia

ORAL/INTRAVENOUS DRUGS

- Analgesia
- Antidepressants
- Anticonvulsants
- NMDA (*N*-methyl-D-aspartate) receptor antagonists
- Methadone

TOPICAL/SUBCUTANEOUS TREATMENT

- Capsaicin cream
- Topical lidocaine
- Subcutaneous lidocaine
- Subcutaneous steroids

INTERVENTIONS

- Stellate ganglion blocks (sympathetic blocks).
- Epidural local anaesthetic within 24 days of rash (good).
- Epidural steroid at the level of the affected dorsal root ganglion is said to interrupt the mechanisms producing chronic pain. The steroids forestall the neural damage and therefore the deafferentation because of their anti-inflammatory properties. The local anaesthetic blocks ongoing spinal input from brain stimuli and therefore prevents sensitization. Local anaesthetic blocks the sympathetic nerves, blocking the neuropathic pain modulation.
- PENS (percutaneous electrical nerve stimulation).
- Intrapleural local anaesthetic.
- DREZ lesions (dorsal root entry zone) can provide good short-term relief but poor long-term (26 per cent) relief at 18 months.
- The results of spinal cord stimulation are poor for PHN.

The quality of most studies is poor and not controlled. More work is needed to improve the management of these patients and establish the best methods available.

DIABETIC NEUROPATHY

Pathophysiology

- The polyol pathway leads to sorbitol accumulation, myoinositol reduction, structural nerve damage, epineural vessel structural disease including arteriovenous shunting which then leads to endoneural hypoxia and proliferation of new leaky vessels.
- Vascular insufficiency.
- Loss of growth factor trophism.
- Autoimmune destruction of small unmyelinated nerves (C fibres).

Incidence

- 43–53 per cent of patients with diabetes have pain in feet or legs.
- An increased incidence is seen with:
  - increased age
  - hypertension
  - long duration of diabetes
  - poor control of blood sugar
  - dyslipidaemia

– smoking
– heavy alcohol intake
– human leucocyte antigen (HLA)-DR3/4 phenotype
– tall height.

Presentation

Symptoms begin in the hands and feet or legs in a 'glove and stocking' distribution. The pain is described as burning, tingling, muscle pain, cramps or a band-like or drawing sensation and it is accompanied by allodynia and hyperalgesia.

Treatment

Rapid changes in glycaemic control have been implicated as a trigger to the neuropathy but this is still unproved. A continuous infusion of subcutaneous insulin has led to amelioration of painful symptoms and improved motor conduction velocity so it is important to aim for excellent control of blood sugar levels in all these patients.

Drug treatment

- NSAIDs
- Capsaicin
- Analgesics
- Tricyclic antidepressants
- SSRIs are not as good as the tricyclic drugs. Paroxetine 20 mg daily is the drug of choice
- Anticonvulsants such as gabapentin. Doses above 1800 mg per day may be required but have produced good pain relief
- Local anaesthetics orally such as mexiletine may help
- Amantadine – 200 mg weekly as intravenous infusion has been shown to be 10 times better than placebo. Improvement is sustained for at least a week
- 10 mg twice daily oxycodone hydrochloride (OxyContin®) can be helpful

TOPICAL TREATMENT

- Capsaicin
- Lidocaine
- Opsite

Other treatments

- TENS – 52 per cent have reduced pain
- PENS – may be useful
- Acupuncture is safe and effective and up to 66 per cent of patients reduce their medication

- Spinal cord stimulation is good but is an invasive technique
- Physiotherapy
- Relaxation
- Warm baths
- Walking regularly
- Elastic stockings
- Counselling and psychological therapy have a limited effect

COMPLEX REGIONAL PAIN SYNDROME

Complex Regional Pain Syndrome (CRPS) has been defined by International Association of the Study of Pain as the 'presence of continuing pain, allodynia or hyperalgesia. The pain is disproportionate to any associated oedema, skin blood flow changes and/or sweating.' There are two types:

- **Type 1** – nerve not damaged (reflex sympathetic dystrophy)
- **Type 2** – nerve damaged (causalgia)

Incidence

The CRPS follows 1:2000 accidents, and it occurs in about 5 per cent of cases of trauma. It may result from blunt trauma, inflammation, laceration, surgery, soft tissue injury, injection, angina, vascular disease, myocardial infarction, stroke, cervical osteoarthritis, degenerative joint disease, frostbite and burns. It may occur spontaneously but the incidence has not been established.

Pathophysiology

The pathophysiology of CRPS is not well understood. There may be local demyelination due to damage to the Schwann cells by injury or inflammation. Peripheral nerve injury leads to maladaptive compensatory changes in the peripheral nervous system. Sensory motor and autonomic symptoms may be due to a disrupted body scheme in central representation (i.e. due to a mismatch between sensory and motor representation involving the pre-motor and motor cortical networks). It may involve cortical abnormalities similar to those observed in phantom limb pain and stroke. There is shrinkage of the cortical representation of the affected limb in the somatosensory cortex and disrupted body schema. Certain individuals may have a genetic susceptibility to developing CRPS.

Symptoms

Symptoms spread distally and proximally. Most patients will present with a selection of these symptoms and they may be transient, permanent, migratory, recurrent, bilateral or widespread:

- spontaneous pain, hyperalgesia, allodynia and increased pain with movement
- active and passive movement disorders
- abnormal regulation of blood flow causing altered skin temperature
- abnormal sweating
- oedema
- trophic changes.

Box 13.2 shows the changes in various stages of the syndrome.

Management

Many patients will improve spontaneously. Vitamin C 500 mg given to patients with a fractured wrist has been

---

> **BOX 13.2 Signs and symptoms in CRPS**
>
> **Acute phase changes – two to five months**
> - Aching and burning pain disproportionate to the trauma
> - Hyperpathia
> - Hyperaesthesia
> - Skin is warm, red and dry, with oedema, because of cutaneous vasodilatation
> - Hypertrichosis and overgrowth of nails
>
> **Three to six months**
> - Pain spreads proximally and distally
> - Hair growth slows
> - Nails become deformed
> - Joints thicken and range of movement reduces
> - Osteoporosis develops
>
> **Chronic changes – after six months**
> - Pain may lessen
> - Skin becomes cool, pale and cyanotic, smooth and glossy
> - Tapering digits
> - Contractures
> - Variable changes in sweating
> - Cutaneous vasoconstriction
> - Allodynia
> - Hyperalgesia
> - Intermittent swelling

---

shown to reduce the incidence of CRPS from 22 to 7 per cent. Early treatment usually has a better outcome. Analgesia (NSAIDs are often no help and opioids have a limited effect), antidepressants and anticonvulsants have all been tried but usually have a limited effect.

Intravenous regional sympathectomy should be performed using a Biers block technique. The aim of this procedure is to reduce noradrenaline in the postganglionic axon. The procedure is usually done three times and the outcome assessed. If the patient continues to improve further blocks should be given.

- Guanethidine produces noradrenaline release from the peripheral nerves and leads to vasodilatation. The dose is 10–20 mg. The action of guanethidine may be better without local anaesthetic as lidocaine blocks guanethidine uptake.
- Ketanserin is an S2 serotonergic antagonist and has been shown to be effective in some patients with CRPS. The dose is 10 mg for the arm and 20 mg for the leg.
- Bretylium tosylate inhibits the release of noradrenaline at the neurovascular junction leading to an increased blood flow by sympatholysis. Doses of up to 1.5 mg/kg have been shown to improve symptoms in some patients with CRPS but the drug has now been withdrawn in the UK.

Stellate ganglion blocks may be helpful. Bisphosphonates slow down resorption of bone by inhibition of osteoclasts but any pain relief may be due to an action on prostaglandin E_2. Calcitonin – parenteral or intranasal – has been tried, again with limited effect.

Other treatments

- Physiotherapy, particularly in the first few weeks, is important. Patients must be encouraged to move the limb.
- TENS – good.
- Peripheral nerve stimulation – up to 50 per cent of patients will improve.
- Spinal cord stimulation.
- Imagery.

Imagery

Some patients with CRPS 1 have an involuntary neurological neglect-like condition and may have to focus their visual and mental attention in order to move the limb leading to a learned disuse. Movement of the limb or even the thought of moving the limb induces severe pain but the limb must be moved in order to reverse the cortical changes. An imagery programme training the patient to recognize the limb has been shown to lead to a significant improvement of symptoms compared to passive immobilization.

Hand laterality recognition: The patient is given photographs of a left or right hand in varying positions in a random order and presses a button as soon as possible corresponding to the correct hand three times each waking hour (about 10 minutes). This activates the brain areas involved in higher order aspects of motor output (pre-motor cortex). It has been shown that patients generally take longer to do this than controls and there appears to be a relation between the duration of CRPS and response time.

Imagined hand movements: The patient is then given photographs of the hands and asked to imagine their hand in that position three times each waking hour (about 15 minutes). The emphasis is on accuracy.

Mirror therapy: A cardboard mirror box 300 mm × 300 mm is separated into two compartments by a vertical mirror, and 20 photographs are given to the patient. Each waking hour the patient is asked to slowly and smoothly adopt the posture shown in each picture with both hands 10 times. The emphasis is on watching the reflection of the unaffected hand in the mirror. The visual feedback of the affected hand is replaced with that of the (reflected) unaffected hand. It is thought to reconcile motor output and sensory feedback and activate pre-motor cortices, which have connections with the visual processing areas. Studies have shown improvement in the following:

- neuropathic pain score
- finger circumference
- response time.

The improvement was maintained for at least 6 weeks and 50 per cent of the patients no longer fulfilled the criteria for CRPS type 1. The NNT for a 50 per cent reduction in neuropathic pain score is about 2. There is a relation between the posture of each hand and the response time for the picture depending on the predicted intensity of pain that would occur if the patient adopted the posture shown. It may be a guarding-type mechanism that impacts on higher-order motor processes.

NERVE ENTRAPMENT SYNDROMES

Causes

Entrapment neuropathies are a group of disorders of the peripheral nerves that are characterized by pain and/or loss of function of the nerves as a result of chronic compression. Chronic injury often involves either a repetitive 'slapping' insult or a 'rubbing/sliding' phenomenon against tight edges with motion at the adjacent joint. Any somatic nerve can become entrapped leading to chronic pain. It may be secondary to trauma, infection, pregnancy, surgery or possible unknown factors.

Pathophysiology

Chronic injury to the nerve can result in ischaemic changes, oedema and structural alterations in membranes in both the myelin sheath and the axon. Focal segmental demyelination is sometimes seen. Whichever nerve is affected, there are similar clinical findings, investigations and treatments available for it.

Symptoms

Symptoms are usually felt at the site of the injury, and also radiate away from the site in the normal distribution of the nerve involved. Detailed anatomical knowledge is required to be able to determine which nerve is involved. The exact signs and symptoms depend on the particular nerve involved but may consist of any or all of the following:

- neuropathic pain (burning, shooting) associated with hypersensitivity, numbness, tingling and muscle weakness depending on whether the nerve involved is purely sensory, purely motor, or mixed sensory/motor
- there may be associated over-activity of the sympathetic nervous system in the area, e.g. excessive sweating, colour changes (blue through to red), and temperature changes (cold through to hot)
- allodynia may be present
- pressure with a finger over the site of the nerve injury will usually reproduce the nerve pain signs and symptoms. Also stretching a damaged nerve will have the same effect
- examination may reveal nerve-specific abnormal sensory and motor function.

Investigations

Where there is doubt about whether nerve function is normal or not, the investigation of choice is electromyography (EMG). It can also be used to assess the recovery of a nerve injury over time, whereas MRI/CT scans can also be useful to assess structural damage to other tissues in the vicinity of the nerve, e.g. bony tunnels, spinal nerve exit foramina.

Treatment

- Analgesia.
- Oral medications including antidepressants, anticonvulsants and antiarrhythmics.

- Topical agents like capsaicin used regularly four times a day may help. Lidocaine patches are also useful.
- Scar desensitization injections repeated three to five times with dilute local anaesthetic and steroid can reduce scar hypersensitivity.
- Intravenous lidocaine infusions are useful for some patients.
- Peripheral nerve blocks on several occasions may help when a peripheral nerve trunk is involved and is easily accessible. Sympathetic nerve blocks (local anaesthetic only) may be useful. Permanent phenol blocks are not advised.
- Surgery may be appropriate to decompress the nerve, and remove suture materials known to increase the risk of scar pain, e.g. nylon.
- Physiotherapy may be appropriate after an injury, but may be difficult due to the presence of pain and sensitivity. A multidisciplinary approach should be tried combining inputs from different specialties.

Common syndromes

CARPAL TUNNEL SYNDROME (CTS)

Carpal tunnel syndrome (CTS) is by far the commonest entrapment neuropathy. Median nerve compression at the wrist is by the transverse carpal ligament. There is a dull, aching pain at the wrist that extends up the forearm to the elbow. The pain typically is worse at night, disturbing sleep. Pain in CTS is often associated with numbness and/or pins and needles in the hand, affecting the thumb, forefinger, middle finger and the half of the ring finger nearest to the thumb. Sensation is decreased at the volar pads of the thumb and index finger.

In longstanding cases, the abductor pollicis brevis is weak and atrophic, causing thinning of the lateral contour of the thenar bulk. Forced wrist flexion causes increasing paraesthesia and pain (Phalen's sign), as does extreme wrist extension. Gentle tapping of the nerve over the flexor retinaculum sets off paraesthesia (Tinel's sign). Surgery is recommended and is associated with a 70–90 per cent rate of improvement in median nerve function.

MERALGIA PARAESTHETICA (LATERAL CUTANEOUS NERVE OF THIGH)

Anatomy

The lateral cutaneous nerve of the thigh arises from the ventral rami of the L1 and L2 nerve roots. The purely sensory nerve is formed just deep to the lateral border of the psoas muscle, then descends in the pelvis over the iliacus muscle deep to the iliacus fascia. The nerve exits the pelvis by passing through the deep and superficial bands of the inguinal ligament as they attach to the anterior superior iliac spine. The nerve is almost horizontal while still within the pelvis before it passes the inguinal ligament, but then takes a vertical course out to the surface of the thigh, deep to the fascia lata causing an almost 90° kink of the nerve. The angulation of the nerve also is exaggerated with extension of the thigh and relaxed with flexion.

Differential diagnosis

- An L3 root lesion is associated with muscle weakness (vastus lateralis, ilio-psoas and/or thigh adductors) or absent or unilaterally decreased knee jerk.
- Lumbar disc herniation at the L1/2 or L2/3 levels.
- Few other conditions can cause the same symptoms.

Symptoms

- Numbness, tingling, burning and painful hypersensitivity in the distribution of the lateral femoral cutaneous nerve, usually in the anterolateral thigh down to the upper patella region.
- Decreased appreciation of pinprick.
- Hyperpathic reaction to touch and persistent, spontaneous tingling after touch.
- Poor tolerance to touch and clothes, or anything that rubs against the thigh.
- Mothers (or fathers) may experience pain or burning with children sitting on their lap.
- It is usually unilateral.
- Symptoms are always present with no night/day preference.
- Symptoms are often accentuated with walking down slopes and stairs, prolonged standing in the erect posture and lying flat in bed.
- Placing a pillow behind the thighs and assuming a slightly hunched posture while standing may relieve symptoms.
- Onset is usually gradual over days or weeks but sometimes it is sudden.

Risk factors

- A protruding, pendulous abdomen, as seen in obesity and pregnancy, pushes the inguinal ligament forward and downward and drags the nerve with it over the kink. Therefore, it is common to encounter meralgia paraesthetica in individuals who are obese and in women during their last trimester of pregnancy.
- Diabetes.
- Family history of diabetes.
- Alcoholism.

- Occupational or nutritional causes of neuropathies.
- Human immunodeficiency virus (HIV) infection.
- Obesity.
- Tight undergarments or clothing in the inguinal area.

Examination

There is decreased sensation over upper and lateral area of thigh. Sometimes sensation is reduced all the way to the patella. It can be difficult to examine the patient because of pain or burning induced by touching or rubbing. Deep digital pressure medial to the anterior superior iliac spine may set off shooting paraesthesia down the lateral thigh. Strength is normal and there is no atrophy of the thigh muscles. Knee jerk is preserved.

EMG

The lateral cutaneous nerve of the thigh is a pure sensory branch. Response may be absent or significantly (<50 per cent) smaller than healthy side.

Treatment

- Conservative management
- Weight loss
- Avoid all constrictive garments
- Postural modification
- Analgesia
- Antidepressants
- Anticonvulsants

Serial injections of local anaesthesia and steroid (0.5 per cent bupivacaine and 40 mg depomedrone injected a finger's breadth medial to the anterior superior iliac spine) may afford long-term control in some patients. Overall, conservative measures are successful in more than 50 per cent of patients. Surgical decompression is very effective, but the recurrence rate is 15–20 per cent.

INTERCOSTAL NEURALGIA

In intercostal neuralgia pain occurs in one or several intercostal spaces, sometimes with a belt-like distribution. It is intensified with coughing or deep breathing. It feels like a sharp pricking or electric shock sensation. The pain may radiate to the lumbo-dorsal region of the affected side, with hyperaesthesia of the skin of the corresponding area and tenderness on pressure at the borders of the ribs. The left side is affected more than the right, and intercostal neuralgia is commoner in women than in men. It is more common with poor health. The painful points are chiefly at the beginning of the nerve as it arises from the spinal canal, and

towards the front of the body, where it breaks up into filaments which ramify in the skin.

Treatment

- Acupuncture
- Injection with local anaesthetic and steroid
- Radio-frequency lesioning/cryotherapy

Other nerve entrapment syndromes

See Table 13.3.

POSTSURGICAL NEURALGIA

Painful hypertrophic scars

Painful scars are common but underestimated and undertreated.

PATHOPHYSIOLOGY

All scars whether surgical or traumatic are capable of producing neuropathic pain in the skin. It is unknown whether the pain is caused by nerve transection, constriction, crushing or inflammation, and it is not completely understood but it seems that in some people superficial skin nerves may become entrapped in scar tissue during the healing process. These scars are more common after a wound infection, or when there is delayed healing. Continuing pain during the healing phase may cause sensitization of the dorsal horn in the spinal cord.

An increase in substance P and CGRP is seen at the base of the epidermis. Increased numbers of cells produce NGF and inflammation leading to hyper-innervation and hyperalgesia. Allodynia and hyperalgesia adjacent to the scar are likely to be the result of central changes driven by afferents within the scar tissue.

Symptoms

- The pain is burning, tingling, shooting or aching in nature and is continuous or paroxysmal.
- Persistent pain in a healed scar of >3 months' duration with allodynia and hyperalgesia to the scar with no sensory loss other than over the scar itself.
- The scar may be hyperaesthetic, itchy and erythematous.

Risk factors

- Young age
- High body mass index (BMI)

- Female sex
- Pain score high one day after surgery

incidence of post-thoracotomy pain from 22–67 per cent to 12 per cent.

Management

There are few studies on the management of postoperative neuralgia so treatment is similar to the treatment of other neuropathic conditions. Prevention should play a major role as treatment can be very difficult. Optimum perioperative pain relief may reduce the problem. Using epidural anal-gesia for thoracotomies has reduced the

DRUG TREATMENT

- Antidepressants
- Anticonvulsants
- Opioids
- NMDA receptor antagonists
- Lidocaine
- Adenosine
- Capsaicin

Table 13.3 *Nerve entrapment syndromes*

Syndrome	Symptoms and management
Occipital neuralgia	Sensory branches of C2 and C3
	Pain in the occipital region to the top of the head
	Complete pain relief with local anaesthetic blockade of the occipital nerve
	Injections of steroids or cryoneurolysis may provide prolonged analgesia
Ilioinguinal nerve	Treat with local anaesthetic blockade
Neuralgia of the genital branch of the genitofemoral nerve	Pain starting in the low back or abdomen radiating into the groin
	Frequently increased with movement of the lower abdominal and upper quadriceps muscle groups
Neuralgia of the infrapatellar branch of the saphenous nerve	May occur weeks to years after blunt injury to the tibial plateau or following total knee replacement
	Dull pain below the knee joint and aching below the knee
	Pain with pressure between the lateral malleolus and extensor retinaculum
Superficial and deep peroneal neuralgia	May occur in diabetic patients who are vulnerable to compression injury
	It is less commonly associated with a blunt injury to the dorsum of the foot
	A dull pain in the great toe made worse with prolonged standing
	Pain with pressure between the first and second metatarsal heads
Superior gluteal neuralgia	Shearing of the nerve between the gluteal musculature with forced external rotation of the leg and extension of the hip under mechanical load
	Rarely, this occurs with forced extension of the hip from head-on automobile collision as the knee extends in anticipation of impact
	Sharp pain in the low back, dull pain in the buttock, and a vague pain in the popliteal fossa
	Aggravated with prolonged sitting, leaning forward, or twisting to contralateral side
	The leg may give way
Supraorbital neuralgia	Deceleration injury, e.g. head striking an automobile windshield
	Presents as a throbbing frontal headache with blurred vision, nausea and photophobia
	Typically worsens with time
Infraorbital neuralgia	Trauma to the zygoma
	Exacerbated by smiling
	Referred to the teeth
	Differential diagnosis – maxillary sinusitis
Auriculotemporal neuralgia	Temporal and retro-orbital pain and referred pain to the teeth
	Patients awaken at night with temporal headache
	Throbbing, aching or pounding
	Differential diagnosis – temporal arteritis
Posterior auricular neuralgia	Pain in the ear with a feeling of fullness and tenderness

Specific

- Agents such as local anaesthetics and steroids usually produce dramatic and rapid relief of the adjacent hyperalgesia when injected carefully within the scar and may produce longlasting relief.
- Nerve blocks with phenol.

- Thermal interventions such as radio-frequency lesions or cryotherapy.
- Peripheral and spinal cord stimulation.

Other postoperative neuropathies

See Table 13.4.

Table 13.4 *Postoperative neuropathies*

Neuropathy	Symptoms	Treatment
After neck/laryngeal surgery/DXRT Superficial cervical plexus injury	Pain in front of throat and over the clavicle, behind the ear and towards the back of the neck Tight, burning sensation in the area of the lower cranial nerves and electric shock-like pain Musculoskeletal pain may occur due to drooped shoulder syndrome	Cervical nerve blocks on several occasions may help
Post-mastectomy pain	Tight, constricting, burning pain in the posterior arm, axilla, and anterior chest wall Pain exacerbated by arm movement, possibly due to musculoskeletal dysfunction or oedema	

Brachial plexus
  Metastatic breast cancer
  Traction injuries to the upper limb
  Incorrect arm positioning during surgery – arm abducted >90°
	Pain radiates to all or part of the upper limb in the C5, C6, C7, C8, T1 dermatomes depending on the part of the plexus affected
	Weakness and numbness in the arm and hand may also be present
		Brachial plexus nerve blocks on several occasions may be useful

Intercostobrachial neuralgia Surgery where lymph glands have been removed from the axilla	Symptoms radiate down the inside of the arm to the elbow (T1), and also around the upper chest (T2)	Radiographic-guided first and second rib intercostal nerve blocks can be helpful
Dorsal radial branch neuralgia Sensory nerve that supplies sensation to back of the hand, fingers and thumb. It can be injured after a Colles' fracture	Symptoms radiate from the lower forearm into the back of the hand and fingers. This may mimic complex regional pain syndrome	Dorsal radial branch nerve blocks may help
Ulnar neuritis The nerve can be injured by direct blows to the elbow or direct pressure during surgery	Pain in the forearm and tingling in the fourth and fifth fingers	Ulnar nerve blocks may be useful. Great care is required not to injure the nerve with the needle
Digital neuralgia Can follow an injury to the fingers	Each finger has four digital nerves. Two larger nerves supply the palmar surface, and two smaller ones supply the back of the finger	Digital nerve blocks may be useful
After thoracotomy Intercostal nerves can be affected either by removal of a rib, or by direct injury caused by surgical instruments. Neuroma formation may occur at the point that the nerve is severed.	Pain recurs or persists along the thoracotomy scar Often delayed Aching/burning Extends beyond the scar Aggravated by temperature change, touch, pressure and emotion The incidence of pain is 70–80% at three months and 41–61% at one year	Intercostal nerve blocks repeated on several occasions can be useful Also targeting the neuroma at the end of the cut rib and nerve can also be helpful Paravertebral **trigger point injections** may also be useful

(continued)

Table 13.4 *(continued)*

	Symptoms	Treatment
After nephrectomy The 11th or 12th intercostal nerves can be affected either by removal of the 11th or 12th ribs, or by direct injury by surgical instruments Neuroma formation may occur at the point that the nerve is severed	11th or 12th intercostal neuralgia with referred pain coming around the chest to the lower abdomen Numbness fullness or heaviness in the anterior abdomen and groin	Intercostal nerve blocks repeated on several occasions can be useful Targeting the neuroma can also be helpful Paravertebral **trigger point injections** may help
After hernia repair Herniorraphy can result in injury to the iliohypogastric, ilioinguinal and genitofemoral nerves The iliohypogastric nerve can also be injured by lower abdominal incisions, e.g. after hysterectomy	Pain in the groin and inner thigh in the T12 and L1 dermatomes 19–54% at 1–3 years postoperatively 5% severe	Iliohypogastric and genitofemoral nerve blocks on several occasions can be useful Infiltrating around the pubic tubercle is also useful when pubic osteitis is suspected
Femoral neuralgia Direct injuries After surgery in the groin region Femoral angiography Vascular graft surgery for poor circulation in the legs Varicose vein surgery	Pain often radiates from the groin into the front of the thigh and inner shin as far as the ankle. Weakness of the quadriceps muscles may cause the knee to give way	Femoral nerve blocks on several occasions may help
Arthroscopy This injures the medial and lateral patellar nerves in front of the knee just below the patella	Pain and sensitivity is felt around the arthroscopy incisions and several inches below the knee on either side of the upper shin There may also be over-activity of the **sympathetic nervous system** in the area	Full thickness scar infiltrations on several occasions can be very useful
Varicose vein surgery Saphenous nerve at the upper tibial level over the medial side knee Sural nerve at the outside ankle joint. Common peroneal nerve deep in the space behind the knee joint (rarely)	Symptoms radiate from the knee down the inner shin to the level of the ankle Symptoms radiate from the ankle to the foot	Appropriate nerve blocks may help
Ankle and foot injuries	May cause pain in the foot depending on injured nerve	
Removal of third molar teeth May be delayed onset	0–23% incidence of pain from the lingual and inferior alveolar nerves	
Sternotomy	Incidence 28–30%. 4–13% severe. Stable over time	

BREAST PAIN

Breast pain occurs following:

- Mastectomy – at three years the incidence of pain is 27 per cent but this does fall with time
- Lumpectomy
- Augmentation and reduction surgery

Pain may occur in the chest or arm or it may be a phantom pain. In a study of 39 patients with unilateral mastectomy, 20 reported phantom sensations. Nine had pain and 11 had non-painful sensations. The sensation was of persistence of the entire breast or parts of it. Onset may occur up to a year after amputation and affects the entire breast more often than the nipple. The prevalence of painful phantom breast is 23 per cent and of non-painful phantom breast is

28 per cent. The incidence of breast pain can be reduced by giving 1200 mg gabapentin preoperatively.

AMPUTATION

Phantom pain

Phantom sensations occur in children born without a limb, suggesting our perception of our limbs is 'hard-wired' into our brains (the neuromatrix). Phantom pain is pain referred to a surgically removed limb or portion of that limb. Although it can also occur after the loss of a tooth, nose, eye, tongue, breast, bladder, penis and scrotum, 78–85 per cent of patients have phantom pain after amputation. The pain varies from constant pain to intermitting stabbing pain.

Stump pain

Stump pain is pain at the site of an extremity amputation. It is important to differentiate between stump pain and phantom pain as they may respond differently to treatment. Patients may have both types of pain or just stump or phantom pain.

Predictive factors

- Preoperative pain
- Repeat surgery
- Surgical approach
- Acute and severe postoperative pain
- Radiation
- Chemotherapy
- Psychological and depressive symptoms

Pathophysiology

- Damaged nerve endings.
- Erroneous regrowth of nerve endings.
- Abnormal central connections.
- Abnormal brain activity secondary to loss of sensory input from the limb.
- A disordered input from the limb sensory systems, combined with a disrupted motor signal back to the limb generates a mismatch between the brain's built-in map of the body and what is perceived, and it may be this that is responsible for pain.

Treatment for phantom pain

Phantom pain often does not respond well to treatment especially when it has been present for some time. Attempts to prevent its occurrence are therefore important. Management should begin at the time of amputation if possible. The role of preoperative epidural analgesia is unclear as studies have produced opposite outcomes but preoperative pain management should be optimal where possible. Good analgesia should be provided at all times. If a patient complains of phantom feelings immediately after amputation all efforts should be made to control it at this stage as early treatment may have a more successful outcome. The possibility of phantom pain should be discussed with the patient prior to surgery.

Treatment should include analgesia, antidepressants, anticonvulsants and antiarrhythmics as for other neuropathic pains. Other treatments include NMDA antagonists and TENS. Fitting the patient with a prosthetic limb as soon as possible will also help reduce the incidence of phantom pain. Spinal cord stimulation does not work well for phantom pain, and DREZ lesions do not work well for phantom pain.

NEW TREATMENTS

- An electrical prosthetic limb moved by signals from the patient's muscles reduces pain if used for several hours per day. It is dependent on reversion of the sensory cortex to the original state.
- Repeated touching of the skin over the stump improves sensory discrimination.
- Motor cortex stimulation and deep brain stimulation.
- Mirror box – the patient places the normal limb in a box divided into two compartments by a mirror. The brain is fooled into thinking the amputated limb is still present and the ability to move this 'phantom' can reduce some of the painful sensations.
- Virtual reality movement.

The above are all attempts to link the visual and motor systems and recreate a coherent body image and a shift in emphasis away from the site of the damage to the brain.

Treatment of stump pain

Treatment of stump pain is similar to the management of phantom pain but local anaesthetic and steroid infiltration to the tender points may reduce pain as may cryotherapy or pulsed radio-frequency lesioning.

JOINT PAIN

Osteoarthritis

Osteoarthritis is the commonest cause of arthritis in the UK.

SYMPTOMS AND SIGNS

- Pain is worse with weight bearing and activity.
- Pain improves with rest.
- Morning stiffness.
- Gelling of involved joint after periods of inactivity.
- Tenderness of joint.
- Bony enlargement.
- Crepitus on motion.
- Limitation of joint motion.
- Inflammation if present is mild and limited.

CAUSE OF PAIN IN DEGENERATIVE BONE AND JOINT DISEASE

Very little is known about the mechanism of pain and the nerve endings in the articular surfaces and bone. The efferent innervation of the cortex and medulla of bones may be primarily nociceptive in function and may play an important role in chronic pain of degenerative bone and joint disease. Articular cartilage is not innervated, but when it wears away, nociceptors in bone are activated by biomechanical forces associated with weight bearing. Inflammatory mediators in synovial fluid or bone interior may exacerbate pain by sensitizing nerve endings in subchondral bone.

Genetic factors are probably also involved. There is no evidence that an active lifestyle such as running increases the likelihood of osteoarthritis occurring.

Quadriceps weakness is common among patients with osteoarthritis of the knee. It may develop because of unloading of the painful extremity, but it can also be seen in patients with radiographic changes of osteoarthritis but with no history of knee pain. Quadriceps weakness may be a risk factor for the development of osteoarthritis by decreasing the stability of the knee and reducing the shock-attenuating capacity of the muscle.

GOALS OF TREATMENT

- Control pain.
- Improve function.
- Improve health-related quality of life.
- Avoid toxic effects of therapy.

There is no known cure for osteoarthritis. See Box 13.3 for issues related to management of osteoarthritis.

BOX 13.3 Recommendations from the Expert Standing Committee for International Clinical Studies including Therapeutic Trials (ESCIST)

Management of osteoarthritis of the knee depends on:
- knee risk factors – obesity and physical activity
- general risk factors – age, polypharmacy
- pain and disability
- inflammation and effusion
- location and degree of structural damage

Assessment
- Symptom assessment
- Functional assessment
- Physical examination

Non-pharmacological treatment
- Patient and family education
- Self-management programme
- Physiotherapy – range of motion exercises, muscle-strengthening exercises
- Appliances – in-soles, sticks, knee brace, weight reduction
- The use of a cane in the hand contralateral to the affected knee reduces loading forces on the joint and can improve function
- Appropriate footwear including lateral wedged in-soles for genu varum
- Occupational therapy

Pharmacological management
- Paracetamol should be taken regularly
- NSAIDs can be useful for an episode of inflammation causing increased pain but they are not useful for long-term pain relief. Because most of the patients are elderly, routine use of regular NSAIDS should be avoided
- NSAID gels and capsaicin – there are no published studies comparing topical and oral NSAIDs
- Gastrointestinal prophylaxis should be given when NSAIDs are prescribed
- Tramadol
- Opioids
- Glucosamine sulphate and chondroitin sulphate may be helpful in the early stages of the disease
- Injection of steroid into a painful joint. The duration of action may exceed the synovial half life of the drug so the mechanism of action is unclear
- Joint replacement

Rheumatoid arthritis

Rheumatoid arthritis is an autoimmune disorder of unknown aetiology characterized by symmetrical erosive synovitis and sometimes multisystem involvement. Most patients exhibit a chronic fluctuating course of disease that if left untreated results in progressive joint destruction, deformity, disability and premature death. Rheumatoid arthritis affects about 1 per cent of the adult population. There is no known cure or means of preventing it. Optimal management requires timely introduction of agents that reduce the probability of irreversible joint damage. Patients with active polyarticular, rheumatoid factor positive-rheumatoid arthritis have a >70 per cent probability of developing joint damage or erosions within 2 years of the onset of the disease.

Rheumatoid arthritis is a chronic pain syndrome but it is obviously normally managed by rheumatologists. However it is important that pain clinicians have some understanding of the management of rheumatoid arthritis because these patients may present to the pain clinic when their pain is uncontrolled by conventional treatment. The aim of treatment is to induce complete remission but this is a rare occurrence.

GOALS OF MANAGEMENT (FIG. 13.2)

- Control disease activity.
- Alleviate pain.
- Maintain function for essential activities of daily living and work.
- Maximize quality of life.
- Slow the rate of joint damage.

DRUG THERAPY FOR RHEUMATOID ARTHRITIS

Paracetamol

Paracetamol is given for analgesia.

NSAIDs and cyclo-oxygenase-2

These reduce pain and swelling and improve function. They do not alter the course of the disease and there are no significant differences between the drugs. Only 80 per cent of patients will respond to a specific anti-inflammatory drug so it is worth trying two or three different drugs. The choice depends on duration of action and patient preference. Effects are immediate but it may take one or two weeks for signs of inflammation to reduce.

Disease modifying antirheumatic drugs (DMARDs)

All patients whose disease remains active despite adequate treatment with NSAIDs are candidates for treatment with

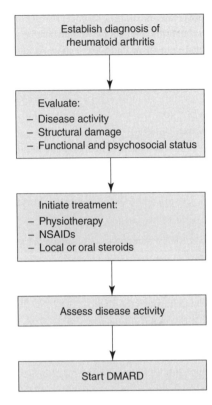

Figure 13.2 *Algorithm for management of rheumatoid arthritis. NSAID, non-steroidal anti-inflammatory drug; DMARD, disease modifying antirheumatic drug*

DMARDs (Box 13.4). These drugs have the potential to reduce or prevent joint damage.

DMARDs have common characteristics. All are relatively slow acting, with a delay of one to six months before a clinical response is evident. Efficacy cannot be predicted for the individual patient, but up to two-thirds of patients may have a response to these agents. Each DMARD has specific toxicity that requires careful monitoring. The decision to start a DMARD must be preceded by a discussion with the patient about the expectations of risks versus benefits of the treatment. It is not known which is the best initial DMARD for patients with rheumatoid arthritis but within one to six months, the response to these agents should be apparent and the need for a change in therapy may be determined.

Glucocorticoids

Oral

Low-dose oral glucocorticoids (≤10 mg prednisone daily or equivalent) and injections of glucocorticoids into the joints are highly effective for relieving symptoms in patients with active rheumatoid arthritis. Low-dose glucocorticoids appear to slow the rate of joint damage. For uncomplicated rheumatoid arthritis, prednisone should not be given at a dosage higher than 10 mg daily. Every effort should be made to limit its use to a short course or, if maintenance treatment is necessary, to use the lowest possible dosage.

Joint injection

Glucocorticoid injection of joints and periarticular structures is safe and effective. Injecting one or a few of the most involved joints in a patient early in the course of rheumatoid arthritis may provide local and even systemic benefit. The effects are sometimes dramatic, but are usually temporary. They may also allow the patient to participate more fully in rehabilitation programmes to restore lost joint function.

In general, the same joint should not be injected more than once within three months. The need for repeated joint injections in the same joint or for multiple joint injections indicates the need to reassess the adequacy of the overall treatment programme.

BOX 13.4 Use of DMARDs for rheumatoid arthritis

Goal

- Remission or optimal control of inflammatory joint disease

Limitations

- May not prevent damage in spite of apparent clinical control
- May not have lasting efficacy
- May not be tolerated due to toxicity

Drugs (see Table 13.5)

- Hydroxychloroquine
- Sulfasalazine
- Methotrexate
- Gold salts
- D-penicillamine
- Azathioprine

Infliximab in rheumatoid arthritis

Infliximab and etanercept are partially humanized monoclonal antibodies aiming to reduce the actions of circulating tumour necrosis factor (TNF). Both exert their effects by removing TNF from the circulation, and consequently interrupt the inflammatory process. Treatment with infliximab for up to 12 months significantly reduces rheumatoid arthritis activity and is safe. Radiographic scores improve and fewer patients show radiographic progression.

PERIPHERAL VASCULAR DISEASE

The pain of peripheral vascular disease is multifactorial and includes claudication pain, ischaemic pain, pain from ulcers and there are also peripheral neuropathic elements. The pain is described as numb, burning, tingling or lancinating.

Table 13.5 *Disease modifying antirheumatic drugs used in the treatment of rheumatoid arthritis*

Drug	Approximate time to benefit	Usual maintenance dose	Toxicity
Hydroxychloroquine	2–4 months	200 mg twice daily	Infrequent rash, diarrhoea, rare retinal toxicity
Sulfasalazine	1–2 months	1000 mg twice or three times daily	Rash, infrequent myelosuppression, gastrointestinal intolerance, gastrointestinal symptoms, stomatitis, rash, alopecia
Methotrexate	1–2 months	7.5–15 mg/week	Myelosuppression, hepatotoxicity, rare but serious (even life-threatening) pulmonary toxicity
Injectable gold salts	3–6 months	25–50 mg IM every 2–4 weeks	Rash, stomatitis, myelosuppression, thrombocytopenia, proteinuria
Oral gold	4–6 months	3 mg daily or twice daily	Same as injectable gold but less frequent, plus frequent diarrhoea
Azathioprine	2–3 months	50–150 mg daily	Myelosuppression, infrequent hepatotoxicity, early 'flu-like' illness with fever, gastrointestinal symptoms, elevated LFTs
D-penicillamine	3–6 months	250–750 mg daily	Rash, stomatitis, proteinuria, myelosuppression, infrequent but serious autoimmune disease

IM, intramuscular; LFT, liver function test

Treatment

Management of pain secondary to peripheral vascular disease can be very difficult and very little research has been done in this area. Analgesia should always be prescribed but is often not effective. Paracetamol and opioids should be given along with tricyclic drugs and anticonvulsants. As the patients tend to be elderly, side effects of drug therapy often limits their usefulness. Other treatments that should be considered include:

- Lumbar sympathetic block – blocking the sympathetic nerves will produce maximal vasodilatation and improve blood flow to a painful limb. Unfortunately patients with peripheral vascular disease already have maximal vasodilatation or the vessels are calcified and unable to dilate any further. As pain fibres travel with the sympathetic nerves the block may produce pain relief in the absence of vasodilatation but it may not have any effect on blood flow to an ischaemic region.
- Spinal cord stimulation can produce both pain relief and restore oxygen delivery and blood flow to an ischaemic limb. Healing of ulcers is often seen and it has been shown to reduce the need for amputation (see Chapter 11).

HUMAN IMMUNODEFICIENCY VIRUS INFECTION AND PAIN

Many different types of pain are seen with HIV disease and pain can also occur as the result of therapy. Each different pain may respond to different treatments.

Muscle stiffness

This occurs particularly in the legs due to a vacuolar myelopathy of the spinal cord. It is associated with weakness in the legs as well. It affects about 5 per cent of patients with HIV.

TREATMENT

- Baclofen
- Dantrolene
- Exercise

Peripheral neuropathy

The cause of the peripheral neuropathy in HIV is unknown. Symptoms comprise numbness and tingling as with other neuropathies. Pain occurs in the feet and less commonly in the hands. The symptoms are usually mild but they can be disturbing. Some inflammation can be seen in nerves along with a loss of nerve fibres. Some drugs used to control HIV can produce the same symptoms (DDC, DDI). Didanosine (DDI) and zalcitabine (DDC) are anti-HIV drugs that reduce the amount of virus in the body. Peripheral neuropathy a common side effect of DDI, which can causes numbness, tingling or pain. It occurs more frequently when taken by people with advanced HIV infection. It usually goes away if the drug is stopped, and treatment may be resumed at a lower dose without recurrence of the neuropathy.

TREATMENT

- Analgesia
- Antidepressants
- Anticonvulsants

Polymyositis

In polymyositis, symptoms occur mainly around the shoulders and hips producing muscle pain and aching. Zidovudine may also produce muscle pain and it often improves if the drug is stopped. Steroids may help relieve the symptoms.

INVESTIGATIONS

- EMG
- Nerve conduction studies
- Nerve/muscle biopsy

NON-CARDIAC CHEST PAIN

About 50 per cent of patients with chest pain have no obvious cardiac abnormality and about 50 per cent of these are unable to work. It is commoner in younger age groups and in the female sex. Thirty per cent have associated panic disorder (normal = 1–2 per cent of the population) and they have a high incidence of autonomic symptoms. Stimulation of periaqueductal grey matter causes autonomic symptoms and ST depression in animals with renal vasoconstriction and decreased vascular resistance in skeletal muscle but no change in coronary resistance. This may be a sympathetically mediated effect as it is blocked by metoprolol.

Hypothesis of mechanism

A dysfunctional responsiveness of the coronary vasculature causing localized ischaemia or a primary malfunction in the neuronal circuitry that regulates the excitability of the periaqueductal grey matter.

TENNIS ELBOW

There is pain and tenderness over the lateral epicondyle of the humerus and pain on resisted dorsiflexion of the wrist, middle finger or both, and gripping. It is a syndrome of overuse and is commonest in those in their forties.

Treatment

- Avoid provoking activities.
- Topical NSAIDS and oral NSAIDs have minimal effect but are the only treatments shown to have any effect at all.
- Corticosteroid injections – there is limited evidence that these are useful but they are very painful.

The effectiveness of the following is unknown:

- Acupuncture
- Exercise and mobilization
- Extracorporeal shock wave treatment
- Brace
- Surgery – release of extensor tendon at origin

CASE SCENARIO

A 75-year-old woman presents with pain over the first division of the trigeminal nerve. Six months previously she had a vesicular rash in the same area that was diagnosed as shingles but she did not receive antiviral treatment. Now the pain is constant. It is burning in nature and very severe particularly in windy weather. She also has shooting pain behind the eye and she is unable to sleep well because of the pain. On examination there is some scarring in the area and there is marked allodynia over the forehead.

MANAGEMENT

Simple analgesia

- Paracetamol
- NSAID of choice
- Codeine or tramadol with the paracetamol

Antidepressants

- Start with 10 mg of amitriptyline about an hour before bedtime
- If this leads to significant side effects the tablet can be scored and broken in half. If the patient is drowsy in the morning they should take the tablet earlier in the evening. They should be advised that the side effects should diminish with time
- If there is no effect the dose can be increased at intervals of three days to one week to a maximum of 50 mg
- If side effects prevent use amitriptyline can be changed to nortriptyline (same dose) or dosulepin 25–50 mg nocte
- If problems still occur consider imipramine

Anticonvulsants

- Sodium valproate 200 mg twice daily to three times daily
- Gabapentin start at 100 mg three times daily and increase weekly to a maximum of 800 mg three times daily. The anticonvulsant should be added to the antidepressant
- Other anticonvulsants that can be considered if there is no response to these are topiramate, lamotrigine and pregabalin

Topical treatment can include:

- Capsaicin 0.075 per cent applied four times a day but the patient must be very careful applying the cream around the eye because it will burn
- Lidocaine ointment 5 per cent applied to the painful area three times a day
- EMLA cream may help but it must be completely occluded for it to work. It should only be worn for an hour at a time or the skin may break down. Lidoderm patches have proved to be successful in many patients. The patch is worn for six hours a day for up to one week and if there are no skin reactions it can be worn for 12 hours at a time

Other treatments to consider

- Subcutaneous infiltration of 1 per cent lidocaine above the eyebrow
- Intravenous lidocaine
- Intravenous ketamine and possibly oral ketamine
- Intravenous amantidine
- Oral mexiletine
- Opioids
- Oxycodone and methadone often prove more effective than other opioids in treating the pain of post-herpetic neuralgia
- TENS can be used but most patients do not like wearing it on their forehead and it is rarely effective in post-herpetic neuralgia

14 Chronic Pain: Back and Neck Pain

INTRODUCTION

Pain in or connected with the spine is usually the most frequent problem presenting in a pain clinic. It is also one of the most frequent complaints in orthopaedic clinics, neurosurgical clinics, rheumatology clinics and general practice surgeries. The size of the problem is enormous and has a major impact on our social and economic structure (see Chapter 6). When pain has persisted for more than three months, or episodes of debilitating pain recur frequently, it is usually described as 'chronic', although the definition cannot be as precise as this. Chronic back and neck pain, and their associated syndromes of referred pain and nerve root pain, are difficult to treat effectively, not only because in most instances it is not possibly to be absolutely certain as to the physiological or pathological cause of the pain, but also because of the wide-reaching effect that these conditions tend to have on the whole person, in their behaviour, their employment and social activities, their relationships with family and friends, and the complex emotions related to somatic awareness and ill-health.

Many patients presenting with chronic spinal pain will have a long history of previous medical intervention. Those presenting to a chronic pain service are those in whom previous interventions such as spinal surgery or simple physical therapies have presumably been insufficient to provide adequate control of their symptoms. A good history is essential in the assessment of chronic back and neck pain.

- When did the pain start?
- Was it related to trauma or previous surgery?
- Is pain continuous or intermittent and is it related to specific postures, activities or movements?
- Is pain localized, and if so, where and what is its pattern of radiation or referral?
- Is pain present at rest, and does it interfere with sleep? Is there any diurnal pattern to the pain?
- Does pain follow any nerve root distribution and does it have any qualities suggesting a neurogenic component of pain, such as numbness, allodynia, paraesthesia or other abnormal sensations?
- What treatments, including medication, have been previously tried and with what effect?
- What effects do the symptoms have on the patient's life and activities, and what are their expectations?

The information gathered in the history taking is often the most useful in helping to form an idea about the pain, its possible causes, and the most effective means of managing the pain.

Physical examination elicits the effect that the pain has on the patient's movement and behaviour, as well as checking for physical signs. Observe how the patient moves to the examination area and how they respond to the examination. A simple physical examination may check mobility of the spine, areas of tenderness or abnormal sensory function, weakness, altered reflexes and sensory function.

MANAGEMENT OF CHRONIC SPINAL PAIN

Although the cause of most back and neck pain may not be proved, it is important to form some idea of the nature of the pain symptoms to plan appropriate management. Many patients attending a pain clinic will already have been investigated, with radiographs, scans and possibly blood tests to exclude major pathology. Following a careful history taking and examination it may be possible to form an idea of the areas that may be amenable to treatment for relief of pain and improved function.

Problems to consider in the management of back/neck pain

- Nerve root pain
- Neurogenic pain
- Disc-related pain
- Facet joint pain
- Mechanical/structural problems
- Soft-tissue pain
- Behavioural aspects of back pain

NERVE ROOT PAIN

Pain from compression of spinal nerve roots may be suggested from the symptoms and often the signs on examination. Pain is expected to be segmental, following a recognized dermatomal distribution that corresponds with the associated level of nerve root involvement. Examination may demonstrate muscle weakness, numbness or altered sensory function, loss of reflexes, and an indication by the patient of pain in this area. Any, all or none of these signs may be apparent.

Imaging investigations (ideally magnetic resonance imaging (MRI)) may reveal evidence of prolapsed intervertebral disc, or at least some protrusion of disc material which is impinging on the nerve root. There may be evidence of bony compression of nerve roots with foraminal stenosis caused by local degenerative changes and joint hypertrophy, or scar tissue arising from previous surgery/trauma which is compressing nerve tissue. Often clear symptoms and signs of nerve root dysfunction are present but no physical interference with the nerve root is demonstrated on imaging. This problem may be explained by a number of possibilities: it may be that there is an intermittent mechanical interference with the nerve root during activity, extruded disc material results in chemical irritation and can produce an inflammatory response in the nerve root, or previous mechanical/chemical irritation of the nerve root has resulted in long-term damage to nerve tissue either within the nerve root itself or in the spinal cord, resulting in a chronic radiculopathy.

When compression of nerve roots causes major impairment of function, intractable pain or other neuropathic responses, and it can be clearly related to demonstrable structural changes such as disc prolapse, bony structural defects or foraminal stenosis, surgical intervention may be appropriate, and advice should be sought from a neurosurgeon or spinal orthopaedic surgeon. If surgery is not appropriate because the likely benefits are outweighed by the potential risks, or there is no clearly demonstrated relation between symptoms and structural changes, symptomatic treatment aimed at improving pain relief and function is indicated (Box 14.1).

BOX 14.1 Treatment for nerve root pain

- Steroid injection around nerve root
- Medication to reduce neuropathic pain
- Stimulatory techniques
- General rehabilitation

Epidural steroids

Epidural injection of steroids has long been a common procedure for treating sciatica: pain from compression of lumbar nerve roots by prolapsed disc material. It has also been used in the cervical and thoracic regions of the spine. The procedure continues to be controversial; the benefits are not universally accepted or proved, and there have been some concerns over the safety of the procedure. The evidence for long-term benefits of epidural steroid injections is thin, but there is some acceptance of the fact that particularly in acute situations where there is firm evidence of disc prolapse, then epidural steroid injections may produce a more rapid resolution of pain than a completely conservative form of management, and therefore allow earlier mobilization and restoration of function. This may have indirect benefits for long-term prognosis. Details of the procedure are discussed more fully in Chapter 8.

Nerve root block

When symptoms and signs of nerve root pain are clearly associated with an identifiable nerve root, a more specific approach is to perform a radiologically guided nerve root block. This may produce a more specific and effective response than an epidural injection. The technique allows a smaller dose and volume of injected drugs to be used and may reduce some of the possible hazards of epidural injection. The nerve root block can be performed at any level of the spine and details of the technique are described in Chapter 8.

Epidural or nerve root injections of steroid frequently provide relief of nerve root pain, which may be temporary or longlasting, depending on the nature of the underlying problem. The mechanism of pain relief is only speculative. When there is chemical irritation or direct mechanical compression of a nerve root, resulting in swelling and inflammatory response in perineural structures, then it seems reasonable to expect that steroids will help to alleviate this process. Relief of pain when there is long-term compression of neural structures, such as with foraminal stenosis, may have a number of possible explanations. Steroids may cause some atrophy of surrounding connective tissue and fibrous scar tissue resulting in less compression of neural structures within a confined bony space, but this remains speculative. There is evidence that steroids have an effect in blocking transmission in C fibres, but not in Aβ fibres, so that there is a direct effect on pain transmission. The anti-inflammatory effects of steroids may not be of any particular significance in this situation.

Medication for treatment of nerve root pain

Radicular pain does not always respond to steroid injection, and this is particularly likely when the pain is not clearly related to a structural problem or is longstanding. It is likely that persistent injury has resulted in long-term changes to nerve structure and function peripherally and within the central nervous system with the development of chronic neuropathic pain. Neuropathic pain should be treated with a tricyclic antidepressant drug, an anticonvulsant, or a combination of these groups, occasionally with the addition of other drugs such as opioid analgesics and baclofen.

ANTIDEPRESSANTS

The tricyclic drug of first choice is usually amitriptyline. This 'old antidepressant' drug has many effects on neurotransmitters within the central nervous system and therefore has a relatively high side effect profile. It may cause unacceptable daytime somnolence. Other troublesome side effects are dry mouth, occasional nightmares, and urinary retention in those who may already be compromised in this area, and increased risks in patients with ischaemic heart disease. Beneficial effects include improved sleep and relaxation, which can be very useful for chronic pain sufferers. Start the patient on a single night-time dose of 10–25 mg. If this is well tolerated the dose can be increased in increments. Most patients will achieve maximum benefit from doses of 75 mg or less; rarely is it necessary to increase the dose to a maximum of 150 mg.

If excessive sedation is a problem with amitriptyline, an alternative is to prescribe nortriptyline 10–75 mg. This has the same effect on neuropathic pain as amitriptyline, but is much less sedative and better tolerated. Other tricyclic drugs which can be used in the management of neuropathic pain include dosulepin, desipramine, doxepin and imipramine. Other antidepressant drugs do not have the same effects in managing neuropathic pain, and no great efficacy has been demonstrated for serotonin selective reuptake inhibitor (SSRI) drugs in this specific indication.

ANTICONVULSANTS

Neurogenic pain may respond to anticonvulsant drugs, either alone, or in combination with tricyclic antidepressants. The term 'anticonvulsant' broadly describes the class of drugs considered and does not imply that there is necessarily an anticonvulsant action involved in providing analgesia. For many years carbamazepine and sodium valproate have been the agents most frequently used for managing neurogenic pain. Tolerance to these drugs is unpredictable and age of the patient is not a clear guide to the prevalence of side effects.

Carbamazepine can be started at as low a dose as 100 mg daily and increased as tolerated to 400 mg three times daily if necessary. Sedation, ataxia and gastrointestinal upset are common side effects at higher doses. Long-term use has occasionally been associated with blood dyscrasias. Sodium valproate may be better tolerated. Doses can start at 100 mg three times daily increasing to 600 mg three times daily if tolerated. Again, gastrointestinal upset, dizziness and sedation are common side effects which may limit optimal use. Hepatic dysfunction can occur with long-term valproate and routine measurement of liver enzymes may be advisable. Alopecia is a rare side effect of valproate use. This distressing effect is usually reversible on cessation of the drug, although it has been known for previously straight hair to regrow curly!

Phenytoin was one of the earliest drugs for managing neuropathic pain. Its membrane-stabilizing properties suggest that it should be helpful in managing pain that has a shooting or lancinating quality. It has a narrow therapeutic range and its troublesome side effect profile has led to the declining use of this drug. Clonazepam, a benzodiazepine anticonvulsant, can be a useful adjuvant in managing sharp neurogenic pain, particularly when there is a major sleep disturbance. Start with a single night-time dose of 0.5 mg and increase to a maximum of 4 mg. Clonazepam is rarely a first choice for neurogenic pain. As a benzodiazepine, it rapidly creates dependence and may produce an unacceptable level of somnolence.

Clobazam, flecainide and mexiletine are among other drugs which have been used for treating sharp, shooting neuropathic pain, but lack of clear evidence of efficacy and troublesome side effects limit their value.

Gabapentin has now become one of the most successful and widely used drugs for treating neuropathic pain. It is generally well tolerated and has few contraindications, either for its effect on coincident disease, or interaction with other medications. It can be used in combination with tricyclic drugs or opiate analgesics. Tolerance is improved by starting at a low dose of 300 mg (100 mg if the patient seems particularly sensitive to medication) once a day. The dose is then increased at intervals of four to five days to 300 mg three times daily, and then again in increments every few days to reach an effective dose, or until unacceptable side effects are encountered. The maximum recommended dose is 1800 mg per day, but it is sometimes necessary to increase this, and doses up to 5200 mg per day have been reported. Some patients are unpredictably sensitive to side effects, which most commonly present as dizziness, ataxia and somnolence. As with most anticonvulsant drugs, if a decision is made to discontinue treatment, the drug should be decreased over several days before stopping completely. Pregabalin is a recent introduction. It seems to have all the beneficial effects of gabapentin in the management of neuropathic pain, but has a more favourable side effect profile. It is usually possible to start on a dose of 75 mg twice daily, doubling this dose if necessary.

OPIOID ANALGESICS

Although neurogenic pain is generally regarded as being relatively unresponsive to opioid analgesics, this is a relative effect, and some patients with severe neuropathic pain do achieve partial relief of their symptoms in this way. The decision to prescribe potent opioid analgesics to patients with a non-life-threatening chronic condition is sometimes controversial and is always subject to careful consideration as to suitability of the patient and the likely benefits of chronic opiate use. When other means of pain relief have been proved inadequate and if a useful analgesic effect can be demonstrated, then this course of action may be considered. Long-acting oral (or transdermal) analgesics should be prescribed on a timed basis. The regular use of short-acting analgesics, as required, is more likely to lead to an apparent 'drug habit' with less effectiveness of analgesia. Although there is usually some development of physical dependency it is rare for patients to develop addictive behaviour when opioids are used in this way.

Tramadol, as a moderate strength opioid, is believed to have some effect in managing neurogenic pain, and should be tried first. **Buprenorphine** is available as a sublingual tablet of 200 μg. It is often poorly tolerated, producing a high incidence of nausea, vomiting and dizziness. It is now available as a 3-day release transdermal patch in three doses: 35 μg/h, 52 μg/h and 70 μg/h. The transdermal route may be associated with a reduced level of unpleasant side effects and is better tolerated.

If a more potent drug is required, **sustained release morphine** (starting at 10 mg twice daily and titrated up depending on effect) or oxycodone SR (again starting at 10 mg twice daily) are suitable choices. **Transdermal fentanyl** patches are used in similar circumstances. The 3-day interval of application may improve compliance and fentanyl may be associated with less constipation than morphine. It is usual to start with the 25 μg/h strength of patch and increase to 50 or 75 μg/h depending on response.

Nerve root pain associated with spinal disease may be very resistant to treatment and become quite disabling. Drugs may be ineffective and further surgery unhelpful or even detrimental. When such pain is unremitting and yet is clearly attributable to specific nerve roots, it may be possible to provide some relief with the use of an implanted spinal cord stimulator. This treatment is generally more effective for nerve root pain and will rarely be helpful for straightforward back or neck pain. The procedure is highly invasive, very expensive,

and requires long-term maintenance and management of potential complications. Correct selection of patients for this system of analgesia is important in maximizing effectiveness and reducing complications, but in the right situations can provide long-term and effective pain relief, enabling a return to a more normal lifestyle. The procedure is described in Chapter 11.

PAIN RELATED TO DISC DEGENERATION

The intervertebral disc undergoes some degenerative process throughout adult life. The 'normal' process involves a dehydration of disc material with shrinkage of disc space. Degenerative changes may include prolapse of nucleus pulposus through the annulus fibrosis as an acute or chronic process, or there may be degenerative changes within the annulus, which appear as annular tears on imaging. Apart from the pain produced from a prolapse impinging on nerve roots, the disc is itself pain-sensitive, and there is a rich network of nerve fibres within the annulus. As some degree of disc degeneration is virtually universal, it is not understood why this process causes pain in some individuals only and is asymptomatic in most.

A painful disc can cause pain in the back, sometimes radiating into the legs, although not necessarily in a clear dermatomal pattern. The persistent back pain may be aggravated by spinal flexion or partially alleviated on extension or distraction, but signs are inconsistent and not specifically diagnostic. Spinal surgeons often use a discogram as a confirmatory diagnostic test for discal pain. A radiograph-guided intradiscal injection is usually painful and the test is considered confirmatory if the patient complains of pain which replicates their usual symptoms. If there is a positive confirmation, this is sometimes taken as an indication to offer a spinal fusion to the patient with a view to relieving their pain. Such surgery is a major procedure and the results are unpredictable. The most experienced spinal surgeons recognize that a proportion of patients who undergo spinal fusion procedures may not have their symptoms relieved, and a small number may experience more severe pain symptoms after surgery. The success rate appears to reduce when there is more than one level of disc degeneration involved. The selection of patients for such procedures is difficult and requires careful consideration.

Management of disc pain

The pain of degenerative intervertebral discs is often managed conservatively. A full range of rehabilitation processes should be offered to the patient. Physiotherapy and possibly some forms of manipulation should be considered in the early stages, with the aim of improving back strength and mobility. Regular analgesics, starting with paracetamol with or without a weak opiate analgesic, should be provided, adding a non-steroidal anti-inflammatory drug (NSAID) unless contraindicated. Transcutaneous electrical nerve stimulation (TENS) and acupuncture may provide further help with pain relief. In the long term consideration should be given to techniques of pain management, including participation in a full pain management programme.

Intradiscal electrothermal therapy

It is difficult to reduce sensory stimulation of the intervertebral disc. The nerve supply is difficult to access and most efforts have concentrated on the network of sensory fibres within the annulus. Intradiscal lesions can be produced using a system called intradiscal electrothermal therapy (IDET). Under radiological control, a flexible electrode is inserted percutaneously to enter the central disc space where it adopts a circular conformation. A heat lesion is produced around the inner surface of the annulus with a view to blocking sensory fibres within the annulus. Great success in relieving discogenic pain has been claimed for this procedure. Considerable potential morbidity remains associated with IDET and the procedure is not yet universally accepted.

Dorsal root ganglion block

Current opinion suggests that some of the afferent innervation of the lumbar discs enters the central nervous system with the sympathetic fibres at the second lumbar root. A lesion produced in the dorsal root ganglion of the L2 root therefore may reduce some discogenic pain. In practice, most practitioners would be reluctant to make a destructive lesion for this purpose, but a pulsed radio-frequency lesion may produce some pain relief without causing permanent loss of nerve function. Under radiographic guidance, an electrode is positioned in the intervertebral foramen adjacent to the dorsal root ganglion. A radio-frequency current is applied in pulses over three minutes, so that the temperature of the tissues does not exceed 42°C. This temperature is not neurolytic but the energy field has an effect on neural function within the dorsal root ganglion and analgesia lasting for several months can result without loss of normal function.

FACET JOINT PAIN

The articular facets of the spine are synovial joints, prone to arthritic and degenerative processes in the same way as other joints. When affected in this way the joints can become hypertrophied and sclerotic, with loss of joint space and, it is postulated, that they become painful on movement and stress. In addition, hypertrophied joints may impinge on the adjacent nerve root foramen and cause symptoms and signs of foraminal stenosis. Facet joint pain may result from primary degenerative/arthritic changes within the joints, or this may be secondary to abnormal stresses on the joints, as seems to occur following surgery or trauma to adjacent discs (perhaps the joint then becomes more weight bearing); surgical fusion of adjacent levels (resulting in increased stress at the joints immediately adjacent to the immobile segment); or in various congenital and developmental abnormalities of the spine that have caused abnormal gait or other movements with resulting excessive stresses on the joints.

Whether pain arising from facet joints can present a recognizable syndrome is debatable and not universally accepted. However, there is a widespread belief that the facet joints can be a site of pain generation within the spine. The main divergence of opinion is about whether this results in specific symptoms and whether the current treatments can be proved effective.

Diagnosing facet joint pain

The diagnosis of facet joint pain syndrome relies first on clinical examination. The patient complains of back pain (usually low back) which often radiates in a non-dermatomal pattern. The pain is often felt in the buttocks, thighs as far down as the knees, and sometimes the groin. This appears to be referred pain as opposed to a dermatomal nerve root pain distribution. Pain is often troublesome on prolonged sitting or standing and may be easier when the patient is able to move around or even walk short distances. On examination low back pain is typically provoked by extension of the lumbar spine and may be easier on flexion. The soft tissues overlying the affected joints are frequently tender. Straight leg raising may provoke more back pain than leg pain. Unfortunately none of these symptoms or signs is consistent and the diagnosis of facet joint pain remains imprecise.

Management of facet joint pain

The management of pain supposedly arising from facet joints is poorly supported by evidence-based medicine. Good controlled trials are difficult, partly because of the poor definition of the condition being treated. A number of physical interventions are widely used and their practitioners claim that a substantial number of patients appear to benefit from pain relief following intervention:

- Facet joint pain can be partly alleviated by more conservative techniques. It is always worth considering improvement of back strength and mobility with physiotherapy. Gentle manipulation by appropriately trained practitioners of the various manual therapy professions is frequently claimed to have great benefits for this type of back pain.
- Acupuncture and TENS are also useful means of relieving or controlling back pain arising in the posterior compartment of the spine.
- Invasive techniques to relieve facet joint pain follow two main routes:
  - Injection of local anaesthetic and depot steroid into the joint space must be done under radiographic guidance, as the joints are too small to be accurately targeted without vision. The technique is described in Chapter 9. If this relieves pain, the relief may develop gradually over a period of four to six weeks and may last for anything between a month and two years. The result is unpredictable. The proof of efficacy is complicated further by the fact that it is often reported that equally good pain relief can be achieved when the injection is sited in the joint capsule, or alongside the joint or around the nerve supply to the joint.
  - Denervation of the painful facet joint may be performed as a primary procedure following diagnosis of facet joint pain, or following an injection procedure where good but temporary pain relief has been achieved. Denervation is intended to produce a more sustained result. Radiofrequency thermocoagulation of the nerve supply to the facet joint is described in Chapter 9.

Pain arising from the cervical facet joints can be treated in the same way, although it is less usual to inject into the cervical facet joints. Injections are aimed at the medial branch of the posterior ramus of the nerve supplying the joint.

Following both injection and denervation of facet joints there is often a period when the patient experiences moderate pain in the back. The patient should be warned about this and be told that any discomfort may last for between one and 14 days with gradual resolution. Pain relief may develop gradually over a period of up to six weeks. Relief of back pain from either procedure is unpredictable; this may only last for a few weeks, or can result in excellent symptom control for two years.

Mechanical and structural problems

The spine is a complex piece of structural engineering and small defects in structural integrity can cause pain and

dysfunction in the whole. Destruction of bone by metastases or vertebral collapse from osteoporosis or trauma may cause back pain from a direct effect on the structural unit, or indirectly by localized pressure on nerve roots or central neural tissue. Loss of integrity of intervertebral discs and ligaments can cause spondylolisthesis, with pain from surrounding tissues under strain or compression of nerve roots. In addition to the structural defects resulting from degenerative change or trauma, congenital variations in spinal development and structure may cause longstanding postural problems with chronic painful degenerative processes being accelerated. These conditions should be managed according to the nature of the underlying structural problems if possible or symptomatically if correction of the structural problem is not an option. When compression of nerve roots is a part of the problem, injection of steroid to the nerve root foramen or epidural space may be considered as a means of relieving symptoms.

SOFT-TISSUE PAIN

Back pain and neck pain frequently present in the absence of any evidence of neuropathic or skeletal abnormality. Sometimes such pain is characterized by either localized or widespread tenderness over the paraspinal tissues. This may be a manifestation of underlying joint disorder or may be seen as a primary soft-tissue problem. Soft-tissue pain may be associated with the ligaments and capsules of spinal joints, as is believed to be the case in some 'whiplash injuries'. Alternatively it can involve the paraspinal muscles and the muscles of the shoulder and pelvic girdles, either in discrete points as are found in a myofascial pain syndrome, or over a wide area involving many groups of muscles, as in a fibromyalgia. Both of these syndromes can develop following trauma or may be completely spontaneous and apparently unrelated to any specific insult.

Treatment of soft-tissue pain

The pain of whiplash injury or spinal ligament/capsule pain may respond to injection with local anaesthetic and steroid to the nerve supply of the spinal joints. Relief, if obtained in this way, may be prolonged by the use of radio-frequency lesioning of nerves to the spinal facet joints.

When pain is localized to discrete areas of tension within the muscles, called 'trigger points', a series of trigger point injections may help to reduce pain. This may be done using local anaesthetic, local anaesthetic and steroid, or even just insertion of needles to the point of maximum tenderness, so-called 'dry needling'. Acupuncture is an alternative method of reducing trigger points. Resistant trigger points may be treated by injection with botulinum toxin. The measured quantities of toxin are injected into the points of tension/tenderness in the muscle. Patients may experience some temporary systemic malaise after such injections and pain relief may take several days to develop. Beneficial effects of botulinum toxin injections last up to three months, when a repeat treatment may be required. The sleep disturbance that frequently accompanies this condition can be improved by prescribing a tricyclic antidepressant drug at night. Amitriptyline 10–75 mg or dosulepin 25–75 mg are suitable choices.

The widespread pain of fibromyalgia rarely responds to localized injections. The cause of this condition is not understood, and some doubt the physical nature of the condition. It seems unlikely that there is any primary muscular disorder and theories suggest a dysfunction of central nociceptive processing, among other possibilities. Tricyclic antidepressants may offer some help, and drugs which alter central pain augmentation, such as gabapentin or ketamine, have been tried with variable degrees of success claimed. Transcutaneous electrical nerve stimulation is usually unhelpful and patients often claim that this tends to aggravate their pain. Treatment more often tends to rely on a pain management approach with graded exercise programmes and training in cognitive and behavioural aspects (see Chapter 13).

BEHAVIOURAL ASPECTS OF MANAGING BACK PAIN

In the majority of cases, there is no clear proved cause for back and neck pain. It therefore follows that most forms of treatment suggested either using an orthodox medical model of disease or through the multiple alternative and complementary therapies available will only provide satisfactory pain relief in a limited number of those who suffer from these complaints. Back and neck pain are rarely simple entities and the widespread effect on behaviour, activity and quality of life can be profound. The psychological effects of chronic pain and disability, with loss of self-esteem, family, social and economic aspects of life, all contribute to the resultant suffering and interfere with the long-term rehabilitation and management of back pain. Prolonged immobility becomes a self-defeating process, contributing to weakened, shortened muscles and stiff painful joints.

When the medical model for treating a condition which is so poorly defined can be no longer sustained, it is in the patient's best interests to be helped to come to terms with this fact and adopt a more active approach to managing their symptoms, discarding the purely passive role of regarding treatment as something which is done to them. Some physical interventions may be seen as giving a temporary respite from pain and so encourage a more active phase to begin, but the emphasis should be on improving mobility, fitness and the skills required to cope with pain. Many patients equate pain with disability and it is important to develop means of maximizing activity potential within the patient's range of abilities despite the continuing presence of pain. A graded exercise programme may not reduce pain, but an improvement in mobility and confidence usually improves the ability to cope with pain and reduces suffering and disability. This may take the form of a full pain management programme involving a multidisciplinary team with input from a clinical psychologist, physiotherapist and occupational therapist; or more individual programmes of rehabilitation can be organized around individual patients.

CASE SCENARIO

John, a 46-year-old man who works as a sales manager, is referred to the pain service by his general practitioner. Two years previously he developed acute back pain and sciatica after lifting his computer at work. He was initially treated in primary care with analgesics and encouraged to return to normal activities as soon as possible. His symptoms persisted and he developed weakness and changes in sensation in the fifth lumbar nerve distribution. An MRI revealed a large prolapse of the right L5/S1 disc. After 12 weeks he underwent a microdiscectomy. This resulted in immediate relief of his severe sciatic pain, but three months later he was still complaining of back pain and some numbness and paraesthesiae in his right leg. He had been unable to return to work.

When he was seen in the pain clinic, John admitted that he was becoming increasingly desperate about his situation. He was worried that his employment would be terminated and that this would lead to severe financial difficulties for his family. He was taking a full dose of co-codamol analgesic which seemed to have little benefit. He had withdrawn from most of his social activities and was feeling both angry and frustrated at the way in which his life had deteriorated.

Physical assessment demonstrated painful restricted mobility of the lumbar spine, but no clearly identifiable painful focus. There was loss of ankle reflex on the right with demonstration of pain and altered sensitivity in the distribution of L5.

John was given amitriptyline 50 mg to take at night. This was to help him to relax and sleep more effectively as well as modifying the neuropathic pain in his leg. Under radiographic guidance, a nerve root block to the right L5/S1 foramen under local anaesthetic and steroid was performed. Following these interventions, John reported that the pain and abnormal sensations in his leg improved considerably but he was still incapacitated by his back pain and felt that all attempts to engage in increased activity resulted in an exacerbation of his back pain. The amitriptyline was helpful, but produced a disagreeable degree of mental impairment the following morning. A change was made to gabapentin 300 mg three times daily which was again helpful for the neuropathic pain, but without the unpleasant sedation associated with the amitriptyline.

John continued to find that his back pain dominated his life, preventing a return to work and normal social activity. He was assessed for a pain management programme and it was felt that he would be likely to gain much in improving the way he paced his physical activities and coped with his pain symptoms. He took part in an 8-week outpatient pain management programme during which he improved his understanding of his back pain and was able to overcome his fear of damaging himself to increase his physical capacity through a graded exercise programme. He also learnt skills to cope with his ongoing pain and to regain some control over his life which had previously been dictated by his pain. Although John described his pain as being about the same as previously, he felt that he could continue to build up his physical activity and think more confidently about a phased return to work.

Section Four

15 Pain in Malignant Disease

INTRODUCTION

There are many aspects of caring for the dying patient that must be considered as well as the management of pain, and these will be discussed briefly in this chapter. The World Health Organization (WHO) definition of palliative care (1992) is as follows:

Palliative care is the active, total care of the patient with life-threatening disease and it provides an interdisciplinary model for continuing management of quality of life concerns, including control of symptoms, maintenance of function, psychosocial and spiritual support for the patient and family and comprehensive care at the end of life.

PAIN MANAGEMENT

Pain associated with cancer is frequently under-treated. Pain and associated symptoms cannot always be entirely eliminated but appropriate use of available therapies can effectively relieve pain in the great majority of patients. Pain management improves the patient's quality of life throughout all stages of the disease.

The prevalence of moderate to severe pain is about 30–50 per cent among patients with cancer who are undergoing active treatment for a solid tumour and 70–90 per cent among those with advanced disease. In general about 35 per cent of the pain is somatic in origin, 17 per cent is visceral, 9 per cent is neuropathic and the remainder is of mixed origin. Ninety per cent of patients should attain adequate relief with simple drug therapies, but this success rate is not achieved in routine practice. Inadequate management of pain is the result of various issues that include:

- under-treatment by clinicians with insufficient knowledge of pain assessment and therapy
- inappropriate concerns about opioid side effects and addiction
- a tendency to give lower priority to symptom control than to disease management
- patients' under-reporting of pain
- non-compliance with therapy.

Patients often believe that pain is inevitable and will become uncontrollable but there is no therapeutic ceiling for morphine so extremely large dosages can be used safely and effectively if the drug is titrated properly. Flexibility is the key to managing cancer pain. As diagnosis, stage of disease, responses to pain and interventions, and personal preferences all vary among patients, so must pain management. Effective pain management is best achieved by a team approach involving patients, their families and healthcare providers. Three principles underlie the treatment of cancer pain:

1 modify the source of pain
2 alter the central perception of pain
3 block the transmission of pain to the central nervous system.

PAIN ASSESSMENT

Continual assessment of cancer pain is crucial and changes in the pattern of pain or the development of new pain should lead to changes in treatment. A comprehensive assessment should address the relation between the pain and the disease, and the impact of the pain and related symptoms on the patient's quality of life. The information elicited from the patient should focus on:

- Temporal features – onset, pattern, and course
- Location – primary sites and patterns of radiation
- Severity – usually measured with a verbal rating scale, e.g. mild, moderate, or severe, or a 0–10 numeric scale
- Quality
- Factors that exacerbate or relieve the pain.

The goals of the initial assessment of pain are to:

- characterize the pathophysiology of the pain
- determine the intensity of the pain and its impact on the patient's ability to function.

Worsening pain is often a sign of worsening disease. Therefore, patients may tolerate increasing pain in order to deny their worsening condition. It is important to clarify whether each escalation of the opioid dosage is due to tolerance, worsening illness or inappropriate usage. Patients with a strong fear of opioid tolerance have been found to have higher pain intensity. Factors that may influence analgesic response and result in persistent pain include changing nociception due to disease progression, intractable side effects, tolerance, neuropathic pain, and opioid metabolites.

Most patients with cancer who experience chronic pain also develop other physical and psychological symptoms. Apart from pain, fatigue and psychological distress are the most common symptoms in patients with cancer. A broad assessment of symptoms is an essential part of the management of cancer pain but it must also include assessment of the difficulties that arise in the quality of life. The following are essential to initial assessment:

- detailed history
- physical examination
- psychosocial assessment
- diagnostic evaluation.

Physical pain can have visceral, somatic and neuropathic origins and the role of each should be determined in each patient. Assessment should occur:

- at regular intervals after initiation of treatment
- at each new report of pain.

An increase in pain intensity following a stable period should result in a new evaluation of the underlying aetiology and pain syndrome. The assessment of pain is discussed in Chapter 2.

Assessment of the outcomes of pain management

The aims of good pain management are to achieve:

- Decreased pain intensity
- Improvement in psychosocial functioning.

Using rating scales of pain intensity at its worst and on average can help monitor outcomes. Measurement of the percentage of pain relief is also useful, though measuring patient satisfaction is less useful because of the low expectations patients sometimes hold of pain control.

Cultural differences

Catholic, Jewish and Islamic teachings support the relief of pain in the dying. Buddhists may feel that clouding of the senses interferes with the work the dying need to complete and they may refuse opioids. Distinct cultural influences need to be incorporated into a multidimensional assessment of pain.

PATHOPHYSIOLOGY OF CANCER PAIN

Identifying the aetiology of pain is essential to its management. The available treatments are not fully effective because the underlying mechanisms that are causing pain are not understood. Patients with the same tumour type often have variable pain scores. Metastatic spread to bone is the commonest cause of pain due to:

- chemical or mechanical signalling from tumour cells to nociceptors in bone or the periosteum
- tumour infiltration of sensory nerves
- destruction of bone
- microfractures
- periosteal involvement.

Other causes of cancer pain include:

- infiltration of nerves by the tumour
- activation of nociceptors by tumour-derived mediators. Malignant cells secrete prostaglandins, cytokines, epidermal growth factor, transforming growth factor and platelet-derived growth factor, all of which can excite primary afferent nociceptors
- nociceptor sensitization – peripheral or central
- activation of silent nociceptors.

Other factors may exacerbate the pain experience by causing stress. Anxiety, depression and opioid-related delirium can all exacerbate pain. Patients can no longer get pleasure from activities, they may feel worthless, guilty, hopeless and helpless (Box 15.1).

Specific causes of pain – cancer pain syndromes

Recognition of pain syndromes (see Box 15.2) is essential to identify the specific aetiology responsible for the pain and introduction of the most appropriate therapy. The syndromes can be divided into those occurring as a direct effect of the tumour, those that result from therapy and those that are unrelated to the disease. Recognition of symptoms may allow intervention that will prevent major complications such as spinal cord compression presenting as back pain.

BOX 15.1 Types of distress

Social distress

- Financial and personal resources
- Sources of support
- Coping skills and styles
- Family dynamics and tension

Psychological distress

- Loss of friends and activities
- Unable to support family
- Lose of sense of self
- Poor concentration with drugs

Spiritual distress

- Wondering what you have done to be punished so much, and anger with God

---

BOX 15.2 Differential diagnosis of pain

Acute pain

- Procedural pain
- Therapeutic pain
- Postoperative pain
- Bone pain
- Obstruction of a hollow viscus
- Bleed into tumour
- Infection
- Shingles – five times the incidence in the normal population

Tumour-related chronic pain

- Bone pain, e.g. pathological fracture
- Joint pain
- Soft tissue pain – myalgia
- Paraneoplastic pain, e.g. hypertrophic osteoarthropathy
- Neoplastic involvement of the viscera
- Headache – raised intracranial pressure
- Neuropathic pain – nerve infiltration by tumour, etc.

Treatment-related pain

- Hormonal therapy, e.g. painful gynaecomastia
- Chemotherapy – commonly associated with the vinca alkaloids, cisplatin and paclitaxel
- Immunotherapy
- Amputation and phantom pain
- Radiotherapy, e.g. radiation-induced osteonecrosis
- Radiation-induced fibrosis can damage a peripheral nerve or nerves and cause neuropathic pain; symptoms usually occur months to years after treatment

---

TUMOUR-RELATED NOCICEPTIVE PAIN SYNDROMES

Bone pain syndromes are the most common. Only a small proportion of bone metastases become painful, and the factors that convert a painless lesion into a painful one are unknown. The spine is the commonest site of bone metastases and many patients with cancer have back pain. Pain can also be caused by obstruction, infiltration or compression of visceral structures, including hollow viscus and supporting connective tissues.

TUMOUR-RELATED NEUROPATHIC PAIN SYNDROMES

Neuropathic pain syndromes may be caused by tumour infiltration or compression of nerve, plexus or roots, or by the remote effects of malignant disease on peripheral nerves. The syndromes are highly variable; patients may have aching pains or dysaesthesiae anywhere in the dermatomal region innervated by the damaged neural structure.

PAIN CONTROL

Identify the cause and provide specific treatment where available. Principles of pharmacologic therapy begin with the WHO ladder (see also Chapter 4):

- Paracetamol $\pm$ non-steroidal anti-inflammatory drug (NSAID)
- Weak opioid $\pm$ NSAID
- Strong opioid $\pm$ NSAID
- Other.

Even within the same family of analgesic drugs, individual variations in effects and side effects are well recognized. Substitution of drugs within a category should be tried before switching therapy:

1 Use the simplest dosage schedules and least invasive pain management modalities first.
2 For mild to moderate pain, use (unless contraindicated) paracetamol and an NSAID.
3 When pain persists or increases, add a weak opioid.
4 If pain increases, increase the opioid potency or dose.
5 Give all analgesic drugs regularly (i.e. 'by the clock') to maintain the level of drug that will help prevent recurrence of pain.
6 Administer additional doses 'as needed' for breakthrough pain.

Opioids in cancer pain

It is important to tailor the dose and delivery route to the individual in opioid therapy. The goal is to achieve a favourable balance between analgesia and side effects.

PRINCIPLES OF MORPHINE TREATMENT

- Use an individual treatment plan.
- The appropriate dose is the dose that relieves pain throughout the prescribed dosing interval without causing unmanageable side effects.
- Use the appropriate route – oral where possible.
- Minimize the total number of daily doses.
- Use 'around the clock' dosing with rescue doses of immediate release opioid for breakthrough pain.
- Anticipate and manage side effects.
- Use co-analgesics where necessary.
- Collaboration between interdisciplinary teams.
- Do not use agonist/antagonist drugs or partial agonists (buprenorphine).
- Prescribe a laxative – sodium docusate or Movical®.
- Patients may feel drowsy on initial opioid doses. They should be advised not to drive for one week.
- Medication doses should be titrated promptly to achieve effective pain relief, i.e. every 24–48 hours. Morphine doses can be safely increased by 50 per cent every 24 hours until a satisfactory response is obtained and can be reduced by 50–75 per cent every 24 hours without causing withdrawal symptoms.
- Few patients need >600 mg morphine to control pain.

The European Association for Palliative Care has drawn up recommendations for the use of morphine in cancer pain (Box 15.3).

> **BOX 15.3 European Association for Palliative Care recommendations for use of morphine in cancer pain**
>
> - Optimal route of administration of morphine is by mouth. It is convenient and inexpensive. Ideally two types of formulation are required – immediate release for dose titration and controlled release for maintenance treatment. In general the response to several opioids is advisable before abandoning the oral route because of side effects.
> - The simplest method of dose titration is with immediate release morphine (mean bioavailability = 35 per cent; plasma half-life = 3–4 hours) given every four hours and the same dose for breakthrough pain. This rescue dose may be given as often as required and the total daily dose is then reviewed. The dose must be titrated individually for each patient. When morphine is first started the dose is 10 mg four hourly. Steady state is reached within 24 hours so assessment and dosage change can be made after this time.
> - Increase by 30–50 per cent increments every other day.

Rescue doses

- There is no logic in using a smaller dose for rescue analgesia than the full dose being used – the full dose is more likely to be affective. When a patient is stabilized on controlled release morphine the breakthrough dose should be one-third of the regular dose.
- Pain returns consistently before the next regular dose – the regular dose should be increased. The aim should be only for four hourly dosing.
- For patients receiving immediate release morphine every four hours a double dose at bedtime is a simple and effective way of avoiding being woken by pain.

Conversion to slow release morphine (MST)

- When pain is controlled on four hourly immediate release morphine convert to 12 hourly slow release morphine (onset = 1 hour; peak = 2–3 hours; duration = 12 hours).
- Calculate the total daily dose of immediate release morphine that has controlled the pain. Divide the dose into two and give this dose twice a day.
- Also provide a PRN rescue dose of Oramorph or similar. The dose should be a third of MST 12 hourly dose.
- The breakthrough dose must be increased as the twice daily dose increases.

Increase MST if patient needs >2 doses extra per day and increase the rescue dose to remain at 1/3 MST dose. The size of each dose increment is usually either the total of the rescue doses consumed during the previous 24 hours or 30–50 per cent of the current daily dose.

Occasionally controlled release morphine needs to be given eight hourly and not 12 hourly. There is no evidence there is any difference between formulations of morphine. Crushing controlled release morphine tablets alters their dissolution and absorption characteristics and should be avoided. Liquid preparations are available and capsules containing granules can be broken and the granules sprinkled on food.

Other routes of administration of morphine

Rectal morphine

If patients are unable to take drugs orally the preferred alternative routes are rectal and subcutaneous. Rectal morphine is safe, inexpensive and effective when patients have nausea and vomiting. The rectal route should not be used in the presence of diarrhoea, anal or rectal lesions, mucositis, thrombocytopenia and neutropenia. The bioavailability of morphine by rectal and oral routes is the same and the duration of analgesia is the same. It also has a similar duration of action. The relative potency of oral morphine: rectal morphine is 1:1.

Subcutaneous morphine

Morphine can be given subcutaneously either as a bolus every four hours or by continuous infusion using an ambulatory infusion pump. The relative potency of oral morphine to subcutaneous morphine is about 1:2, but this varies according to circumstances in which the morphine is used and among individual patients. Exact figures cannot be given but guidelines recommend the following: to convert oral to subcutaneous morphine, divide the dose by 2 (somewhere between 1:2 and 1:3). Drugs other than morphine may be preferred to be given subcutaneously because of their greater solubility. Only 1.6 mL of water is needed to dissolve 1 g of diamorphine, but 1 g of morphine requires 20 mL water.

Subcutaneous administration is not practical in:

- generalized oedema
- erythema, soreness or sterile abscess development at site of administration
- coagulation disorders
- very poor peripheral perfusion.

The buccal, sublingual and nebulized routes are not recommended because there is no evidence of clinical advantage over conventional routes and the absorption of morphine by these routes is unpredictable so should be avoided.

INTRATHECAL OR EPIDURAL OPIOIDS

Intrathecal or epidural opioids are second-line treatment for managing cancer pain. This route should be considered for patients who develop intractable pain or intolerable side effects with other routes. The main indication for long-term administration of intraspinal opioids is intractable pain in the lower part of the body, particularly bilateral or midline pain. Profound analgesia is possible without motor, sensory or sympathetic blockade. Local anaesthetics may be combined with opioids for intraspinal administration.

ROLE OF OTHER OPIOID DRUGS IN PALLIATIVE CARE

The use of oral, rectal and subcutaneous morphine produces effective pain control in about 80 per cent of patients. In the remaining 20 per cent other methods must be considered. Sublingual or transdermal use of other opioids may be an alternative to subcutaneous injection. Highly lipophilic drugs like methadone, fentanyl and buprenorphine are well absorbed sublingually.

Transdermal administration (fentanyl)

Patches currently available are formulated to provide analgesia lasting up to 72 hours. They can be used when the oral route is compromised but they are not suitable for rapid dose titration because of the slow onset of analgesia. They should be used for relatively stable analgesic requirement when rapid increases or decreases in dosage are not likely to be needed. The patches may be less constipating than other opioids and generally seem to be associated with greater patient satisfaction.

Problems with the fentanyl patch

- Fever increases drug absorption because of vasodilatation.
- Sweating reduces absorption because the patch does not stick properly.
- 5 per cent get erythema/pruritus from the patch. To relieve this, spray the skin with steroid (beclomethasone inhaler 50 μg dose).

Transmucosal administration (fentanyl)

Oral transmucosal fentanyl citrate can be used for the relief of breakthrough pain. The lipid solubility of fentanyl allows rapid onset of pain relief that is faster than the oral route. Side effects are consistent with other opioid therapies, including sedation, constipation and nausea.

Sublingual fentanyl

- 25 μ/h = 45–134 mg oral morphine/day

Oral fentanyl

- Bioavailability = 25 per cent buccal, 25 per cent oral
- Onset = 5–10 minutes
- Duration = 60–120 minutes

Fentanyl lozenges

- Pain relief in 5–10 minutes, maximum 20–40 minutes.
- Place lozenge in mouth and constantly move and suck and finish within 15 minutes.
- Initial dose = 200 μg.
- After 15 minutes can use a second dose but no more thereafter.
- Use a larger dose after three to four attempts.
- No more than four doses per day.
- Duration = 1–3 hours.
- Bioavailability about 50 per cent.
- 25 per cent of patients have no pain relief with the fentanyl lozenge.

Intermittent injection or continuous infusion

Intravenous and subcutaneous routes provide effective opioid delivery. Methadone may cause skin irritation when infused subcutaneously or intravenously. Intravenous administration provides a rapid onset of analgesia, but the duration of analgesia after a bolus dose is shorter than with other routes. In patients requiring continuous intravenous access for other purposes, this route of administration may be the most cost effective and provides a consistent level of analgesia. When there is no intravenous access, subcutaneous opioid infusion is a practical alternative for the home setting.

PATIENT-CONTROLLED ANALGESIA (PCA)

Use PCA to help the patient maintain independence and control by matching drug delivery to the need for analgesia. The opioid may be administered orally or via a dedicated portable pump to deliver the drug intravenously, subcutaneously or intraspinally.

CESSATION OF OPIOIDS

When a patient becomes pain free as a result of cancer treatment or palliation (e.g. nerve destruction), gradually decrease the opioid to avoid withdrawal.

Other opioids

For the patient who experiences dose-limiting side effects with one oral opioid (e.g. hallucinations, nightmares, dysphoria, nausea or mental clouding), other oral opioids should be tried before abandoning one route in favour of another.

Changing one opioid drug for another

The dose of the new drug should be reduced by 30–50 per cent because of the different bioavailability of each drug. If the new drug is methadone the dose may need to be reduced by up to 90 per cent (Chapter 3).

METHADONE

Methadone is a very useful second- or third-line opioid for cancer pain management. It can be given orally, intravenously and by suppository. It is a synthetic opioid agonist that has a number of unique characteristics.

- Excellent oral and rectal absorption
- No known active metabolites
- Prolonged duration of action resulting in longer administration intervals
- Low cost.

Methadone used for chronic pain management demonstrates a much higher potency than the 1:1 or 1:2 methadone to morphine ratio that is generally reported in tables of opioid equivalence. Methadone is 5–15 times more potent than

---

> **BOX 15.4   Rotation to methadone**
>
> **Day 1**
>
> The total 24-hour opioid dose is decreased by 30 per cent. This is replaced by a dose of methadone calculated at a ratio of 10:1 compared to a morphine-equivalent dose (methadone given at one-tenth the morphine-equivalent dose), given on an 8-hour schedule. Patients are followed closely, with inpatient monitoring preferred.
>
> **Day 2**
>
> The original opioid is decreased by a further 30 per cent, and the methadone dose increased by 10 per cent to 30 per cent, based on clinical assessments of patient's analgesic requirements. If the patient is drowsy or shows respiratory depression, the methadone dose should not be increased, and the original opioid dose may be decreased by a further 30 per cent.
>
> **Day 3**
>
> If the patient is not sedated and respiration is not compromised, the original opioid is discontinued and the methadone dose increased by up to 30 per cent as determined by the clinical assessment. At this point, the rescue dose of opioid is also switched to methadone, calculated at 10 per cent of the 24-hour dose. Daily assessment should be continued on days 4 through 7, watching for sedation, respiratory depression and analgesic efficacy. Despite using this cautious approach, respiratory depression has been observed, requiring intervention with subcutaneous naloxone.

morphine. Patients on high opioid doses but achieving inadequate pain control and significant opioid-related toxicity have achieved good pain control with methadone. A careful method of rotation to methadone over a 1-week period has been proposed (Box 15.4).

SIDE EFFECTS OF OPIOIDS

Side effects should be anticipated and where possible treatment given to prevent their occurrence.

Constipation

Constipation is dose related, but there is marked variability among patients.

Mechanism

- Opioid-receptor mediated via both central and peripheral mechanisms.

- Opioids extend the gastrointestinal transit time.
- Opioids compromise gastrointestinal tract peristaltic function so the stool within the gut lumen becomes excessively dehydrated.

At an extreme it may be present as a severe ileus and pseudo-bowel obstruction. Rapid resolution can occur within days of complete withdrawal of opioids but this is rarely possible in patients with cancer-related pain. The use of orally administered opioid antagonists such as naloxone may be helpful.

Unlike nausea, complete tolerance to this effect does not generally develop, and most patients require laxative/stool softener therapy for as long as they take opioids. Opioid-induced constipation is a frequent cause of chronic nausea and is observed in 40–70 per cent of patients receiving opioids.

Management
- Keep well hydrated.
- Prescribed a scheduled regimen of stool softening agents (e.g. docusate sodium).
- Add where necessary:
  - mild osmotic agent (e.g. 70 per cent sorbitol solution, lactulose, milk of magnesia)
  - lubricants (e.g. mineral oil)
  - bulk-forming laxatives (e.g. psyllium)
  - mild cathartic laxatives (e.g. casanthrol, senna)
  - stimulant cathartics (e.g. senna, bisacodyl).

A recent study has demonstrated decreased laxative use in patients on transdermal fentanyl compared with patients on oral morphine treatment. Whether this decrease is clinically significant or not, however, and whether the decrease in laxative usage relates to the route of administration instead of the opioid type, needs to be demonstrated.

Nausea and vomiting

Nausea and vomiting occurs in approximately one-third to two-thirds of patients taking opioids. It is a common complication of early exposure to opioids and usually disappears within the first week of treatment. Appropriate antiemetic coverage during the opioid-initiation phase is usually effective in limiting this adverse effect. Nausea may be experienced when an opioid dose is significantly increased.

Three main mechanisms underlie this opioid-related adverse effect:

- stimulation of the chemoreceptor trigger zone, where dopamine is the main neurotransmitter
- reduced gastrointestinal motility, including delayed gastric emptying

- nausea via increased vestibular sensitivity, which is uncommon.

Metoclopramide or domperidone are generally recommended as first-line agents because they improve gastrointestinal motility and are antidopaminergic. The antihistamines act on the histamine receptors in the vomiting centre and on vestibular afferents. They are generally reserved for cases where vestibular sensitivity, often manifesting as motion-induced nausea, is suspected or where bowel obstruction precludes the use of gastrointestinal prokinetic agents.

There appear to be differences among individual patients in the extent to which different opioids cause nausea. This forms the basis for the strategy of switching from one opioid to another when a particular opioid produces persistent nausea.

Cognitive effects of opioids

Most patients become tolerant of the sedating effects that accompany either the initiation of opioid therapy or dose increases and patients should be able to continue to drive in the early stages. Reaction times are not significantly reduced with opioids. Mild opioid-induced cognitive impairment often resolves on changing the opioid.

Delirium affects 80 per cent of dying patients. The contribution of opioids to the delirium is often difficult to determine because of the associated multisystem impairment, and the concurrent administration of other psychotropic agents. The aetiology is multifactorial but there is no doubt medication contributes. High doses of opioids especially if increased quickly can cause central nervous system toxicity, hyperalgesia and hypersensitivity to touch, myoclonus and delirium. The patient presents with:

- Hallucinations
- Distraction
- Inability to concentrate
- Insomnia
- Daytime somnolence
- Nightmares
- Confusion
- Restlessness
- Agitation
- Anxiety.

Delirium often presents as rapidly escalating pain. Decreased brain cholinergic activity is recognized as one of the potential underlying pathophysiological mechanisms of delirium. The potential role of morphine metabolites, in particular the ratio of 3-glucuronide to 6-glucuronide in the development of opioid-related toxicity, has been reported but there has been conflicting evidence regarding the role and ratios of the metabolites in patients exhibiting both a poor response to increasing morphine doses and associated toxicity.

Management of delirium

When delirium develops, adjuvant analgesics should be considered if not already being used. The opioid dose should be reduced if possible and the opioid-related side effects managed with medical treatment. Any contributing metabolic abnormalities need to be corrected. The specific management approach to opioid-induced delirium involves either a dose reduction or an opioid switch. Also consider haloperidol or levomepromazine.

Opioid switching

If symptoms persist it appears that opioid switching does have a useful role when pain control remains inadequate with escalating opioid doses, and the opioid results in unacceptable opioid-related side effects.

Treatment of opioid-induced myoclonus

- Change opioid (see Box 15.5)
- Clonazepam 0.5–1 mg nocte to three times daily
- Baclofen 5 mg – 20 mg three times daily
- Intravenous midazolam 1–7 mg/h

Respiratory depression

Patients receiving long-term opioid therapy generally develop tolerance to the respiratory depressant effects of these agents.

Other opioid side effects

- Dry mouth
- Urinary retention
- Pruritus
- Dysphoria
- Euphoria
- Sleep disturbances
- Inappropriate secretion of antidiuretic hormone

BOX 15.5   Opioid conversion doses

Converting from oral morphine to subcutaneous diamorphine

- Divide the total 24-hour oral morphine dose by 3 and give over 24 hours
- Morphine 3 mg PO $\equiv$ diamorphine 1 mg subcutaneously
- Increase by 25–50 per cent increments as required

CONVERTING FROM MORPHINE TO FENTANYL

The conversion of morphine to fentanyl can lead to a modified withdrawal syndrome with symptoms including shivering, diarrhoea, bowel cramps, sweating and restlessness, although pain relief is maintained. These symptoms can be relieved with morphine PRN for a few days:

1   Start with a 25 μg patch (releases 25 μg/h fentanyl = 600 μg/24 h).
2   25 μg patch $\equiv$ 10 mg morphine orally four hourly $\equiv$ 30–40 mg morphine subcutaneous infusion over 24 hours.
3   Therapeutic blood levels are reached in 12–24 hours and a steady state at 72 hours.
4   Give last dose of 12 hourly morphine when applying patch, or give three more doses of morphine elixir.
5   Continue with morphine as required for withdrawal symptoms.
6   The patch should be changed every 72 hours and applied to a different site but up to 25 per cent of patients need a patch change every 48 hours.
7   To convert a 25 μg patch to subcutaneous fentanyl use 500 μg/24 h to start with.

OXYCODONE

- Bioavailability = 65 per cent
- The modified release preparation has an onset time of 1/2 hour with peak action at one hour and a duration of 12 hours
- The immediate release four hourly dose is 1/3 the modified release dose.

Morphine-resistant pain

- Pain responds to morphine but side effects limit the dose.
- Equivocal response but side effects are unacceptable.
- Pain is unresponsive to increased doses of opioid:
  - neuropathic pain
  - bony pain.
- Try methadone and other treatments given below.

Metastatic bone pain or hypercalcaemia

Tumours that are most likely to metastasize to bone are:

- Breast
- Prostate
- Lung
- Kidney
- Multiple myeloma

SYMPTOMS OF HYPERCALCAEMIA

- Drowsiness
- Nausea and vomiting
- Bone pain
- Dehydration

TREATMENT OF HYPERCALCAEMIA

- 0.9 per cent saline 1 L every six hours for 24 hours
- Calcitonin. Dose = 800 U/24 hours for 48 hours

MANAGEMENT OF PAIN

- Analgesia
- Treatment of the tumour (hormones or chemotherapy)
- Treatment of the bony metastases (radiotherapy or bisphosphonates)

Radiotherapy

Radiotherapy leads to pain reduction in 60 per cent of patients with complete pain relief in 33 per cent; 80 per cent of patients will not need to repeat the treatment after the first dose.

Bisphosphonates

Most patients have multiple bony metastases at presentation and therefore systemic treatment may be better than radiotherapy. Bisphosphonates are potent inhibitors of normal and pathological bone resorption. Regular bisphosphonates will:

- reduce the progression of bony metastases
- reduce the incidence of pathological fracture and therefore orthopaedic surgery
- reduce pain
- reduce the need for palliative radiotherapy
- reduce the risk of hypercalcaemia.

Bisphosphonates do not reduce the risk of spinal cord compression.

Indications
- Bone pain and metastases.
- Myeloma.
- Prognosis >2 months.
- Hypercalcaemia (corrected Ca^{2+} >2.8 nmol/L).
- Prevention of steroid-induced hypercalcaemia.
- Previous pathological fracture or risk of pathological fracture such as the presence of lytic lesions or vertebral collapse.

Doses
Intravenous treatment is more effective and better tolerated than oral therapy and the outcome is more predictable because oral absorption is variable.

- Pamidronate – 90 mg intravenous infusion in 500 mL saline over two to four hours. An effect is seen in 14 days and lasts four to eight weeks. It should be given every four weeks.
- Clodronate – intravenous infusion 1500 mg every three weeks.
- Clodronate 800 mg twice daily orally.

Side effects
- Myalgia
- Fever
- Uveitis
- Scleritis
- Transient increase in bone pain
- Gastrointestinal irritability

Adjuvant analgesics

NEUROPATHIC PAIN

Up to 40 per cent of cancer patients may have a neuropathic mechanism underlying their pain, for example from erosion of a nerve by the tumour. Stop each drug after a trial period if there is no clear response so patient does not take unnecessary drugs. Use opioids as first line (Table 15.1) because there is often coexisting nociceptive pain. Opioids alone help some neuropathic pain.

Antidepressants

The tricyclic drugs are useful in the management of neuropathic pain. The most widely reported experience has been with amitriptyline and this should be the tricyclic agent of choice. Onset of action usually takes one to seven days but it may be delayed four to six weeks. It may increase the bioavailability of morphine. The serotonin selective reuptake inhibitors (SSRIs) are less effective than the older agents for the management of neuropathic pain.

Table 15.1 *Treatments for neuropathic pain*

First line	Second line
Opioids	Ketamine
Non-steroidal anti-inflammatory drugs	Spinal/epidural
Transcutaneous electrical nerve stimulation	Methadone
Radiotherapy	Lidocaine infusion
Steroids 8 mg once daily – 3–5 day trial	Mexiletine
Tricyclic antidepressants	Flecainide
Anticonvulsants	Neurolytic procedures
	Capsaicin

Anticonvulsants

These agents are particularly indicated for the management of lancinating or burning pain. Some agents must be used with caution in cancer patients undergoing marrow-suppressant therapies, such as chemotherapy and radiation therapy. There are no data to compare the efficacy of different drugs, but they include clonazepam, phenytoin, valproate, carbamazepine, gabapentin and topiramate. All these agents have different sites of action so it is worth changing them around if there is no response to the first drug tried.

Local anaesthetics

Local anaesthetics can used to treat neuropathic pain. Side effects include gastrointestinal upset. A careful cardiac evaluation is required as these drugs should not be used in patients with heart block or other dysrhythmias.

Mexiletine (oral)

Start with 100–200 mg/day and increase slowly up to 625 mg/day. It is not well tolerated – causes transient palpitations and tachycardia. It undergoes CYP2D6 metabolism so it will have different effects in different people.

Contraindications

- Second- and third-degree heart block, arrhythmias
- Avoid other drugs affecting cardiac conduction – tricyclics. Take an electrocardiogram (ECG) before use.

Corticosteroids

Steroids reduce inflammatory sensitization of nerves and reduce pressure on nerves by oedema. A dose of 8 mg/day will work in one to three days and the dose can then be reduced rapidly to maintain benefit. Corticosteroids are multipurpose drugs and are used commonly in patients with advanced disease to improve pain, anorexia, nausea and malaise. They provide a range of effects including transient mood elevation, anti-inflammatory activity, antiemetic activity and appetite stimulation. They may be beneficial in the management of cachexia and anorexia.

α2 adrenergic agonists

Clonidine 25 μg three times daily increasing to 100 mg three times daily.

Neuroleptics

- Levomepromazine (methotrimeprazine) – up to 12.5–50 mg every four hours orally.
- Levomepromazine lacks the opioid-inhibiting effects on gut motility and may be useful for treating opioid-induced intractable constipation or other dose-limiting side effects. It also has antiemetic and anxiolytic effects. It is sedating and may cause hypotension if administered by rapid intravenous injection.

NMDA (N-methyl-D-aspartate) antagonists

Ketamine and amantidine are the two NMDA receptor antagonists available but hallucinations and other cognitive changes may limit their use.

Ketamine

- Oral bioavailability is 20 per cent and the onset of action is 30 minutes.
- Absorption is better when given sublingually.
- Duration of action orally is four to six hours.
- Subcutaneous dose – 10–360 mg in 24 hours.
- Sublingual dose – start at 10 mg four times daily and increase by 10 mg increments daily up to 50 mg four times daily.

Ketamine is metabolized to the active metabolite (nor-ketamine) which has a similar analgesic potency to ketamine. Nor-ketamine may be the main analgesic component in chronic use. It has been shown to relieve pain in up to 67 per cent of patients. Less than 10 per cent is excreted unchanged. Long-term use leads to hepatic enzyme induction.

Amantadine

- 200 mg/24 h then 100 mg once daily for two weeks – may last six months.

Miscellaneous

Baclofen up to 60 mg/day can be helpful for paroxysmal pain.

Topical agents

- Local anaesthetics
- NSAIDs
- Capsaicin

Other available treatments

TOPICAL OPIOID FOR SKIN ULCERS

Morphine or diamorphine 10 mg is mixed with sterile aqueous gel and applied one to three times daily. Fentanyl has been used in the same way.

ANTI-NEOPLASTIC INTERVENTIONS FOR PAIN RELIEF

Radiotherapy

Local, half-body or whole-body radiation enhances the effectiveness of analgesic drugs and other non-invasive therapy by directly affecting the cause of pain (i.e. reducing primary and metastatic tumour bulk). A single intravenous injection of β particle-emitting agents such as iodine-131, phosphorus-32-orthophosphate and strontium-89, as well as the investigational new drugs rhenium-186 and samarium-153, can relieve pain of widespread bony metastases. Half the patients so treated respond to a second treatment if pain recurs.

SURGERY

Curative excision or palliative debulking of a tumour has potential to reduce pain directly, relieve symptoms of obstruction or compression, and improve prognosis, even increasing long-term survival.

PHYSICAL MODALITIES

Generalized weakness, deconditioning and musculoskeletal pain associated with cancer diagnosis and therapy may be treated by:

- Heat – avoid burns by wrapping the heat source (e.g. hot pack or heating pad) in a towel. A timing device is useful to prevent burns from an electrical heating pad. The use of heat on recently irradiated tissue is contraindicated.
- Cold – use ice packs that conform to body contours for less than 15 minutes. Cold treatment reduces swelling and may provide longer-lasting relief than heat but should be used cautiously in patients with peripheral vascular disease and on tissue damaged by radiation therapy.
- Massage, pressure and vibration – physical stimulation techniques have direct mechanical effects on tissues and enhance relaxation when applied gently. Tumour masses should not be aggressively manipulated.
- Exercise – exercise strengthens weak muscles, mobilizes stiff joints, helps restore coordination and balance, and provides cardiovascular conditioning. Therapists and trained family or other caregivers can assist the functionally limited patient with range-of-motion exercises to help preserve strength and joint function. During acute pain, exercise should be limited to self-administered range-of-motion. Weight-bearing exercise should be avoided when bone fracture is likely.
- Stimulation techniques – patients with mild to moderate pain may benefit from a trial of transcutaneous electrical nerve stimulation (TENS) to see if it is effective in reducing the pain or from acupuncture.
- Psychology – stress and anxiety are often associated with poor pain relief. Some patients benefit from short-term psychotherapy provided by trained professionals. Reduction in stress and anxiety can greatly improve pain relief.
- Cognitive behavioural interventions – interventions introduced early in the course of illness are more likely to succeed because they can be learned and practised by patients while they have sufficient strength and energy. Patients and their families should be given information about and encouraged to try several strategies, and to select one or more of these cognitive behavioural techniques to use regularly.
- Physical and psychosocial interventions – patients should be encouraged to remain active and participate in self-care when possible. Non invasive physical and psychosocial modalities can be used concurrently with drugs and other interventions to manage pain during all phases of treatment. The effectiveness of these modalities depends on the patient's participation and communication of which methods best alleviate pain.
- Relaxation and imagery – simple relaxation techniques should be used for episodes of brief pain (e.g. during procedures). Brief and simple techniques are preferred when the patient's ability to concentrate is compromised by severe pain, a high level of anxiety, or fatigue.
- Hypnosis – hypnotic techniques may be used to induce relaxation and may be combined with other cognitive behavioural strategies. Hypnosis is effective in relieving pain in individuals who can concentrate well, use imagery, and who are motivated to practise.
- Cognitive distraction and reframing – focusing attention on stimuli other than pain or negative emotions accompanying pain may involve distractions that are internal (e.g. counting, praying, or making self-statements such as 'I can cope'), external (e.g. music, television, talking, listening to someone read or the use of a visual focal point). In the related technique – cognitive reappraisal – patients learn to monitor and evaluate negative thoughts and replace them with more positive thoughts and images.

Management of procedural pain

Many diagnostic and therapeutic procedures are painful to patients. Treat anticipated procedure-related pain prophylactically and integrate pharmacologic and non-pharmacologic interventions in a complementary style. Use local anaesthetics and short-acting opioids to manage procedure-related pain, allowing adequate time for the drug to achieve full therapeutic effect. Anxiolytics and sedatives may be used to reduce anxiety or to produce sedation. Cognitive behavioural interventions, such as imagery or relaxation, are useful in managing procedure-related pain and anxiety. Patients generally tolerate procedures better when they are informed of what to expect.

PAIN IN MALIGNANT DISEASE: INVASIVE PROCEDURES

- Indications for invasive techniques of pain relief
- Role of the anaesthetically trained practitioner

- Nerve blocks
- Spinal and epidural drug delivery
- Cordotomy

Indications for invasive procedures for pain relief

Pain in cancer is not always adequately managed with analgesic drugs, although the appropriate use of analgesics is nearly always the first choice of therapy. The required dose of opiate may be of such a level that it is impossible to avoid intolerable side effects. Some pains are relatively unresponsive to opioid analgesics, so that neurogenic pain may be inadequately controlled with acceptable levels of opioid and other drugs. The pain of movement, incident pain, which often accompanies skeletal invasion, is rarely satisfactorily controlled with analgesic drugs. In these situations it may be appropriate to consider specialized modes of delivery of analgesic, specifically via the epidural or spinal route, or in some cases, a neuroablative procedure may be appropriate.

The use of epidural or spinal delivery of drugs can result in a major improvement in pain relief while minimizing the side effects of opioids. Small doses are used, delivered in close proximity to the central nervous system. The adverse side is that the procedure is invasive, requiring a fair degree of cooperation from the patient and involving implantation and maintenance of a delivery system with the potential complications of mechanical failure, displacement and infection.

Nerve or plexus blocking or ablation is used when no other satisfactory means of pain relief is available. The procedure must aim at a specific target to denervate, so that the source of pain must be clearly identified and localized. The neuroablation must be possible without causing damage to other nerve tracts or only in exceptional circumstances where the potential damage to other nerves is considered an acceptable price for achieving analgesia. Destruction of nerve tracts always has some deleterious effects on sensory function, and the beneficial effects may have a limited duration.

The practitioner who frequently has the most experience of performing nerve blocks or inserting catheters into the epidural and subarachnoid compartments has trained as an anaesthetist and may be called upon to assist palliative care physicians in the performance of these techniques. This is a logical extension of the anaesthetist's role in providing pain relief, so although this is an area in which some anaesthetists specialize, some of the procedures should be within the experience of the generalist.

Epidural and intrathecal analgesia

Opioid drugs placed in the epidural or subarachnoid space can provide potent analgesia. The dose of opioid required is much smaller than the dose given systemically and the improved analgesia is generally accompanied by fewer side effects, such as sedation, nausea and constipation. Epidural and spinal opioids can produce respiratory depression, and in the acute postoperative situation this can be a serious problem. In chronic pain associated with malignant disease, the patient is often opioid tolerant and respiratory depression is less of a hazard. Once the epidural or spinal delivery of opioid has been established, it is usually possible to decrease the oral or parenteral dose of opioid quite rapidly with consequent improvement in the patient's general quality of life.

When pain on movement, incident pain, is a particular problem, local anaesthetic can be added to the opioid infusion. Volumes of local anaesthetic are small, so that hypotension is not usually a problem and motor block is minimal. The resulting pain relief on movement can produce an improvement in mobility which more than compensates for any slight sensory and motor loss.

TECHNIQUE – EPIDURAL

An epidural catheter is inserted using standard techniques, preferably at a site as close as possible to the segmental level of pain. Placement should be with full aseptic technique to avoid the possible introduction of infection to the epidural space. This is not only potentially damaging to the central nervous system but will necessitate removal of the catheter. The catheter will normally be expected to remain in place for a considerable time (weeks or months). It should be tunnelled subcutaneously to a point away from the level of spinal entry. This allows a more convenient site for injection or infusion, and reduces the risk of infection.

Silicone catheters designed for long-term use are more suitable than the standard epidural catheters. They are less likely to kink or cause local reactions and are often provided with a Dacron cuff which fixes in the subcutaneous tunnel and reduces the risk of displacement. The catheter can be externalized and used for intermittent injection or continuous infusion for many weeks, provided there is careful protection of the entry site beneath a waterproof dressing. Alternatively the catheter is connected to an implanted injection port/reservoir or an infusion pump which is buried in a subcutaneous pouch. Implantation is more comfortable and convenient for the patient and reduces the risk of infection. However, should the catheter become blocked, displaced or infected, replacement is a more complicated procedure.

TECHNIQUE – INTRATHECAL

A fine catheter can be introduced directly into the subarachnoid space, and again tunnelled subcutaneously to an external or implanted port or infusion device. This can produce a superior quality of analgesia to epidural infusion and the dose of drugs is even lower. The subarachnoid route also avoids the development of epidural fibrosis which can develop around the tip of an epidural catheter, limiting its useful life. Subarachnoid infusions may be complicated by leakage of cerebrospinal fluid (CSF) and the risk of infection is potentially more serious.

DOSES

A patient who is already on oral opioid drugs and is changing to an infusion can be started with a dose of about 5–15 per cent of the equivalent daily oral dose for an epidural infusion or 0.25–0.5 per cent of oral dose for an intrathecal infusion. The opioid of choice in the UK is usually diamorphine, which is highly soluble and is available as a preservative-free preparation.

Some recommend assessing the dose by allowing the patient to use a PCA delivery of opioid to the epidural infusion after stopping the oral dose. Allow administration of 1 mg diamorphine on demand with a 20-minute patient lockout. When the demand rate is established, the total can be infused over 24 hours in a volume of 20 mL.

An intrathecal infusion is usually started at 0.25–0.5 per cent of the total daily oral dose of opioid given over 24 hours. The analgesia should be reassessed at 24 hours and the rate of infusion adjusted as necessary. If local anaesthetic is to be included in the infusion, the volume can be made up with 0.125–0.25 per cent bupivacaine.

Nerve blocks in the management of pain in malignant disease

ABDOMINAL PAIN

The pain of visceral cancer may not be adequately managed with analgesic drugs, or only partially controlled with high doses of opioid analgesics, resulting in an unacceptable degree of sedation. Pain from pancreatic tumours usually develops rapidly, with epigastric pain, often radiating through to the back.

Neurolytic injection of the coeliac plexus may completely relieve pain from pancreatic and other upper abdominal tumours, or at least reduce pain to a level which is more easily controlled with smaller doses of opioid analgesics.

INDICATIONS FOR COELIAC PLEXUS BLOCK

- Unrelieved upper abdominal pain.
- Limited life expectancy where the potential morbidity of the procedure is considered an acceptable risk in order to achieve pain control.

- Informed patient consent from a patient who is able to cooperate with the procedure and tolerate positioning and possible sedation or general anaesthesia to allow accurate injection.

Practical details of coeliac plexus block are provided in Chapter 8. Following a successful procedure it is usually possible to plan a phased reduction in the patient's opioid dose. If coeliac plexus block is effective in relieving pain, the patient's regular dose of opioid may suddenly become excessive when the stimulus of pain has been removed, and care should be taken to monitor sedation and respiratory depression in case this relative overdose of opioid should occur, requiring withdrawal or antagonism of opioid analgesics.

Analgesia usually develops over the 24 hours following a coeliac plexus block, but the effects may diminish after a few weeks. When the patient outlives the duration of analgesia, a repeat coeliac plexus block may be considered.

LUMBAR SYMPATHETIC BLOCK

Blockade of the lumbar sympathetic chain is most often performed for the relief of rest pain and improvement of skin perfusion in peripheral vascular disease. However, some pain from lower abdominal viscera and pelvic organs may be transmitted via the sympathetic system, and lumbar sympathetic block may be helpful in managing pain from these organs when affected by malignant disease and medication has proved inadequate. If pelvic pain is due to invasion of skeletal structures or involvement of pelvic nerves, then sympathetic block is not likely to be effective. The procedure is described in detail in Chapter 8.

SEGMENTAL NERVE BLOCK

Blocking the segmental nerve roots, mainly in the thoracic and lumbar regions, may be considered as a means of controlling pain arising in the body wall, where pain has a peripheral origin and is primarily nociceptive. A prognostic paravertebral block is helpful in determining whether this approach will provide pain relief. The addition of steroid to the local anaesthetic will often provide a more prolonged analgesic effect. If a destructive nerve lesion is considered appropriate for intractable pain in debilitated patients, it is occasionally justified to use 6 per cent aqueous phenol (2–3 mL) in the nerve block. The use of neurolytic agents in this situation can result in motor weakness and the development of dysaesthetic neuropathic pain.

Intractable pain that has a clear segmental origin which can be relieved by local anaesthetic block of the segmental nerve can be effectively managed by producing a lesion in the dorsal root ganglion. This is usually effected with a selective radio-frequency thermal lesion performed under radiographic control (Chapter 8). This procedure is more selective than a chemical neurolysis and has less risk of producing a motor lesion or causing post-injection neuropathic pain. The lesion requires accurate localization using radiographic screening and sensory testing. This means that very sick or debilitated patients may not be able to provide enough cooperation to allow the procedure to be performed safely and effectively. However, it can be a very effective means of relieving pain in a defined nerve root distribution in a patient who is otherwise mobile and has a life expectancy of a few weeks or more.

SUBARACHNOID BLOCK

Subarachnoid neurolysis was one of the most important techniques for relieving intractable pain in patients with late-stage cancer in the earlier days of pain medicine. Thirty years ago, the use of opioid analgesics was more guarded than nowadays and epidural and intrathecal drug delivery systems were largely undeveloped. Intrathecal injection of neurolytic agents was one of the most effective measures available and became widely used. It was a technique in which anaesthetists had skills and experience. As less destructive analgesic methods have become more widely available, intrathecal neurolysis has become less used although there is still an occasional indication in late-stage disease when all other methods of providing pain relief have proved ineffective or impractical. The potential morbidity of intrathecal neurolysis, motor paralysis and loss of sphincter control can be devastating and the indications for subjecting the patient to these risks should be clearly defined.

Indications include the presence of severe uncontrolled pain, which is not managed with doses of opioid drugs which are consistent with acceptable levels of sedation or other side effects. The pain should be well defined and located to an area supplied by identifiable nerve roots. In the low lumbar and sacral areas, the high risk of affecting sphincter control means that the procedure may be more likely to be considered in patients who are already suffering from incontinence.

Radiographic imaging of intrathecal neurolytic injection makes the procedure safer and more accurate. Occasionally the injection may be performed as a bedside procedure in the terminal stages of illness when pain relief is paramount, and potential morbidity of the procedure is unlikely to substantially alter the quality of life.

Technique

Neurolytic solutions used include hyperbaric phenol 5 per cent in glycerin, and dehydrated alcohol. Alcohol is hypobaric and this means that the patient can be positioned with the painful side uppermost during injection. This may be an advantage, but phenol is more often employed as its hyperbaricity makes the spread of the block more predictable and the quality of the block may be preferable.

For a subarachnoid block in the thoracic or lumbar regions, using hyperbaric phenol, the patient lies in a lateral position with the painful side dependent. Lumbar puncture is performed using a 20 g bevelled spinal needle at a level corresponding to the nerve roots to be blocked. The vertebral level does not correspond with the spinal cord level but an injection at the vertebral level produces the greatest concentration of solution at the region where the posterior roots enter the dura and therefore results in an effective block.

When the needle reaches CSF it is withdrawn as far as possible while a slight flow of CSF is maintained. This position ensures that the subsequent injection is placed as far posteriorly as possible and therefore as far away from the anterior roots. Inject 5 per cent phenol in glycerin, using a volume of up to 1 mL in the lumbar region, and up to 1.5 mL in the thoracic region. Before the needle is withdrawn it should be flushed with a minimal amount of saline so as to avoid leaving a track of phenol. The patient should be maintained in the lateral position, possibly with a slight posterior tilt, for 20 minutes, to allow the phenol to fix over the posterior roots. If the procedure is performed with radiological screening, injection of radiocontrast medium prior to the phenol will help to predict the spread of the neurolytic solution, and the table can be tilted to control the direction of spread of the neurolytic solution.

Pain in the sacral region is treated with smaller volumes of neurolytic solution to minimize damage to sphincter control. The injection can be made at the L5/S1 level with the patient sitting up, or in the lateral position with a head-up tilt on the table. A volume of 0.5 mL phenol is injected. If analgesia is inadequate, it is better to repeat the procedure on two or three subsequent days rather than increasing the volume of injection.

CORDOTOMY

Percutaneous lesioning of the anterolateral spinothalamic tract may be indicated to provide pain relief in terminal illness in the following situations:

- relief of unilateral pain below the level of the proposed lesion
- other means of pain relief have been inadequate
- the patient has a limited life expectancy, usually of less than one year
- the patient is well enough to tolerate the procedure
- appropriate facilities and operator skills are available or are easily accessible.

Percutaneous cordotomy (described in Chapter 8) is a procedure which requires special training and regular experience of the operator. It is therefore best performed in a limited number of centres where the number of procedures will enable the operator to maintain skills and experience.

SYMPTOM CONTROL IN MALIGNANT DISEASE

Along with pain relief, it is important to address all other symptoms that can accompany malignant disease to optimize the quality of life at this time. Such symptoms include:

- Gastrointestinal symptoms
- Neurological and psychiatric symptoms
- Infection
- Endocrine problems
- Metabolic symptoms
- Nutrition and hydration
- Skin care
- Sweats/hot flushes
- Complementary therapy.

Some of the commoner symptoms and their management will be discussed here briefly but for a more comprehensive review of symptom management in palliative care, the reader should refer to the text in the section on Further reading.

Gastrointestinal symptoms

NAUSEA AND VOMITING

There are many causes, such as opioid analgesia, bowel involvement of tumour, other treatment, etc. Management should begin with assessment of possible cause in each individual patient and the most appropriate antiemetic prescribed. If the patient is no better after 24 hours the antiemetic should be changed. It is often necessary to use more than one antiemetic and when this is the case a drug from a different class should be used, for example, cyclizine and ondansetron. Antiemetics should be given regularly, along with regular reassessment of the patient.

CONSTIPATION

The causes are immobility, dehydration and drug therapy. A patient receiving opioid analgesia should always be given prophylactic laxatives. Initially a stimulant laxative (e.g. senna) should be given along with a softener/osmotic laxative (e.g. lactulose). Alternatively Movicol (polyethylene glycol) can be used. Fluid intake should be encouraged.

ANOREXIA

Dexamethasone 4 mg once daily may improve appetite.

Respiratory system

Dyspnoea can occur frequently and can be a very unpleasant symptom. Assessment should include identifying a cause where possible, for example, lung tissue destruction, airway obstruction or pulmonary fibrosis. Where possible treatment should be aimed at the cause, but if there is no specific treatment, reducing the sensation of breathlessness will make the patient more comfortable:

- Give oxygen when SaO_2 is <90 per cent
- Sit the patient up (symptoms are often worse lying down)
- Give a bronchodilator
- Cool humidified air where possible
- Morphine 2.5 mg four hourly or 25–100 per cent of the four hourly dose already prescribed
- Diazepam 2 mg three times daily
- Lorazepam 1 mg sublingually.

Neurological/psychiatric symptoms

ANXIETY

- Diazepam
- Lorazepam
- Propranolol

DEPRESSION

Depression should be managed with SSRIs unless otherwise indicated. The response to treatment may take up to four weeks.

- Mirtazapine – noradrenaline and specific serotoninergic antidepressant
- Lofepramine – for frail and elderly 70 mg nocte and increase to twice daily on days 5–7
- Sertraline – 12.5–25 mg up to 200 mg
- Fluoxetine – 5–10 mg, maximum 60 mg
- Citalopram – 20 mg, maximum 60 mg
- Venlafaxine – 37.5 mg twice daily to 375 mg.

The addition of psychostimulants or steroids may also help reduce depression. Consider dextroamphetamine or methyltrimeprazine (levomepromazine).

See Table 15.2 for other symptoms, their causes and treatment.

Table 15.2 *Other symptoms of malignant disease*

Symptom	Cause and treatment
Pathological fractures	Radiotherapy/surgery
Smooth muscle colic	Antimuscarinic agents (opioids ineffective)
Infection	Antibiotics
Raised intracranial pressure	Steroids
Visceral	Tumour infiltration
	Constant, dull, poorly localized
	Usually responds well to opioids
Liver	Stretching of liver capsule
	Try dexamethasone 4–6 mg once daily
Central nervous system	
Cerebral metastases	
↑ Intracranial pressure	Stretching meninges. Try dexamethasone
Pancreatic	Retroperitoneal nerve involvement. May not respond to opioids. Coeliac plexus block has 80% success rate, or try octreotide
Malignant bowel obstruction – can be difficult to treat	Scopolamine
	Glycopyrrolate
	Octreotide
Musculoskeletal/general debility	NSAID/opioid
Soft tissue	E.g. chest wall, breast or lung carcinoma
	Dexamethasone, NSAID, radiotherapy
Odynophagia (painful dysphagia)	Painful mouth, radiotherapy-induced oesophagitis, candidiasis, oesophageal spasm (nifedipine or GTN)
Ischaemia	Spinal with local anaesthetic is best
	Emla cream over affected part
	LA subcutaneous infusion
	Ketamine or methadone
Pleuritic pain	Steroid, intercostal nerve block, interpleural infusion
Other pharmacotherapy	Chemotherapy
	Hormone therapy
	Antibiotic therapy

NSAID, non-steroidal anti-inflammatory drug; GTN, glyceryl trinitrate; LA, local anaesthetic

Syringe drivers

Syringe drivers provide a continuous infusion of drugs to control symptoms of malignant disease.

INDICATIONS

- Severe persistent nausea and vomiting.
- Severe dysphagia.
- Inability to swallow.
- Patient too weak to take oral drugs.
- Poor gastrointestinal absorption.
- Doubts about or problems with compliance.

The use of syringe drivers does not provide better analgesia than the oral route. The oral route should always be the first line of management.

ADVANTAGES

- Constant blood levels of drug.
- More comfortable than the intravenous or intramuscular route.
- The patient can continue to be mobile.
- Good drug absorption.

THE PUMPS

Many pumps are available but they usually provide a 24-hour dose of the drug so the syringe needs to be changed daily. Drug delivery is usually in mm/h or mm/day and delivers 0.2 mm/h. The 24-hour dose is diluted into 48 mm. A paediatric butterfly needle should be inserted into the skin at a 45° angle. The 'butterfly' is then connected to a 1 m extension tube that is in turn attached to the syringe.

SITES FOR INFUSION

- Intercostal space
- The outer arm
- Upper thigh
- Abdomen

Avoid:

- oedematous areas
- the chest wall in very cachectic patients
- the upper abdomen in patients with an enlarged liver
- bony prominences
- joints
- the abdomen in patients with ascites
- previously irradiated skin.

Drugs used:

- Diamorphine
- Cyclizine
- Haloperidol

- Metoclopramide
- Hyoscine
- Levopromeprazine

Drugs that should not be used:

- Diazepam
- Prochlorperazine
- Chlorpromazine.

SUMMARY

Pain management must be optimized using a combination of available methods to keep patients with malignant disease as comfortable as possible. However, most patients are willing to tolerate pain, even when substantial. Among patients who are dying, other factors are often more important than pain relief, and other symptoms should be managed aggressively. The treatment of pain is important, but the prevalence of pain itself might not be the best outcome measure for the assessment of the quality of end-of-life care.

CASE SCENARIO 1

A 63-year-old man develops upper abdominal pain and jaundice. Investigations demonstrate a tumour in the head of the pancreas causing biliary obstruction. Surgical resection is not considered possible but a stent is inserted to relieve the obstruction. He continues to experience epigastric pain which radiates through to his back and is prescribed oral morphine in sustained release formulation. Initially his pain is well controlled on morphine 60 mg twice daily, but as his disease progresses this becomes inadequate within three weeks. The dose of morphine is increased to 120 mg twice daily but pain control remains incomplete while he finds the increased dose of morphine makes him feel disorientated and sleepy. He is admitted to a palliative care unit where higher doses of alternative opioid analgesics are tried. Eventually some moderate control of pain is achieved using intravenous alfentanil by infusion. The man is bed-bound and tends to sleep between episodes of increased pain and additional analgesia.

The palliative care physician requests help from the pain clinic anaesthetist who agrees to offer the patient a coeliac plexus block. It is explained to the patient that the procedure will probably relieve most, but not all, of his pain, although there are possible risks associated with the procedure.

Although worried about the block, the patient agrees to the procedure, providing that it can be done under a general anaesthetic. The anaesthetist considers that the patient's general status is acceptable for an anaesthetic and that this will enable the block to be done without causing further distress.

The following day, the patient is taken to theatre and, under general anaesthesia, turned prone. Using an image intensifier for radiographic guidance, bilateral injections are made to the coeliac plexus, using 15 mL of a 50:50 mixture of absolute alcohol and 0.5 per cent bupivacaine. After injection the patient remains prone under anaesthesia for 20 minutes before being turned supine and woken.

The patient remains in bed for the next 12 hours while his blood pressure is carefully monitored. His dose of opioid analgesic is gradually reduced while his respiration and conscious levels are observed regularly. He remains slightly hypotensive but claims to be almost pain free over the subsequent 24 hours. An increased fluid load is given and the patient is advised to get up gradually in stages, to minimize postural hypotension.

Over the following three days the patient manages to mobilize freely without intolerable postural hypotension and is comfortable without the opioid infusion. He is discharged from the palliative care unit with a requirement for occasional tramadol 50 mg for a little residual back ache.

CASE SCENARIO 2

Colin is a 48-year-old man who presents on a neurosurgical unit. He underwent surgical treatment for bowel cancer two years previously. Eighteen months later he developed back pain which radiated to his left iliac crest and lower abdominal wall. Investigations revealed a metastatic tumour invading the eleventh vertebral body. Surgical removal of tumour with repair and stabilization of the vertebral body was undertaken.

Colin now presented with persisting severe pain on movement in the distribution of the eleventh thoracic nerve. Transdermal fentanyl maintained him reasonably pain free at rest, but mobilization was almost impossible.

Colin was assessed by the pain clinician and it was decided that a nerve blocking procedure might relieve pain on movement. He was taken to theatre, and under radiographic guidance an electrode was positioned in the posterior section of the T11/12 intervertebral foramen, adjacent to the dorsal root ganglion. Stimulation at this point resulted in the patient identifying this as being the area coincident with his pain. After injecting local anaesthetic, a thermal lesion was produced at this point, using the radio-frequency lesion generator set at 70°C for 60 seconds.

Following this procedure Colin was able to move without severe pain, while continuing his use of transdermal fentanyl. The pain relief lasted for three months.

FURTHER READING

Back IN. *Palliative Medicine Handbook*, 3rd edn. Cardiff: BPM Books.

Index

Please note: page numbers in **bold** type refer to material in tables or figures.